WELLNESS, NOT WEIGHT

HEALTH AT EVERY SIZE AND MOTIVATIONAL INTERVIEWING

Ann Yang

Edited by Ellen R. Glovsky, PhD, RD, LDN
Northeastern University
Training with Dr. Ellen

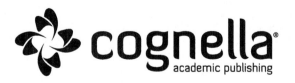

cognella®
academic publishing

Bassim Hamadeh, CEO and Publisher
Michael Simpson, Vice President of Acquisitions
Jamie Giganti, Managing Editor
Jess Busch, Graphic Design Supervisor
John Remington, Acquisitions Editor
Brian Fahey, Licensing Associate
Mandy Licata, Interior Designer

First published in the United States of America in 2014 by Cognella, Inc.

Trademark Notice: Product or corporate names may be trademarks or registered trademarks, and are used only for identification and explanation without intent to infringe.

Cover images
- Copyright © 2012 by Depositphotos / Rolfgeorg Brenner.
- Copyright © 2011 by Depositphotos / Natalia Artemjeva.
- Copyright © 2012 by Depositphotos / Bobby Wijaya.

Printed in the United States of America

ISBN: 978-1-62131-092-1 (pbk) / 978-1-62131-091-4 (br)

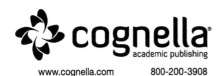

www.cognella.com   800-200-3908

CONTENTS

COMMUNICATING A NON-DIET APPROACH TO PATIENTS/CLIENTS

CONTRIBUTORS

Siddhartha Angadi, PhD received his doctorate in physical activity, nutrition and wellness at Arizona State University in 2012. His dissertation research focused on the effects of high-intensity interval exercise training in patients with diastolic heart failure. Following his graduation, he was a post-doctoral scholar at UCLA before joining the Exercise and Wellness program in the School of Nutrition and Health Promotion at Arizona State University as an assistant professor.

Lucy Aphramor, PhD, RD pioneered the delivery of HAES in the UK National Health Service and developed the HAES course, *Well Now*, which is delivered internationally. Lucy is recognized for her research and publications across weight science, critical dietetics, and HAES. Her co-authored article stating the case for a paradigm shift in weight management, written with HAES expert Linda Bacon, is widely regarded as a leading review in the field.

Linda Bacon, PhD is a researcher on weight regulation science—a scientist whose three graduate degrees, research, and clinical expertise uniquely prepare her to understand and translate the physiological, psychological, and socio-cultural underpinnings of weight control. She is currently a nutrition professor at City College of San Francisco and an associate nutritionist at the University of California, Davis. An internationally recognized authority on weight and health, Dr. Bacon has published her work in top scientific journals as well as the highly acclaimed bestseller, *Health at Every Size: The Surprising Truth About Your Weight* (Ben Bella Books, 2008).

Dharini Bhammar, PhD, MBBS went to medical school in India and then came to the United States to pursue a master's degree in exercise and wellness at Arizona State University. She went on to complete her doctor of philosophy in 2013 in the physical activity, nutrition and wellness program at ASU, where she studied the effects of novel exercise protocols on cardiovascular disease risk reduction. She currently is a postdoctoral scholar at the Institute of Exercise and Environmental Medicine in Dallas, Texas.

Mary Ellen Bingham MS, RD, CSSD, CDN is the head sports dietitian at the University of North Carolina, Chapel Hill. She was previously the campus health dietitian and sports nutritionist for St. John's University in New York. Mary Ellen completed her undergraduate studies in nutrition at Boston University and received a master of science in clinical nutrition from New York University. She is credentialed as a registered dietitian (RD) and is a certified specialist in sports dietetics (CSSD).

Dawn Clifford, PhD, RD is an associate professor and director of the Didactic Program in Dietetics at California State University, Chico. She also directs FitU, which is a nutrition and physical activity counseling program for college students. Her peer counselors are trained in both motivational interviewing and the Health at Every Size (HAES®) paradigm.

Rebecca Y. Concepcion, PhD received her doctoral degree in exercise science from Oregon State University. She is an associate professor in the Department of Kinesiology at Saint Mary's College of California where she teaches courses in health promotion and Health at Every Size. Her research has examined personal and social factors that influence physical activity and dietary behaviors as well as the role of weight bias in health behaviors.

Paul Ernsberger, PhD is a medical educator and biomedical researcher and is currently associate professor of nutrition at Case Western Reserve University School of Medicine. He has researched the health effects of yo-yo dieting and the benefits of weight stability. He studies treatments for diseases associated with adiposity, such as hypertension and diabetes, independent of weight loss.

Ellen Frankel, LCSW has specialized in the field of eating disorders for over fifteen years. She is currently writing full-time on topics related to eating, body image issues, and spirituality. Ellen is a co-author of *Beyond a Shadow of a Diet* (2014) and *The Diet Survivor's Handbook: 60 Lessons in Eating, Acceptance and Self-Care* (Sourcebooks, 2006). She is also the author of *Beyond Measure: A Memoir About Short Stature and Inner Growth* (Pearlsong Press, 2006) and *Syd Arthur* (Pearlsong Press, 2011), and is the co-author of *Revolution of Jewish Spirit* (Jewish Lights Publishing, 2012).

Glenn Gaesser, PhD is a professor of exercise physiology in the School of Nutrition and Health Promotion at Arizona State University. He has had prior academic appointments at the University of Virginia and UCLA. He is author of *Big Fat Lies: The Truth About Your Weight and Your Health* (Gurze Books, 2002).

Marsha Hudnall, **MS, RD, CD** is president and co-owner of Green Mountain at Fox Run, a pioneering healthy lifestyle retreat for women. Founded in 1973, Green Mountain offers the country's oldest non-diet residential program to help women establish healthy relationships with food, eating, and their bodies. A nationally known speaker and writer, Marsha sits on the boards of the Binge Eating Disorder Association and the Center for Mindful Eating.

Kathy Kater, LCSW is a psychotherapist, author, speaker, and consultant who has specialized in treatment and prevention of the full spectrum of body image, eating, fitness, and weight-related concerns for 35 years. She is the author of the *Healthy Bodies: Teaching Kids What They Need to Know* (Body Image Health, 2012) curriculum, a weight-stigma-reduction plan designed to inspire boys and girls to care for their bodies from the inside out and appreciate the healthy, diverse sizes and shapes that result. Kater has also published articles in professional journals and the popular press.

Molly Kellogg, RD, LCSW is the author of *Counseling Tips for Nutrition Therapists: Practice Workbook* and has a private nutrition and psychotherapy practice in Philadelphia, Pennsylvania. She is a member of the Motivational Interviewing Network of Trainers and served on the Academy of Nutrition and Dietetics Evidence Analysis Library Nutrition Counseling workgroup. She provides free monthly counseling tips by e-mail subscription.

Karen R. Koenig, LCSW, MEd is a psychotherapist and eating coach who has practiced in the field of eating disorders for 30 years. An expert on the psychology of eating—the *why* and *how*, not the what of it—she is an international author of five books, including *The Food and Feelings Workbook* (Gurze Books, 2007), does Skype and phone coaching, lectures nationally, and has a therapy practice in Sarasota, Florida.

Pam Macdonald, PhD is a research psychologist, coach, and trainer. She is actively involved in supporting carers of people with eating disorders using the principles of motivational interviewing and now supervises carers in becoming peer mentors to other carers. She co-edited *The Clinician's Guide to Collaborative Caring in Eating Disorders: The New Maudsley Method*

(Routledge, 2009) with Janet Treasure and Ulrike Schmidt and has contributed to several peer-reviewed papers in the academic literature.

Judith Matz, LCSW is a therapist and co-author of *The Diet Survivor's Handbook: 60 Lessons in Eating, Acceptance and Self-Care* (2006) and *Beyond a Shadow of a Diet: The Therapist's Guide to Treating Binge Eating Disorder, Compulsive Eating and Emotional Overeating* (2014). Judith is the director of The Chicago Center for Overcoming Overeating, Inc., a frequent presenter at local and national conferences, and has a private practice in Skokie, Illinois. Descriptions of her work have appeared in national publications and media.

Michelle May, MD is the award-winning author of *Eat What You Love, Love What You Eat: How to Break Your Eat-Repent-Repeat Cycle* (Am I Hungry Publishing, 2013) and *Eat What You Love, Love What You Eat with Diabetes* (New Harbinger Publications, Inc., 2012). She is the founder of Am I Hungry?™ Mindful Eating Programs and Training.

Michelle Neyman Morris, PhD, RD is a professor and dietetic internship director in the Department of Nutrition & Food Sciences at California State University, Chico. She is a Ford Foundation Fellow, earned her doctorate in nutrition from the University of California, Davis, and held the CSU-Chico Lantis Endowed Professorship. Her research interests include nutrition education across the lifespan, using the socially just Health at Every Size paradigm. Dr. Neyman Morris advocates for an end to weight-based discrimination and inclusion of the HAES tenets in dietetics education and practice.

Paula Quatromoni, PhD, RD, LDN is a registered dietitian and associate professor of nutrition at Boston University where she pioneered the sports nutrition clinical practice serving student athletes on campus. Dr. Quatromoni is a nutritional epidemiologist who has a funded research program in adult and child obesity. She is an investigator on the world-renowned Framingham Heart Study and a published author.

Jonathan Robison, PhD, MS holds a doctorate in health education/exercise physiology and a master of science in human nutrition from Michigan State University, where he has taught for 15 years in the nutrition and physiology departments as an adjunct Assistant professor. Dr. Robison is also an adjunct associate professor at Western Michigan University, where he teaches in the Holistic Health Care program. He has authored numerous articles on a variety of health-related topics and is a frequent presenter at conferences throughout North America. He is the author of *The Spirit and Science of Holistic Health: More Than Broccoli, Jogging, and Bottled Water…More Than Yoga, Herbs, and Meditation* (AuthorHouse, 2004).

Alice J. Rosen, LMHC has been an educator and therapist for over 25 years and has a private practice in Concord, Massachusetts. She is the former director of Education for Feeding Ourselves and author of *The Feeding Ourselves Method* training CD. She is on the faculty of the Institute for Mindfulness and Psychotherapy and is certified in the Internal Family Systems Model.

Brandon Sawyer, PhD, ATC holds a master's degree in exercise physiology from the University of Virginia and a doctorate in physical activity, nutrition, and wellness from Arizona State University. He is currently an assistant professor in the kinesiology and biology departments at Point Loma Nazarene University in San Diego, California.

Janet Treasure, OBE, PhD, FRCP, FRCPsych is a psychiatrist who has specialized in the treatment of eating disorders for over 30 years. A key figure at the Maudsley Hospital, London, a leading center in clinical management and training of eating disorders, Professor Treasure is also active in research. Throughout her illustrious career, she has edited seven academic texts on eating disorders, authored three self-help books, and has over 300 peer-reviewed papers in print. Among her many accolades, she was awarded the Academy for Eating Disorders (AED) Leadership Award in Research in 2004, which honors an individual who has developed new knowledge of eating disorders through research over a substantial period of time, is internationally respected, and has had a measurable impact in the field. She was awarded the Order of the British Empire (OBE) in early 2013 for her services to the field of eating disorders.

Patti Lou Watkins, **PhD** received her doctoral degree in clinical psychology from Virginia Tech. Currently she is an associate professor in the School of Psychological Science at Oregon State University where she teaches fat studies. Her research has involved promotion of physical activity for fat women from a HAES perspective, examination of interpersonal weight bias and its consequences, and pedagogical approaches to teaching about women, weight, and body image.

INTRODUCTION

I am thrilled to be working with such a strong collection of collaborators on this book, and this has been a dream come true for me. I have been a Registered Dietitian for 40+ years, and, as such I have worked with many people who are trying to change their diet and exercise habits and lose weight. The damage that the traditional approach of *telling people* what to do, and blaming them when they don't, troubled me until I found the ideas in Health At Every Size (HAES) and Motivational Interviewing (MI). Having been a part of the HAES movement, a clinician using Motivational Interviewing, and a MI trainer for many years, I have seen first-hand how much better these approaches are at *helping* rather than harming patients.

A few words about terms used in this book. The expression "non-diet" sounds at first glance as though it is talking about what it is *not*, rather than a description of something that *is*. This term is chosen because there is much evidence that *diets*, both for weight loss and for wellness, are not effective. It is most unfortunate that the current state of the art in medicine and health care has only dietary and "lifestyle" change to offer as a solution to the perceived threat of obesity and overweight. This traditional medical approach assumes that weight loss is the best and only means of achieving health and reducing the risk of chronic illness for people whose weight is above a predetermined level. Since it is clear from the scientific literature that diets do not work to promote weight loss and health, and most people regain the lost weight and more, some practitioners have come to believe that diets are not only *not a good answer, but are also destructive*. Thus, the term "non-diet" was born, and refers instead of restraint, to a mindful, conscious style of eating that focuses on responding to bodily sensations of hunger and fullness to know *when, what, and how much to eat.*

Health At Every Size is a set of ideas that logically follows the ideas of a non-diet approach. HAES posits that people can be healthy at whatever size they are, and that size does not equal health or ill health. There is no room for "dieting" in a HAES approach. All people are encouraged to adopt healthy lifestyle behaviors, including healthy food choices, moving one's body in a way that feels good, visiting a health care provider when needed, and other behaviors that promote health and wellness.

The concepts and techniques of Motivational Interviewing work beautifully with a non-diet and HAES approach. The basic approach of MI is that practitioners enhance motivation for change in health behavior by helping their clients examine their own motivation for change, and then to decide if, when and how they will change. One basic idea in MI is that people have autonomy or *free will* to make decisions for themselves, and that the practitioner is a *guide* who helps them make decisions about change. The concept of guiding works very nicely with the non-diet and HAES approaches as well. In all three sets of ideas, the client is the one who makes decisions about how they will behave regarding lifestyle change.

I know that some practitioners and lay people are sensitive to the terms "client" and "patient" and I am sometimes criticized for my choice of terms. I think the choice of terms depends upon the setting in which practitioners work, and I hope that professionals from many areas will use this book as a resource. Therefore, the terms "patient" and "client" are used interchangeably.

I have divided this book into three parts, which follow in logical order.

Part One includes an overview of each of the three basic ideas described in this book: 1) a Mindful, Non-Diet approach to healing food problems, 2) a Health At Every Size (HAES) approach to wellness, and 3) Motivational Interviewing (MI) as an approach to helping people make decisions about changing behavior. The chapter on MI focuses on using this approach with food problems, but can apply to any behavior change under consideration. The history of the development of a non-diet approach and Health At Every Size is also described here.

Part Two offers more on each topic, further elaborating on these three sets of ideas, and, in some cases, focuses on the scientific underpinnings of the approach.

Part Three includes information on using the non-diet and HAES approach and Motivational Interviewing from a practical, client-centered point of view. This section will also interest the lay public who wish to learn more about a non-diet and HAES approach.

Ellen R. Glovsky, PhD, RD, LDN
Northeastern University
Training with Dr. Ellen

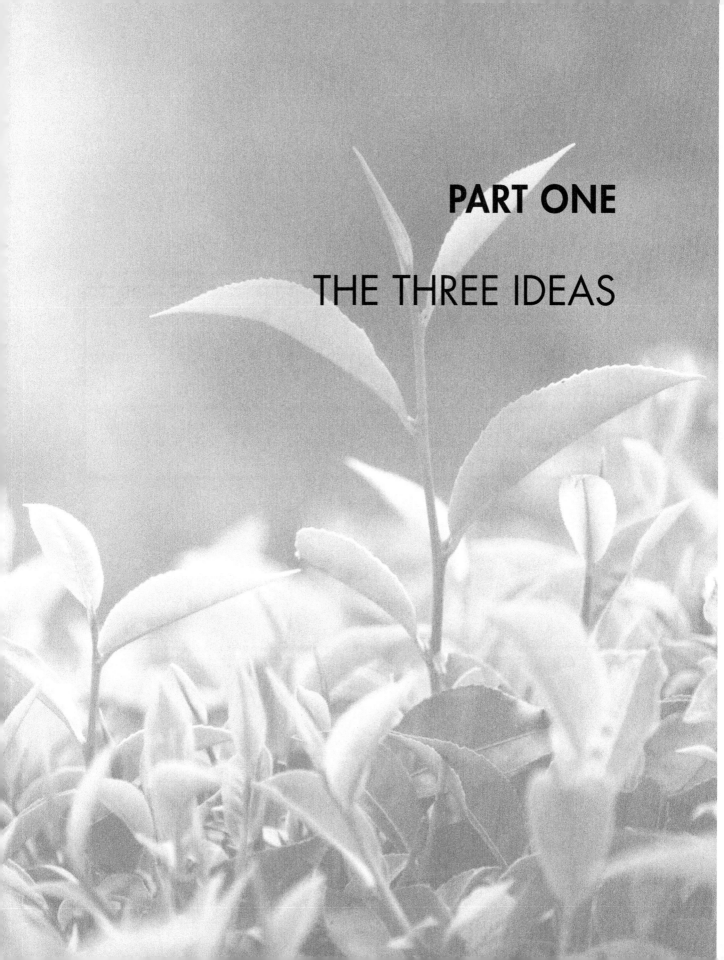

PART ONE

THE THREE IDEAS

SPOTLIGHT

This chapter, by Marsha Hudnall, explores the ideas encompassed in the non-diet approach. She explains the distinctions among a number of terms that have been used to describe such an approach, including mindful eating, intuitive eating, attuned eating, conscious eating, and structured eating. These ideas are related to HAES, in that they emphasize *health*, rather than *weight*, and invite people to tune into their inner signals to know when, what, and how much to eat.

Chapter One

A Mindful, "Non-Diet" Approach to Eating

Marsha Hudnall

O ver the past five decades, the idea of dieting, or changing one's eating habits, has been the cornerstone for the treatment of overweight and obesity. It has been a long process for health professionals and members of the public to understand that dieting does not work for most people to lose weight and keep it off.[1] At long last, the non-diet approach to successful dietary behavior change is gaining momentum. While it is unclear how much the public is aware of or has accepted the concept at the time of this writing, we know that there is a groundswell of support among health professionals. This is evidenced by growing numbers of professionals teaching the principles of mindful eating and intuitive eating in colleges, universities, and training programs for health professionals. We also see the emergence of groups such as the Association for Size Diversity and Health and eating disorder organizations that recognize the deleterious effects of dieting.

WHAT IS THE NON-DIET APPROACH?

The non-diet approach represents a backlash to dieting, and this backlash is definitely warranted, as research shows most people who lose weight through dieting regain it and often end up gaining more.[1] Furthermore, while the etiology of eating disorders is unclear, the development of eating disorders is thought to be exacerbated by the restrictive approach to eating as well as the "thin ideal" that weight-loss dieting supports.[2]

Much more than a reaction to weight-loss dieting, however, the non-diet approach represents a system that utilizes the body's natural homeostatic drive for health, thereby increasing the likelihood of its success in helping individuals eat in a way that supports health. It can be broadly summed up as a body-positive approach to self-care that involves self- and size-acceptance and is based on using internal cues for guidance in eating and physical activity.

From a psychological perspective, body positivity and self- and size-acceptance are essential elements of a non-diet approach.[3] Negative thoughts about self and size are often externally generated, arising from comparisons made based on unrealistic societal standards of acceptability and attractiveness. Accompanying those societal standards are rules about how to achieve the standards, but they are rules that often don't work for the average person. The end result is a conflict between what a person is "supposed" to look like and do and what is within an individual's ability to change, leading to repeated failure to achieve the societal standard. By acknowledging individuality and rejecting the societal standard, individuals can better support their ability to adopt behaviors that support health.

The use of internal cues for hunger and fullness to guide eating is based on the body's homeostatic mechanisms that work to keep the body in balance. Weight-loss diets generally have not considered the individual's level of hunger or satisfaction when eating, relying instead on estimating caloric requirements. This system is based on faulty suppositions, as individual energy utilization and expenditure is complex and cannot be calculated formulaically.[4]

Hunger and fullness cues, however, are part of a complex physiological system that evolved to keep the body in balance and help ensure survival, and involves the interaction of hormones that regulate hunger and appetite.[5] While the exact system has yet to be fully illuminated, it is known that when the body needs fuel, levels of orexigenic hormones produced in the hypothalamus, stomach lining, and pancreas, such as neuropeptide Y, orexen, and ghrelin, increase to produce feelings of hunger. The natural response is to eat, if food is available. That sets in motion natural processes that support the efficient digestion, absorption, and metabolism of the food consumed. It also eventually leads to production of a variety of peptides, proteins, and hormones that signal satiety, stopping food consumption at a point that meets individual needs for energy and nutrients. There is flexibility in the system, allowing for minor under- and overeating as the body balances consumption by signaling hunger sooner in the case of undereating, and increased time to get hungry again in the case of overeating.

Traditional weight-management efforts have focused on encouraging a reduced consumption of food, independent of levels of hunger or satisfaction that an individual may experience at any one moment. Researchers speculate that by ignoring both hunger and fullness cues, homeostasis is disrupted and can actually set the stage for weight gain.[5] Ignoring hunger cues may lead to overproduction of hunger hormones and a resulting intensity of hunger that leads to overeating. This theory is supported by research showing that the frequency of dieting is correlated with a higher body mass index.[6]

In contrast, research supports the effectiveness of a non-diet approach in preventing consistent overeating.[7-9] Further, a non-diet approach is associated with improved nutrient intake, reduction of eating disorder symptomatology, and improved health.[10]

Understanding of physiologic cues for physical activity is not as advanced, but in the non-diet approach, physical activity is encouraged for the mood and health benefits and connection to body that it supports, rather than energy expenditure.[10]

HISTORY OF THE NON-DIET APPROACH

The non-diet approach emerged in the 1970s in the form of two different programs that, while they offered somewhat different methods, both recognized the importance of individual choice in the ability to make intelligent decisions about eating. One program grew out of a professional understanding of the dilemma that dieting for weight loss presented. The other program was the result of personal experience with dieting.

In 1973, Thelma Wayler, a registered dietitian who had worked in the 1950s and 60s in diabetes camps for children, founded Green Mountain at Fox Run, a residential educational center for women, located in Vermont. Wayler had seen the effects of restrictive approaches to eating on eating behavior and subsequent success at diabetes management. As she observed weight-loss diets begin their ascendance as the primary method for weight management, she resolved to found a place where she could educate women in a non-diet approach that would better support them in their efforts toward self-care. She targeted women because, at the time, dieting was more popular among women, and she also recognized women as the gatekeeper to the family's health, passing on beliefs and attitudes about eating, weight, and health to those around them.[11]

Wayler's approach was based on a nutritional framework that ensured regular, balanced eating, and was supplemented by what she called "optioning," which comprised her method of teaching women how to stop and think about if they want to eat, and if so, what they wanted to eat beyond meeting basic nutritional needs. Today, that approach would be more defined as structured eating, which helps ensure an individual eats in a regular and well-balanced manner to support the body's ability to deliver accurate cues as they re-learn how to respond to internal cues for eating. Wayler's approach also addressed physical activity as a way to reduce stress, increase connection to the body, and support well-being, not as a method for burning calories. Additionally, there was a focus on building self-esteem to help a woman "live now, instead of putting her life on hold until she lost weight."[11] Green Mountain still operates today with those principles, although the program has evolved to include a greater focus on emotional healing. As the length of time women have struggled with dieting and weight has increased, Green Mountain has seen the degree of emotional disturbance associated with eating, body image, and life stress also increase.

Around the same time, Carol Munter, now a psychotherapist, began teaching a course titled "Compulsive Eating and Self Image for Women" at a free university in New York City. As someone who had been on many diets, only to continue to struggle with her weight, Munter had been introduced to the idea of weight management without dieting through a consciousness-raising group she was attending. The group of 35 or so women she initially worked with were "able to conclude within a short period of time that to say if we've been on every diet imaginable, and we've all been very, very successful dieters, had lots of willpower and so on, and we're all fatter than we've ever been before, maybe the problem is not with us, maybe the problem is with the diets themselves." Munter went on to author with Jane Hirschmann in 1988 the groundbreaking book *Overcoming Overeating*, which has since gone through several editions, and underlies the work done via the National Center for Overcoming Overeating founded by Munter and Hirschmann.[12]

Munter and Hirschmann's approach relies on exclusively using internal cues to guide eating. She states, "I think Jane and I are perhaps among the most rigorous in terms of how we see this so that we really are on the side of really no outside regulation at all, only internal regulation, internal sensing and figuring out on a day-to-day basis what it is that you need without any thought about anything that the world says about eating."[12]

There have been many, too numerous to mention here, who came after these early leaders in the 40 years since, to add their own experience and understanding to the evolution of the non-diet approach. Collectively, their work has formed a research and practice foundation that offers real solutions in the struggle with overeating and health that has arisen from a reliance on weight-loss diets. One voice, however, does stand out because of the foundational definition of normal eating she penned. Ellyn Satter, MS, RD, LCSW, described normal eating in a way that has been used by countless professionals working in this area to illuminate the variations in normal eating that run counter to many of the rules of dieting.

> *Normal eating is being able to eat when you are hungry and continue eating until you are satisfied. It is being able to choose food you like and eat it and truly get enough of it—not just stop eating because you think you should. Normal eating is being able to use some moderate constraint in your food selection to get the right food, but not being so restrictive that you miss out on pleasurable foods. Normal eating is giving yourself permission to eat sometimes because you are happy, sad or bored, or just because it feels good. Normal eating is three meals a day, most of the time, but it can also be choosing to munch along. It is leaving some cookies on the plate because you know you can have some again tomorrow, or it is eating more now because they taste so wonderful when they are fresh. Normal eating is overeating at times; feeling stuffed and uncomfortable. It is also undereating at times and wishing you had more. Normal eating is trusting*

your body to make up for your mistakes in eating. Normal eating takes up some of your time and attention, but keeps its place as only one area of your life.

In short, normal eating is flexible. It varies in response to your emotions, your schedule, your hunger, and your proximity to food.[13]

MINDFUL EATING VS. INTUITIVE EATING VS. ATTUNED EATING VS. CONSCIOUS EATING VS. STRUCTURED EATING

A number of terms have evolved to describe the process of tuning in to the body for guidance in eating. Although the terms are often used interchangeably, and for the consumer may be enough to use them as such, there is value in understanding some of the nuances of each in order to better grasp the different issues that are often at play in normalizing eating. More terms will likely arise but the current lexicon includes the following.

Mindful Eating

Rooted in ancient meditation practices, mindfulness came to the forefront in the late 1970s with the development of the Mindfulness-Based Stress Reduction approach developed by Jon Kabat-Zinn and colleagues at the University of Massachusetts Medical School.[14] The focus of mindfulness is paying attention to the moment, without judgment, and mindful eating grew out of that focus. See Table 1 for a description of mindful eating from The Center for Mindful Eating.

Intuitive Eating and Attuned Eating

Intuitive eating and attuned eating emphasize eating for physical instead of emotional reasons, relying on internal cues for hunger and satiety, and giving oneself unconditional permission to eat using attunement. While the term "attuned eating" has been in use since the 1980s, the term "intuitive eating" was popularized through the work of Evelyn Tribole, MS, RD, and Elyse Resch, MS, RD. In 1995, they published the book *Intuitive Eating: A Revolutionary Approach That Works*[16] and have over the last two decades worked diligently to communicate their intuitive eating model to registered dietitians and other health professionals. Additionally, the model has been validated through scientific testing.[17] Table 2 lists ten principles that lie at the core of an intuitive eating approach.

Conscious Eating

Although the concept of conscious eating often includes a focus on the quality of food, including the environmental impact of how a food is produced, in the context of normalizing

Table 1. Basics of Mindful Eating

Principles of Mindfulness: • Mindfulness is deliberately paying attention, non-judgmentally. • Mindfulness encompasses both internal processes and external environments. • Mindfulness is being aware of what is present for you mentally, emotionally, and physically in each moment. • With practice, mindfulness cultivates the possibility of freeing yourself of reactive, habitual patterns of thinking, feeling, and acting. • Mindfulness promotes balance, choice, wisdom, and acceptance of what is.
Mindful Eating Is: • Allowing yourself to become aware of the positive and nurturing opportunities that are available through food preparation and consumption by respecting your own inner wisdom. • Choosing to eat food that is both pleasing to you and nourishing to your body by using all your senses to explore, savor, and taste. • Acknowledging responses to food (likes, neutrality, and dislikes) without judgment. • Learning to be aware of physical hunger and satiety cues to guide your decision to begin eating and to stop eating.
Someone Who Eats Mindfully: • Acknowledges that there is no right or wrong way to eat but varying degrees of awareness surrounding the experience of food. • Accepts that his/her eating experiences are unique. • Is an individual who, by choice, directs his/her awareness to all aspects of food and eating on a moment-by-moment basis. • Is an individual who looks at the immediate choices and direct experiences associated with food and eating, not to the distant health outcome of that choice. • Is aware of and reflects on the effects caused by unmindful eating. • Experiences insight about how he/she can act to achieve specific health goals as he/she becomes more attuned to the direct experience of eating and feelings of health. • Becomes aware of the interconnection of earth, living beings, and cultural practices and the impact his/her food choices has on those systems. Developed by The Center for Mindful Eating[15]

eating, the term is frequently used to describe eating in a mindful, intuitive or attuned way. Table 3 lists specific guidelines developed for use in recovery from an eating disorder.

Structured Eating

Within a non-diet approach, structured eating is simply a method by which to put in place a foundation that supports the regulation of hormonal cues that guide eating as well as providing a regular eating schedule to help allay anxieties around food that have arisen from dieting practices. Described as nutritional rehabilitation, it serves as a starting point for people whose

Table 2. Principles of Intuitive Eating

1. Reject the Diet Mentality Throw out the diet books and magazine articles that offer you false hope of losing weight quickly, easily, and permanently. Get angry at the lies that have led you to feel as if you were a failure every time a new diet stopped working and you gained back all of the weight. If you allow even one small hope to linger that a new and better diet might be lurking around the corner, it will prevent you from being free to rediscover Intuitive Eating.
2. Honor Your Hunger Keep your body biologically fed with adequate energy and carbohydrates. Otherwise you can trigger a primal drive to overeat. Once you reach the moment of excessive hunger, all intentions of moderate, conscious eating are fleeting and irrelevant. Learning to honor this first biological signal sets the stage for re-building trust with yourself and food.
3. Make Peace with Food Call a truce, stop the food fight! Give yourself unconditional permission to eat. If you tell yourself that you can't or shouldn't have a particular food, it can lead to intense feelings of deprivation that build into uncontrollable cravings and, often, bingeing. When you finally "give in" to your forbidden food, eating will be experienced with such intensity, it usually results in Last Supper overeating and overwhelming guilt.
4. Challenge the Food Police Scream a loud "NO" to thoughts in your head that declare you're "good" for eating minimal calories or "bad" because you ate a piece of chocolate cake. The Food Police monitor the unreasonable rules that dieting has created. The police station is housed deep in your psyche, and its loudspeaker shouts negative barbs, hopeless phrases, and guilt-provoking indictments. Chasing the Food Police away is a critical step in returning to Intuitive Eating.
5. Respect Your Fullness Listen for the body signals that tell you that you are no longer hungry. Observe the signs that show that you're comfortably full. Pause in the middle of a meal or food and ask yourself how the food tastes, and what your current fullness level is.
6. Discover the Satisfaction Factor The Japanese have the wisdom to promote pleasure as one of their goals of healthy living. In our fury to be thin and healthy, we often overlook one of the most basic gifts of existence—the pleasure and satisfaction that can be found in the eating experience. When you eat what you really want, in an environment that is inviting and conducive, the pleasure you derive will be a powerful force in helping you feel satisfied and content. By providing this experience for yourself, you will find that it takes much less food to decide you've had "enough."
7. Honor Your Feelings Without Using Food Find ways to comfort , nurture, distract, and resolve your issues without using food. Anxiety, loneliness, boredom, anger are emotions we all experience throughout life. Each has its own trigger, and each has its own appeasement. Food won't fix any of these feelings. It may comfort for the short term, distract from the pain, or even numb you into a food hangover. But food won't solve the problem. If anything, eating for an emotional hunger will only make you feel worse in the long run. You'll ultimately have to deal with the source of the emotion, as well as the discomfort of overeating.
8. Respect Your Body Accept your genetic blueprint. Just as a person with a shoe size of eight would not expect to realistically squeeze into a size six, it is equally as futile (and uncomfortable) to have the same expectation with body size. But mostly, respect your body, so you can feel better about who you are. It's hard to reject the diet mentality if you are unrealistic and overly critical about your body shape.
9. Exercise—Feel the Difference Forget militant exercise. Just get active and feel the difference. Shift your focus to how it feels to move your body, rather than the calorie-burning effect of exercise. If you focus on how you feel from working out, such as energized, it can make the difference between rolling out of bed for a brisk morning walk or hitting the snooze alarm. If when you wake up, your only goal is to lose weight, it's usually not a motivating factor in that moment of time.

(continued)

10. Honor Your Health—Gentle Nutrition Make food choices that honor your health and tastebuds while making you feel well. Remember that you don't have to eat a perfect diet to be healthy. You will not suddenly get a nutrient deficiency or gain weight from one snack, one meal, or one day of eating. It's what you eat consistently over time that matters; progress not perfection is what counts.
Source: *Intuitive Eating: A Revolutionary Program That Works*[16]

cues for hunger and satiety don't function well, and is commonly used with people who are in recovery from chronic dieting and/or an eating disorder.[19]

Generally, structured eating consists of regularly eating balanced meals that consist of protein foods, grains/starchy vegetables, and vegetables and/or fruit. The Plate Model is often employed as a schematic to allow for easy understanding of balance, using a 9-inch plate to provide initial portions. Periodically throughout the eating experience, a person is encouraged to assess feelings of hunger, fullness, and satisfaction, generally using a hunger scale. The use of a smaller plate builds in an automatic stopping point where a person has the opportunity to assess if she/he wants more or if she/he is satisfied, thereby consciously making the choice to eat more if so desired. When first working with this model, a person may

Table 3. Conscious Eating Guidelines

1. Be conscious of your hunger. Eat when moderately hungry; don't wait until you are famished.
2. Eat regularly. Do not skip meals, and if possible, don't go over four hours without eating.
3. Allow yourself to eat all foods (unless you are allergic or have some other serious health issue).
4. Eat what you want, while also being conscious of how foods make you feel, what you have already eaten, and relevant health issues (for example, candy may not be a good conscious choice if you have diabetes or if you haven't eaten any protein all day).
5. All calories are equivalent when it comes to weight (that is, a calorie is a calorie).
6. For meals, eat a balance of protein, fat, and carbohydrates. Your body needs all of these to function properly and efficiently. Deprivation of foods or nutrients leads to physical and psychological problems and can actually trigger eating-disorder behaviors.
7. Stay conscious of your fullness and your satisfaction. You can eat a lot and not be satisfied. Texture and taste of food is important for satisfaction and eating enough is important so your body registers the experience of being comfortably full. The goal is to feel full and satisfied, but not physically uncomfortable in any way.
8. If you do overeat (which is normal to do sometimes), reassure yourself that your body can handle the excess food if you simply get back on track. It is OK to wait until you are hungry before eating again, but don't wait too long.
9. Enjoy food and the pleasure of eating. At times, enhance your eating to dining, using candles, nice dishes, and flowers on the table.
10. Make conscious choices to avoid foods that make you physically feel bad after eating them.
Source: *8 Keys to Recovery from an Eating Disorder*[18]

choose to stay with initial portion sizes but as he/she becomes more proficient in understanding cues, he/she works with the therapist to learn how to make choices about when and how much additional to eat.

Eating timing is generally encouraged as breakfast, lunch, and dinner, and snacks between meals, if desired, with no longer than 3–5 hours between eating. As a person becomes more experienced in listening to their body and interpreting the cues, the need for structured eating becomes less important. Eating in response to cues becomes internally driven and less in need of external input.

The ecSatter competent eating model developed by Ellyn Satter, RD, LCSW, author of the above definition of normal eating, emphasizes the importance of structured eating. Satter's definition of structured eating and her complete model have been described and validated in the scientific literature.[20, 21] The four primary components are listed in Table 4. The model has been shown to help people do better nutritionally, medically, emotionally, and socially, and have less body dissatisfaction and fewer other symptoms of eating disorders.[21, 22, 23, 24]

Summary

The non-diet, mindful approach to eating utilizes the body's natural instincts for eating to support health and well-being. Its very name positions it as an approach that runs counter to popular diet notions about how to eat for healthy weights, notions that have not been proven to be valid in the over five decades they have formed the core dietary approach to health and weight management in the U.S. While there may be minor differences in how the non-diet, mindful approach to eating is practiced, and while there may be preliminary interventions that be required before some individuals can successfully practice it, the method essentially relies on using the body's internal cues for guidance about what, when, and how much to eat. A growing body of research supports the effectiveness of this approach, underscoring its

Table 4. Four Components of the ecSatter Model of Eating Competence

- Context: Take time to eat, and provide yourself with rewarding meals and snacks at regular and reliable times.

- Attitude: Cultivate positive attitudes about eating and about food. Emphasize *providing* rather than *depriving*; seeking food rather than avoiding it.

- Food acceptance: Enjoy your eating, eat foods you like, and let yourself be comfortable with and relaxed about what you eat. Enjoying eating supports the natural inclination to seek variety, the keystone of healthful food selection.

- Internal regulation: Pay attention to your sensations of hunger and fullness to determine how much to eat. Go to the table hungry, eat until you feel satisfied, and then stop, knowing another meal or snack is coming soon when you can do it again.

Source: www.EllynSatter.com.

potential as part of the solution to the increasing problems with eating and weight struggles in cultures that experience food abundance.

References

1. Mann T, Tomiyama AJ, Westling E, Lew AM, Samuels B, and Chatman J. **"Medicare's Search for Effective Obesity Treatments: Diets Are Not the Answer."** *Am Psychol* 2007, **62:**220–233.

2. Daníelsdóttir S, Burgard D, and Oliver-Pyatt W. *AED Guidelines for Childhood Obesity Prevention Programs.* Academy of Eating Disorders, 2009.

3. Hirschmann, JR and Munter, CH. *When Women Stop Hating Their Bodies.* Ballantine Books, New York, 1995.

4. "Energy Balance and Its Components: Implications for Body Weight Regulation." *Am J Clin Nutr* April 2012 95: 989–994; doi:10.3945/ajcn.112.036350.

5. Outland L (2012). "Bringing Homeostasis Back into Weight Control." *J Obes Weig Los Ther* 2:115. doi:10.4172/2165-7904.1000115 http://www.omicsgroup.org/journals/2165-7904/2165- 7904-2-115.php?aid= 5108#9.

6. Pietilainen KH, Saarni, SE Kaprio J, and Rissanen A. "Does Dieting Make You Fat? A Twin Study." *Intl Jnl of Obesity* 2012, 36: 456–464.

7. Bacon L, Stern J, Van Loan M, and Keim N. **"Size Acceptance and Intuitive Eating Improve Health for Obese, Female Chronic Dieters."** *J Am Diet Assoc* 2005, **105:**929–936.

8. Rapoport L, Clark M, and Wardle J. **"Evaluation of a Modified Cognitive-Behavioural Programme for Weight Management."** *Int J Obes* 2000, **24:**1726–1737.

9. Provencher V, Begin C, Tremblay A, Mongeau L, Corneau L, Dodin S, Boivin S, and Lemieux S. **"Health-At-Every-Size and Eating Behaviors: 1-Year Follow-up Results of a Size Acceptance Intervention."** *J Am Diet Assoc* 2009, **109:**1854–1861.

10. Bacon L and Aphramor, L. "Weight Science: Evaluating the Evidence for a Paradigm Shift." *Nutrition Journal* 2011, 10:69.

11. Interview with Thelma Wayler, May 2012.

12. Interview with Carol Munter, April 2012.

13. http://www.ellynsatter.com/what-is-normal-eating-i-62.html.

14. http://www.umassmed.edu/cfm/index.aspx.

15. The Center for Mindful Eating, www.tcme.org/principles.htm.

16. Tribole, E and Resch, E. *Intuitive Eating: A Revolutionary Program That Works.* St. Martin's Griffin; Third Edition, August 7, 2012.

17. Tylka TL. "Development and Psychometric Evaluation of a Measure of Intuitive Eating." *Journal of Counseling Psychology,* 53:226–240.

18. Costin, C and Grabb, GS. *8 Keys to Recovery from an Eating Disorder.* W. W. Norton & Company, 2012.

19. Tribole, E. "Intuitive Eating in the Treatment of Eating Disorders: The Journey of Attunement." *BHNewsletter*, Behavioral Health Nutrition dietetic practice group of the Academy for Nutrition and Dietetics, fall 2011.

20. Satter EM. Eating Competence: Definition and Evidence for the Satter Eating Competence Model. *J Nutr Educ Behav.* 2007, 39 (suppl):S142–S153.

21. Lohse B, Satter E, Horacek T, Gebreselassie T, and Oakland MJ. "Measuring Eating Competence: Psychometric Properties and Validity of the ecSatter Inventory." *J Nutr Educ Behav.* 2007, 39 (suppl):S154–S166.

22. Lohse B, Bailey RL, Krall JS, Wall DE, and Mitchell DC. "Diet Quality Is Related to Eating Competence in Cross-Sectional Sample of Low-Income Females Surveyed in Pennsylvania." *Appetite.* Nov 25 2011, 58(2):645–650.

23. Lohse B, Psota T, Estruch R, et al. "Eating Competence of Elderly Spanish Adults Is Associated with a Healthy Diet and a Favorable Cardiovascular Disease Risk Profile." *J Nutr.* Jul 2010, 140(7):1322–1327.

24. Psota T, Lohse B, and West S. "Associations Between Eating Competence and Cardiovascular Disease Biomarkers." *J Nutr Educ Behav.* 2007, 39 (suppl):S171–S178.

SPOTLIGHT

The following chapter, by Jon Robison, describes the Health At Every Size (HAES) movement, its ideas, history, and how it differs from the current weight-centered approach. He makes the cogent argument that our focus on weight as a measure of health is a faulty assumption, since body weight and health are not really related. Instead, the focus on healthy lifestyle including diet, physical activity, stress management, and attention to medical problems when they arise is the core of HAES.

Chapter Two

Weight, Health and Culture: Exposing the Myth, Exploring the Realities

Jon Robison

WEIGHT AND CULTURE: ECONOMIC, SOCIAL, AND POLITICAL ISSUES

An American Obsession

The current American obsession with dieting and slimness is a cultural aberration. Throughout history, most cultures have regarded fatness as a sign of success, health, and beauty.[1] Less than 100 years ago Americans actually equated body fat with affluence and higher socioeconomic status. Excess fat was described as a "snug balance in the body bank and a comfortable reserve in the case of emergencies."[2] Victorian-era women wore corsets to achieve the plump, hourglass figure deemed desirable for the leisure class. This style of dress was advocated by the medical establishment, though it often resulted in constricted lungs, squeezed livers and bladders, and dislocated stomachs.[3-5] A 1908 article in *Harpers Bazaar* advised readers on "how to get plump," saying "fat is force and stored up fat is stored up force."[6] Fashion models were advised to be "far from thin, with no suggestion of hollows in the face or the collar-bones, for the camera seems to accentuate such defects."[7]

Anthropologists point out that the first strong cultural emphasis on weight loss in the United States appeared around the turn of the century. This coincided with women obtaining the right to vote and demanding a more visible and active role in shaping society. As women's power and status improved, the dictates of fashion began to change as well. Medical recommendations for women to lose weight also followed suit. For the next 100 years, medical science would promote a wide variety of potentially dangerous and sometimes lethal diets, drugs, and surgeries to help people reduce their weight in the name of health. A partial chronological list of these recommended treatments is included below.[8]

IN THE NAME OF HEALTH

1893 – Thyroid Extract*	1964 – Total Fasting
1920 – Laxatives *	1969 – Intestinal Bypass**
1933 – Dinitrophenol*	1974 – Jaw Wiring
1937 – Amphetamine*	1977 – Gastric Bypass **
1940 – Atropine*	1985 – Gastric Balloon**
1940 – Digitalis*	1990s – Fen-Phen, Redux, Meridia, Xenical*
1957 – HCG*	2000s and beyond—Gastric Banding**

*Medication
** Surgery

The vast majority of those participating in and suffering the consequences from these "cures" would be women, despite the fact that women's fat confers only a fraction of the health risk of men's and may actually carry with it significant health benefits.[9–11] This legacy continues today, as young girls and women continue to divert significant proportions of their physical, emotional, and financial resources to the pursuit of ideals of body shape and size that are, for the vast majority, neither achievable nor healthy.[12]

It has been suggested that keeping women occupied by continually striving toward an unreachable ideal of perfection serves the purposes of a control-oriented, patriarchal society.[5,13] When women's energies are diverted by the pursuit of dieting and body improvement, they are kept from dealing effectively with the realities of existence in a man's world and from participating more fully in art, politics, literature, and life in general.

Much has been written concerning the historical association of female fat, particularly on the abdomen, buttocks, and breasts, with the "feminine" values of nurturance, compassion, etc.[14–16] Throughout history, soft, rounded hips, thighs, and bellies have been considered ideal for women in the vast majority of cultures.[1] As long as women were content to stay at home and bear children, these associations remained relatively intact. It has been argued convincingly that the obsessive hatred of fat in this country began with the women's equality movement and that the more powerful women become, the more pressure there is to alter the aspects of their bodies that distinguish them from their male counterparts.[15–18] For example, one of the things that women dislike most about their bodies is cellulite (actually a made-up name referring to dimpled fat that some women accumulate as they age), a characteristic of the female body that is rarely found in men. The continuing trend toward an ever-thinner, androgynous ideal for women would also seem to support this view.[19] Thus:

> Taking on the accouterments of the white male world may be experienced by many women themselves as a chance to embody qualities such as detachment, self-containment, self-mastery, and control which are highly valued in this culture.[17]

Since the 1960s, a preference for slenderness also has taken hold in other Western, industrialized nations. However, due to a unique confluence of social, economic, and political developments favoring the desire for thinness, "no other culture suffers from the same wild anxieties about weight, dieting and exercise as we do."[7] It is estimated that approximately 50% of adult American women (versus 25% of adult men) are attempting to lose weight at any one time.[20] Research also suggests that most young women who try to lose weight are already at or below "normal" weight.[21] Even very young children are not spared. Fear of fat, restricted eating, and binge eating are common among girls by age 10.[22] In fact, nearly half of American children between 1st and 3rd grades want to be thinner and half of 9–10-year-old girls are dieting.[23]

The Body as Machine

Traditional treatment approaches to weight management strongly reflect the underlying assumptions of the mechanistic worldview of the scientific revolution of the 17th Century. The human body is seen as a "finely calibrated combustion engine that should weigh a certain amount," and therefore scientists have issued "recommendations about exactly how many calories, calibrated to age, height, and activity levels are needed to achieve this goal."[15] Because body weight has been considered largely a mechanical matter of calories in (diet) and calories out (exercise), weight management is reduced to a measurable numeric equation and it is assumed that everyone can attain their goal by merely adjusting the variables. Furthermore, scientists have determined the exact amount of calories and nutrients needed for health and efficiency, and food therefore has become "an instrument of science, stripped down to a quantity of energy and deprived of all its sensual and emotional aspects."[15] The resulting reductionist view of weight- and eating-related issues "is typical of the medicalization of complex conditions, in which contextual factors are treated as single variables to be overcome."[13]

These premises continue to guide medical weight-management efforts. Yet it is common knowledge that weight, like almost all other human characteristics, varies according to a "normal" distribution, meaning that there is a wide range of weights that are considered to be normal. Furthermore, the existence of different body types (somatotypes in Western medicine, doshas in Ayurveda) is well documented, and it is likely that each has its own range of normally distributed weights and body fat percentages. William Sheldon, MD, originator of the concept of the somatotype, commented in the 1930s on ideal weights such as those set forth by the height and weight tables, saying "this kind of foolishness gives some of our best people inferiority complexes."[19] Strong arguments have been made that these tables are flawed to the point of being relatively meaningless for the majority of people.[19,24] World-renowned researcher Dr. Ancel Keys described them as "arm-chair concoctions starting with questionable assumptions and ending with three sets of standards for 'body frames' which were never measured or even properly defined."[12]

These tables have now been replaced by the Body Mass Index (BMI) as the gold standard for distinguishing "healthy" from "unhealthy" weights. Unfortunately, the BMI is fraught with its own set of problems. It was created in the mid-1850s by a Belgian mathematician as a means of measuring the size of large populations. It was neither intended for health-related use or for use with individuals. In a recent article entitled: Do You Believe in Fairies, Unicorns, or the BMI?; Stanford University Professor and National Public Radio "Math Guy" Dr. Keith Devlin examines these problems in detail, concluding about the BMI as a measure of individual health.

> Since the entire sorry saga of the BMI was started by a mathematician—one of us—I think the onus is on us, as the world's experts on the formulation and application of mathematical formulas, to start to eradicate this nonsense and demand the responsible use of our product. (http://www.maa.org/devlin/devlin_05_09.html)

The view of weight control as a simple mathematical relationship between caloric intake and expenditure has been shown to be inaccurate.[25] Furthermore, the reduction of food to caloric input, devoid of other less-measurable qualities, denies the reality of the complex interaction of emotional, psychological, and cultural variables that determines voluntary food intake.[26] The resulting diet mentality "reinforces the split between the dieter's mind and her body, and asks her to distrust her body, which is seen as the source of sabotage."[27] This separation of mind from body inhibits the development of internally regulated eating in children[28] and contributes to the current epidemic of adult eating disorders, disordered eating, and exercise addiction.[29,30]

Food Industry and Media
Food Advertising and Labeling

In keeping with the larger cultural agenda, today's media images constantly tell us we should control our eating and our weight. We have become so accustomed to this phenomenon that we forget it is relatively new. Fifty years ago our grandparents did not walk down grocery store aisles surrounded by thousands of messages about food products being "low-fat," "cholesterol free," "low sodium," or "high fiber." Concern about removing "undesirable" ingredients from our diet has led to product labeling that categorizes foods as "good/healthy" versus "bad/unhealthy." Many product advertisements even suggest that our food choices reflect our personality characteristics. Some health professionals have observed that this type of labeling by the food industry has contributed to the development of a food- and eating-based morality. More than 20 years ago, the prestigious Tufts University Diet and Nutrition Letter commented on the dangers of this trend, saying:

> Good nutrition is getting a bad name—one that smacks of rigidity, guilt-making and extremism. … Worse still, some eight out of ten (Americans) think foods are inherently good or bad—that is, the decision to eat a particular item has nothing to do with its context in the diet as a whole, but every single bite they take represents an all-or-nothing choice either for or against good health. [For example,] [t]wo out of 10 Americans are even under the false belief that all fat should be eliminated from the diet.[31]

Because our culture encourages us to "think" constantly about our food choices, eating has become an intellectual activity that is increasingly disconnected from the physical body. We no longer know how to eat in response to hunger, fullness, and body cravings because we are intellectually trying to sort out what we should eat, what we shouldn't eat, and how our choices will affect our weight and our health. In his recent book, entitled *The End of Overeating*, former Food and Drug Commissioner Dr. David Kessler suggests eating only foods we can control and avoiding "bad" foods by retraining the brain to think "I'll hate myself if I eat that."[32]

Images of Beauty

While advertising and cultural messages urge us to eliminate fat in foods, fat on our bodies is portrayed as even worse. The media bombard women with female fashion models who project an emaciated, adolescent, androgynous look as the aesthetic ideal. What most women do not realize is that the published images of these models have been airbrushed to remove any flaws (such as wrinkles or visible pores in the skin), photographically elongated to maximize thinness, and, in some cases, generated entirely on a computer.

The content of many of the articles in women's magazines is also unhelpful. The main messages in most articles and ads are (1) Your natural appearance, including your weight, is unacceptable, so buy something to disguise or fix it; and (2) "Good" women nurture other people by preparing delicious recipes for loved ones, but they do not partake in these rich foods themselves.

Not surprisingly, the relentless pressure to conform to unrealistic body shapes and sizes is wreaking havoc with the body image and self-esteem of women of all sizes. An often-quoted survey in *Psychology Today* involving more than 3,400 women in their 30s and 40s, with an average weight of 140 pounds, is illustrative of the problem. Among the findings, 24% of the women said they would give up more than three years of their lives to lose weight, 35% considered pregnancy a major source of body hatred, and 50% reported that they smoked cigarettes in order to control their weight. The author of the article concluded that:

> … the magnitude of self-hatred among women is astonishing. Despite being at a weight that most women would envy they are still plagued by feelings of inadequacy.[33]

A substantial body of literature supports this extreme body dissatisfaction as a "normative discontent" in our culture, especially among young women.[16,34,35]

It is interesting to note that men's health and fitness magazines now routinely feature cover images of young, scantily clad, tan males with washboard abdominals, broad chests, and full heads of hair. Not surprisingly, this new cultural interest in making men sexual objects has gone hand in hand with an alarming increase in eating disorder rates.[36,37]

The "Diet-Pharmaceutical-Industrial Complex"

The tremendous pressure to be thin is driven by diet, fashion, cosmetic, fitness, insurance, and pharmaceutical industries that reap tremendous financial rewards by promoting unattainable expectations, especially for women.[5] In addition, many obesity researchers have economic links to this so-called diet-pharmaceutical-industrial complex, creating powerful incentives for maintaining the status quo. For example, most members of the National Institutes of Health National Task Force on The Prevention and Treatment of Obesity serve as consultants to both commercial weight-loss programs and to pharmaceutical companies involved in the development of weight-loss medications.[38] Furthermore, "obesity research is primarily funded by companies that make money by promoting short-term weight-loss methods," contributing, perhaps, to questionable objectivity in the reporting of research findings.[7]

Medical support for thinness is one of the important developments contributing to the growth of our current obsession. It is interesting to note that only 100 years ago, American physicians were encouraging people to gain weight, believing that "a large number of fat cells was absolutely necessary to achieve a balanced personality."[39] As late as 1926, Dr. Woods Hutchinson, former president of the American Academy of Medicine, warned that "the longed-for slender and boyish figure is becoming a menace, not only for the present, but for future generations."[2] Today, fatness as chronic disease and weight reduction as cure stand as almost universally accepted medical dogma.

> "A focus on approaches that can produce health benefits independently of weight loss may be the best way to improve the physical and psychological health of Americans seeking to lose weight."

> National Institutes of Health, *Annals of Internal Medicine*

History

A dramatically new perspective on resolving weight-related struggles is now emerging. The thinking behind this perspective began in the 1970s as part of the women's movement. At that time feminist activists began to question the way in which women were being targeted differently from men regarding weight and health issues. In addition, in 1979 two major scientific reviews were published that questioned the effectiveness and social appropriateness of traditional weight-loss treatment.[40,41]

Since that time, numerous books and research papers have been written challenging the basic assumptions of the biomedical emphasis on weight loss. Increasingly, the ethics of offering traditional weight-loss programs is being questioned. From the combined work of many women and men from a variety of fields, the Non-Diet/Size Acceptance Movement was born. Over the last 30 years this movement has grown in popularity and developed into what is referred to by those involved as the Health At Every Size® (HAES) approach.

Foundations of HAES®

Although specific approaches within the Health At Every Size® movement vary somewhat depending on the source, the philosophy and emphasis are remarkably similar. The basic conceptual framework includes acceptance of:

1. The natural diversity in body shape and size
2. The ineffectiveness and dangers of dieting
3. The importance of relaxed eating in response to internal body cues
4. The critical contribution of social, emotional, and spiritual, as well as physical factors to health and happiness.

Overall, HAES®® supports a holistic view of health that promotes "feeling good about oneself, eating well in a natural, relaxed way, and being comfortably active."[27] Table 1 below contrast the conceptual bases of traditional weight-management approaches with those of Health At Every Size®.[42]

Components of HAES®®

HAES® provides health professionals with the opportunity to shift how we define and respond to people's food- and weight-related struggles. In exploring the use of HAES®, there are three major components to be aware of. These components are outlined in TABLE 2 and discussed in more detail following the table.

Size- and Self-Acceptance

The most important component of HAES® is self-acceptance. Self-acceptance is not a denial of the importance of self-care but is rather an affirmation that, just as human worth is not based on race, color, or creed, it also is not dependent on body weight, shape, or size. Our obsession with thinness has spawned a culturally accepted prejudice against individuals who do not live up to our unrealistic societal standards. Like racism, sexism, anti-Semitism, and homophobia, this weightism:

Table 1. A Comparison of the Traditional Weight-Loss Paradigm and Health At Every Size

Traditional Weight-Loss Paradigm	Health At Every Size®
Everyone needs to be thin for good health and happiness	Thin is not intrinsically healthy and beautiful, nor is fat intrinsically unhealthy and unappealing.
People who are not thin are "overweight" because they have no willpower, eat too much, and don't move enough.	People naturally have different body shapes and sizes and different preferences for physical activity.
Everyone can be thin, happy, and healthy by dieting.	Dieting usually leads to weight gain, decreased self-esteem, and increased risk for eating problems. Health and happiness are not dependent on weight loss and involve a dynamic interaction among mental, social, spiritual, and physical considerations.

is based on visible cues, i.e., the fat person is discriminated against primarily because of the way she looks ... defines an entire group of people numbering in the millions within a narrow range of negative characteristics and behaviors ... elevates the status of one group of people at the expense of another ... and serves as a vehicle for the bigot's own anxieties, frustrations and resentments.[43]

The result of this prejudice is rampant social, economic, and educational discrimination against larger individuals.[5,7,43–45] In fact, the latest research suggests that weight discrimination is now more prevalent than discrimination based on sexual orientation, nationality/ethnicity, physical disability, and religious beliefs. Indeed, for women, weight discrimination is even more prevalent than racial discrimination.[46]

The cornerstone of HAES®, self-acceptance, involves honoring the natural diversity in the human form and challenging cultural weight prejudice. As health professionals, we must

Table 2. Health At Every Size: Major Components

Self-Acceptance
  Affirmation and reinforcement of human beauty and worth irrespective of differences in weight, physical size, and shape.

Physical Activity
  Support for increasing social, pleasure-based movement for enjoyment and enhanced quality of life. Calorie burning and weight loss are not the goals of the activity.

Normalized Eating
  Support for discarding externally imposed rules and regimens for eating and attaining a more peaceful relationship with food by relearning to eat in response to physiological hunger and fullness cues.

begin by confronting our own prejudices and learning strategies to empower our clients to do the same. Fortunately, materials have been developed to assist health professionals with the process of understanding and combating their own weight prejudice.[47]

Physical Activity

Physical activity is widely recognized as an important element in human health, yet the majority of Americans of all sizes remain sedentary. Part of the problem may lie in traditional approaches used to encourage people to become more active. As Thomas Moore writes in *Care of the Soul*:

> Usually we are told how much time to spend at a certain exercise, what heart rate to aim for, and which muscle to focus on for toning. ... If we could loosen our grip on the mechanical view of our own bodies and the body of the world, many other possibilities might come to light.[48]

HAES® focuses on promoting movement that is social, playful, and pleasurable and includes not just jogging, cycling, and exercise classes, but also activities connected with everyday living such as walking and gardening. Movement is encouraged for enjoyment, camaraderie, and improved quality of life, not calorie burning and weight loss.[49] Much accumulated research supports that physical activity can positively affect health and longevity regardless of weight status.[50,51] Dr. Steven Blair, one of the world's most respected experts on exercise and health, summed up the evidence by saying:

> if you're fit ... being 25 or even 75 pounds overweight is perfectly healthy. And if you aren't fit, being slim gives you no protection whatsoever.[52]

In addition, this alternative paradigm acknowledges the prevalence of sedentary living in our society as largely a cultural phenomenon that can be significantly impacted only by addressing cultural barriers.[53] This is especially true for larger individuals, many of whom are deterred from engaging in physical activity by fear of the ridicule and humiliation that they have endured as a regular, ongoing part of their lives.[54] For many such individuals, discovering movement in a size-friendly environment can be a means of beginning to rediscover and reconnect to the bodies they have been taught to hate and ignore.[55]

Normal Eating

Healthy, balanced eating is generally accepted as an important component of a healthy lifestyle. However, the externally focused, restrictive methods used by diet programs rarely succeed in helping people to become healthy eaters. Traditional wisdom has it that larger people get that way because they eat a lot more than thinner individuals. Contrary to this belief, however, research on the caloric intake of larger individuals does not provide conclusive evidence that they eat more than their thinner counterparts.[54,56,57] In fact, the most recent research suggests that fatter children may actually consume fewer calories than their thinner counterparts beginning as early as age 7.[58]

There is strong evidence that human beings are capable of regulating caloric intake according to internal hunger, satiety, and appetite signals,[59,60] and that chronic food restriction such as dieting interferes with this process and actually increases the likelihood of overeating.[61–63]

HAES® refutes the concept of "good" and "bad" foods and discourages the use of externally focused eating strategies. Instead, all foods are legalized and the focus is placed on reducing anxiety about eating by relearning how to eat in response to internal signals: hunger, appetite, and satiety. This innate ability to regulate our eating is referred to as "normal," "intuitive," "mindful," or "attuned" eating.[64–67] (For more on this topic, see chapter 13.)

As a result of being more aware of internal signals, individuals may or may not decrease their weight. However, promoting internally directed eating is likely to improve people's health by reducing the anxiety, guilt, preoccupation with food, bingeing, weight cycling, and weight gain commonly associated with restricted eating (dieting).[68–75]

HAES® also recognizes that when people are struggling with food- and weight-related issues, it may be symptomatic of underlying distress that cannot be solved merely by delivering nutrition information and advice. Trying to help people with these kinds of issues and being sure to *do no harm* in the process necessitates a compassionate, weight-neutral, compassionate, truly holistic approach.

HAES®: IMPLICATIONS FOR HELPING

Redefining Success

The underlying goal of traditional approaches to weight management is for people to be smaller, i.e., to lose weight. This is an inappropriate and unacceptable goal for at least four important reasons.

- The research linking weight loss to improved health is equivocal at best
- Weight loss is not, at the present time, a sustainable outcome for the vast majority of people
- Most health-related problems can be ameliorated with lifestyle changes without significant weight loss
- There is considerable evidence that promoting weight loss violates the underlying health care principle of "first do no harm."

The goal for health professionals in HAES® is to empower their clients to live healthier, more fulfilled lives by honoring and caring for the bodies they presently have. A healthy weight is therefore defined as the weight at which a person settles when they normalize their eating, accept their body, and turn their attention to creating a more fulfilled and meaningful life. Success with this process can be measured in a variety of ways including:

- Improved quality of life and reduction of medical problems and health risks, with or without weight loss
- Decreased reliance on medications
- Increased involvement with and enjoyment of physical activity
- Body acceptance
- Movement toward increased Normal, Intuitive, Mindful eating
- Improved quality of diet.

Focus on Health

Removing the focus on weight does not imply ignoring health risks and medical problems. On the contrary, the HAES® approach strongly acknowledges that a person's experience with weight and health is part of a complex, dynamic interplay of social, emotional, ecological, and spiritual as well as physical factors.[42] A focus on weight can obscure or even exacerbate these factors, whereas removing this focus enables health professionals to view clients more appropriately as complex "wholes" who are more than the sum of their parts.[76]

HAES® proposes that people create health by healing disturbed relationships with food and making peace with their bodies, not by weight loss. This is a critical distinction between HAES® and traditional approaches. Furthermore, it suggests that an appropriate healthy weight cannot be determined by a set of numbers on an ideal height and weight chart, or associated BMIs or body fat percentages, but only by observing the weight at which an individual's body settles as she stops dieting and strives toward living a fulfilled, meaningful life. The HAES® approach does not suggest that all people are at a weight that is the healthiest for their circumstances. What it strongly suggests is that the movement toward a healthier lifestyle will, over time for most people, produce a weight that is healthy for that person.

Medical Treatment

The HAES® approach does not suggest that health professionals ignore effective health care for large people. When large individuals present with medical problems, health professionals should consider and offer the same approaches that they would for a thin person with similar presenting problems.[27] In the case of a thin person with essential hypertension, for example, conventional medicine suggests dietary changes, increases in aerobic physical activity, and stress management followed by medication, if necessary. Yet a larger individual presenting with the same diagnosis is told to lose weight, despite all that is known about the likely unhealthy consequences of this prescription.

HAES® can be followed regardless of the individual's presenting problems. Even with individuals experiencing serious conditions such as type 2 diabetes, hypertension, and coronary artery disease where weight is commonly seen as such an important risk factor, research shows people's health status and risk can be improved without changes in weight, and even in individuals who remain markedly fat.[77–80]

Summary

Insanity is often defined as "doing the same things over and over again and expecting different results." With their inevitable failure, traditional approaches to helping people with weight-related concerns cause shame and embarrassment and are likely to diminish further seeking of medical care.[81, 82] Continuing to prescribe and promote these approaches is ineffective and potentially harmful. Health professionals should therefore refrain from doing so.

Health professionals and size-acceptance advocates have joined together to form The Association for Size Diversity and Health (ASDAH), which has become the governing body for health professionals involved in promoting the HAES® Approach. Through dissemination of scientific research and political advocacy, this organization is striving to turn around the failed approaches of the past and help people of all sizes make peace with their bodies and their food by learning to love and take care of the bodies they have right now.

References

1. Brown, P. J. "Cultural Perspectives on the Etiology and Treatment of Obesity." In A. J. Stunkard and T. A. Wadden, eds., *Obesity: Theory, and Therapy*. New York: Raven Press, 1993.

2. Hutchinson, W. "Fat and Fashion." *Saturday Evening Post*, August 21, 1926.

3. Bennett, W., and J. Gurin. *The Dieter's Dilemma: Eating Less and Weighing More*. New York: Basic Books, 1982.

4. Brownmiller, S. *Femininity*. New York: Fawcett Columbine, 1984.

5. Rothbloom, E. D. "I'll Die for the Revolution, but Don't Ask Me Not to Diet": Feminism and the Continuing Stigmatization of Obesity." In P. Fallon, M. Katzman, and S. Wooley, eds., *Feminist Perspectives on Eating Disorders*. New York: Guilford, 1994.

6. "How to Stay Plump." *Harpers Bazaar*, August 1908.

7. Fraser, L. *America's Obsession with Weight and the Industry That Feeds on It*. New York: Dutton, 1997.

8. Ernsberger, P., and P. Haskew. "Re-thinking Obesity: An Alternative View of Its Health Implications." *Journal of Obesity and Weight Regulation* 6, no. 2 (1987): 1–81.

9. Schapira, D. V., N. B. Kumar, C. H. Lyman, D. Cavanagh, W. S. Robert, and J. La Polla. "Upper-Body Fat Distribution and Endometrical Cancer Risk." *Journal of the American Medical Association* 266 (1991): 1808–11.

10. Schapira, D. V., N. B. Kumar, C. H. Lyman, and C. E. Cox. "Abdominal Obesity and Breast Cancer." *Annals of Internal Medicine* 112 (1990): 182–86.

11. Terry, R. B., M. L. Stefanick, W. Haskell, and P. H. Wood. "Contributions of Regional Adipose Tissue Depots to Plasma Lipoprotein Concentrations in Overweight Men and Women: Possible Protective Effects of Thigh Fat." *Metabolism* 40 (1991): 733–40.

12. Keys, A. "Overweight, Obesity, Coronary Heart Diseasem and Mortality." *Nutrition Reviews* 38 (1980): 297–307.

13. Allan, J. D. "A Biomedical and Feminist Perspective on Women's Experiences with Weight Management." *Western Journal of Nursing Research* 16, no. 5 (1994): 524–43.

14. Hutchinson, M. G. "Imagining Ourselves Whole: A Feminist Approach to Treating Body Image Disorders." In P. Fallon, M. Katzman, and S. Wooley, eds., *Feminist Perspectives on Eating Disorders*. New York: Guilford, 1994.

15. Seid, R. P. *Never Too Thin: Why Women Are at War with Their Bodies*. New York: Prentice Hall. 1989.

16. Wolf, N. *The Beauty Myth: How Images of Beauty Are Used Against Women*. New York: Morrow, 1991.

17. Bordo, S. "Reading the Slender Body." In M. Jacobs, E. F. Keller, and S. Shuttleworth, eds., *Body/Politics, Women, and the Discourses of Science*. New York: Routledge, Chapman, and Hall, 1990.

18. Hirschmann, J. R., and C. H. Munter. *When Women Stop Hating Their Bodies: Freeing Yourself from Food and Weight Obsession*. New York: Ballantine, 1995.

19. Schroeder, C. R. *Fat Is Not a Four-Letter Word*. Minneapolis: Chronimed, 1992.

20. Market Data Enterprises, Inc. "The U.S. Weight Loss and Diet Control Market." March 9, 2011.

21. Rosen, J. C., B. Tacy, and D. Howell. "Life Stress, Psychological Symptoms, and Weight Reducing Behavior in Adolescent Girls: A Prospective Analysis." *International Journal of Eating Disorders* 9 (1990): 17–26.

22. Mellin, L. M., C. E. Irwin, and S. Scully. "Prevalence of Disordered Eating in Girls: A Survey of Middle-Class Children." *Journal of the American Dietetic Association* 92, no. 7 (1992): 851–53.

23. U.S. Department of Health and Human Services. "Rate of Eating Disorders in Kids Keeps Rising." http://www.healthfinder.gov/news/newsstory.aspx?docID=646574

24. Gaesser, G. A. *Big Fat Lies: The Truth about Your Weight and Your Health*. Rev. ed. Carlsbad, California: Gurze Books, 2002.

25. Hall, K. D., S. B. Heymsfield, J. W. Kemnitz, S. Klein, D. A. Schoeller, and J. R. Speakman. "Energy balance and its components: implications for body weight regulation." *American Journal of Clinical Nutrition* 95, no. 4 (2012):989–994.

26. Thomas, P. R., ed. *Determinants of Food Choice and Prospects for Modifying Attitudes and Behavior*. Washington, DC: National Academy Press, 1991.

27. Burgard, D., and P. Lyons. "Alternatives in Obesity Treatment: Focusing on Health for Fat Women." In P. Fallon, M. Katzman, and S. Wooley, eds., *Feminist Perspectives on Eating Disorders*. New York: Guilford, 1994.

28. Satter, E. M. "Internal Regulation and the Evolution of Normal Growth as the Basis for Prevention of Obesity in Children." *Journal of the American Dietetic Association* 96, no. 9 (1996): 860–64.

29. Kratina, K., N. King, and D. Hayes. *Moving Away from Diets: New Ways to Heal Eating Problems and Exercise Resistance.* Lake Dallas: Helms Seminars, 1996.

30. Wiseman, C. V., J. J. Gray, J. E. Mosimann, and A. H. Ahrens. "Cultural Expectations of Thinness in Women: An Update." *International Journal of Eating Disorders* 11, no. 1 (1992): 85–89.

31. "Just What Is a Balanced Diet, Anyway?" *Tufts University Diet and Nutrition Letter* 9, no. 11 (1992): 3–6.

32. Kessler, D. *The End of Overeating: Taking Control of the Insatiable American Appetite.* Rodale, 2009.

33. Garner, D. M. "The 1997 Body Image Survey Results." *Psychology Today*, January–February 1997.

34. Rodin, J., L. Silberstein, and R. Striegel-Moore. "Women and Weight: A Normative Discontent." In T. B. Sonderegger, ed., *Nebraska Symposium on Motivation: Psycholog, and Gender.* Lincoln: University of Nebraska Press, 1985.

35. *Science Daily.* "Three Out Of Four American Women Have Disordered Eating, Survey Suggests." www.sciencedaily.com/releases/2008/04/080422202514.htm

36. Woodside, B. "Eating Disorders in Men: An Overview." *Healthy Weight Journal* 16, no. 4 (2002): 52–55.

37. Sarkis, S. "Eating Disorders in Men: An Interview With Dr. Roberto Olivardia." *Psychology Today*, May 16, 2012. http://www.psychologytoday.com/blog/here-there-and-everywhere/201205/eating-disorders-in-men-interview-dr-roberto-olivardia

38. National Institutes of Health. "National Task Force on the Prevention and Treatment of Obesity: Long-Term Pharmacotherapy in the Management of Obesity." *Journal of the American Medical Association* 276 (1996): 1907–15.

39. Banner, L. W. *American Beauty.* Chicago: University of Chicago Press, 1983.

40. Stunkard, A. J., and S. B. Penick. "Behavior Modification in the Treatment of Obesity: The Problem of Maintaining Weight Loss." *Archives of General Psychiatry* 36, no. 1 (1979): 801–6.

41. Wooley, O. W., S. C. Wooley, and S. R. Dyrenforth. "Obesity and Women II: A Neglected Feminist Topic." *Women's International Quarterly* 2 (1979): 81–92.

42. Robison, J. I. "Weight Management: Shifting the Paradigm." *Journal of Health Education* 28, no. 10 (1997): 28–34.

43. Goodman, W. C. *The Invisible Women: Confronting Weight Prejudice in America.* Carlsbad, CA: Gurze, 1995.

44. Gortmaker, S., A. Must, J. Perrin, A. Sobol, and W. Dietz. "Social and Economic Consequences of Overweight in Adolescence and Young Adulthood." *New England Journal of Medicine* 329 (1993): 1008–12.

45. Solovay, S. *Tipping the Scales of Justice: Fighting Weight-based Discrimination.* New York: Prometheus, 2000.

46. Puhl, R. M., T. Andreyeva, and K. D. Brownell. "Perceptions of weight discrimination: prevalence and comparison to race and gender discrimination in America." *International Journal of Obesity* 32 (2008): 992–1000.

47. NAAFA. "Guidelines for Healthcare Providers Who Treat Fat Patients." 2011. http://issuu.com/naafa/docs/naafa_healthcarep_guidelines_2011_v06_screencut

48. Moore, T. *Care of the Soul: A Guide for Cultivating Depth and Sacredness in Everyday Life.* New York: Harper Perennial, 1994.

49. Lyons, P., and D. Burgard. *Great Shape: The First Fitness Guide for Large Women.* iUniverse Press, 2000.

50. Gaesser, G. "Fatness, Fitness & Health: A Closer Look At The Evidence." *Absolute Advantage* 5, no. 3 (2006): 18–21.

51. McAuley, B. "Obesity Paradoxes." *Journal of Sports Sciences* 29, no. 8 (2011):773–782.

52. Barlow, C. E., H. W. Kohl, L. W. Gibbons, and S. N. Blair. "Physical Fitness, Mortality, and Obesity." *International Journal of Obesity* 19, suppl. 4 (1995): S41–44.

53. Robison, J. I., and M. A. Rogers. "Adherence to Exercise Programmes: Recommendations." *Sports Medicine* 17, no. 1 (1994): 39–52.

54. Garner, D. M., and S. Wooley. "Confronting the Failure of Behavioral and Dietary Treatments for Obesity." *Clinical Psychology Review* 11 (1991): 729–80.

55. Lyons, P. "Weight and Health: A New Approach for the New Year." *Wellness Management: Newsletter of the National Wellness Association* 11, no. 4 (1995): 1, 5–7.

56. Rolland-Cachera, F., and F. Bellisle. "No Correlation between Adiposity and Food Intake: Why Are Working Class Children Fatter?" *American Journal of Clinical Nutrition* 44 (1986): 779–87.

57. Striegel-Moore, R. H., and J. Rodin. "The Influence of Psychological Variables in Obesity." In K. D. Brownell and J. P. Foreyt, eds. *Handbook of Eating Disorders.* New York: Basic Books, 1986.

58. "Medscape Medical News." May 11, 2011.

59. Davis, C. "Self-Selection of Diet by Newly Weaned Infants: An Experimental Study." *American Journal of Diseases of Children* 36, no. 4 (1928): 650–79.

60. Johnson, S. L., and L. L. Birch. "Parents' and Children's Adiposity and Eating Style." *Pediatrics* 94 (1994): 653–61.

61. Polivy, J. "Psychological Consequences of Feed Restriction." *Journal of the American Dietetic Association* 96, no. 6 (1996): 589–92.

62. Field, A. E., et al. "Relation Between Dieting and Weight Change Among Preadolescents and Adolescents." *Pediatrics* 112 (2003): 900–906.

63. Neumark-Sztainer, D., et al. "Obesity, disordered eating, and eating disorders in a longitudinal study of adolescents: how do dieters fare 5 years later." *Journal of the American Dietetic Association* 112, no. 4 (2006): 900–906.

64. Hirschmann J. R., and C. H. Munter. *When Women Stop Hating Their Bodies: Freeing Yourself from Food and Weight Obsession.* 1st edn. New York: Fawcett Columbine, 1995.

65. Matz, J. and E. Frankel. *The Diet Survivor's Handbook: 60 Lessons in Eating, Acceptance and Self-Care.* Naperville, IL: Sourcebooks, 2006.

66. Satter, E. *Secrets of Feeding a Healthy Family: How to Eat, How to Raise Good Eaters and How to Cook.* Madison, WI: Kelcy Press, 2008.

67. Tribole, E. and E. Resch. *Intuitive Eating: A Revolutionary Program That Works.* 2nd edn. New York: St. Martin's Griffin, 2010.

68. Armstrong, D., and A. King. "Demand Feeding as Diabetes Treatment." *Obesity and Health* 1 (1993): 109–10, 115.

69. Carrier, K. M., M. A. Steinhardt, and S. Bowman. "Rethinking Traditional Weight Management Programs: A Three-Year Follow-up Evaluation of a New Approach." *Journal of Psychology* 128, no. 5 (1993): 517–35.

70. Ciliska, D. K. *Beyond Dieting: Psychoeducational Interventions for Chronically Obese Women.* New York: Brunner/Mazel, 1990.

71. Omichinski, L., and K. R. Harrison. "Reduction of Dieting Attitudes and Practices after Participation in a Non-diet Lifestyle Program." *Journal of the Canadian Dietetic Association* 56, no. 2 (1995): 81–85.

72. Rosen, J. C., P. Orosan, and J. Ritter. "Cognitive Behavior Therapy for Negative Body Image in Obese Women." *Behavior Therapy* 26 (1995): 25–42.

73. Roughan, P., E. Seddon, and J. Vernon-Roberts. "Long-Term Effects of a Psychologically Based Group Programme for Women Preoccupioed with Body Weight and Eating Behavior." *International Journal of Obesity* 14 (1990): 137–47.

74. Bacon, L., N. L. Keim, M. D. Van Loan, M. Derricote, B. Gale, A. Kazakis, and J. S. Stern. "Evaluating a Non-diet Wellness Intervention for Improvement of Matabolic Fitness, Psychological Well-Being, and Eating and Activity Behaviors." *International Journal of Obesity* 26 (2002): 854–65.

75. Provencher, V,. C. Bégin, A. Tremblay, L. Mongeau, S. Boivin, and S. Lemieux. "Short-Term Effects of a 'Health-At-Every-Size' Approach on Eating Behaviors and Appetite Ratings." *Obesity* 15 (2007) :957–966.

76. Robison, J. I., and K. Carrier. *The Spirit and Science of Holistic Health: More Than Broccoli, Jogging and Bottled Water, More Than Yoga, Herbs and Meditation.* Bloomington, Indiana: Authorhouse Books, 2004.

77. Tremblay, A., J. P. Despres, J. Maheux, M. C. Pouliot, A. Nadeau, S. Moorjani, P. J. Lupien, and C. Bouchard. "Normalization of the Metabolic Profile in Obese Women by Exercise and a Low Fat Diet." *Medicine and Science in Sport and Exercise* 23 (1991): 1326–31.

78. Barnard, R. J., T. Jung, and S. B. Inkeles. "Diet and Exercise in the Treatment of Non-Insulin-Dependant Diabetes." *Diabetes Care* 17 (1994): 1469–72.

79. Blankenhorn, D. H., R. L. Johnson, W. J. Mack, H. A. El Zein, and L. I. Vailas. "The Influence of Diet on the Appearance of New Lesions in Human Coronary Arteries." *Journal of the American Medical Association* 263 (1990): 1646–52.

80. Bacon, L., J. Stern, M. Van Loan, and N. Keim. "Size Acceptance and Intuitive Eating Improve Health for Obese, Female Chronic Dieters." *J. Am. Diet. Assoc.* 105 (2005):929–936.

81. Olson, C., H. Schumaker, and B. Yawn. "Overweight Women Delay Medical Care." *Archives of Family Medicine* 3 (1994): 886–92.

82. Amy, N., A. Aalborg, P. Lyons, and L. Keranen. "Barriers to Routine Gynecological Screening for White and African-American Obese Women." *Int. J. Obes. Res. Metab. Disord.* 30 (2006):147–155.

SPOTLIGHT

The next chapter, by Ellen Glovsky, offers an overview of the basic concepts and application of Motivation Interviewing to the HAES and non-diet, mindful eating approach. MI is an evidence-based approach to helping people change their behavior about their health. Based upon the idea that most people already have the skills to successfully modify lifestyle and decrease health-risk, MI uses strategies that will enhance the patient's own motivation for and commitment to change. Motivational Interviewing integrates an empathic, non-confrontational style of counseling with powerful behavioral strategies for helping people convince themselves that they ought to change. Refer to Chapter 14 by Molly Kellogg, "Integrating Motivational Interviewing and a Non-Diet Approach", for an elaboration of these ideas and their application to work with patients and clients.

Chapter Three

Motivational Interviewing: The Basics

Ellen Glovsky

INTRODUCTION

If your work is as a health care provider, or anyone whose job entails advising others on behavior change, you may become frustrated by the fact that your clients often don't take your recommendations about lifestyle change. Your role may be to instruct or tell other people what to do and what changes they must make. You may have been trained to believe that if we just *teach* others what they need to do to change and do it effectively enough, they certainly will do so. We may even think there's something wrong with the other person, since the need for such change is so obvious to us. However, imparting *knowledge* is just a small part of the equation, and misses some very important aspects of the counseling relationship.

An alternative to this top-down approach is Motivational Interviewing (Miller and Rollnick 2013), a style of talking with clients in a constructive manner about health-risk reduction and behavior change. An important idea in Motivational Interviewing (MI) is that most individuals already have at least some of the skills and knowledge they need to be successful in modifying lifestyle and decreasing health risk. MI uses strategies that will enhance the client's own motivation to change. The approach integrates an empathic, non-confrontational style of counseling with powerful behavioral strategies for helping clients *convince themselves* that they ought to change. It is important to note that "MI is not a technique, but a set of integrated interviewing skills" (Miller and Rollnick 2013, 334).

MI combines the two "streams" of a client-centered, empathic approach with adequate direction so that clients can make their own decisions about changes they may wish to make (Miller and Rollnick 2013 DVD set). The empathic "stream" refers to the clinician's relationship or partnership with the client. Direction is provided via the technical skills of MI, which include listening skills and knowing the best response that will move the client in the direction of positive behavior change.

A BRIEF HISTORY OF MI

MI was originally formulated by William Miller and Steven Rollnick. As they tell the story on their 2013 training video, "Motivational Interviewing, Helping People Change," Dr. Miller was on sabbatical in Norway, and was asked by his hosts to demonstrate the "patient-centered" counseling approach he was using in the treatment of addictions. As he demonstrated, they asked him to elaborate on why he was saying certain things and using certain strategies. These conversations caused Miller to reflect on why he had certain "decision rules" in this work. Miller then wrote an article on this "patient-centered" approach (Miller 1983), which Rollnick read. Rollnick began to use and elaborate upon these ideas. Eventually they began working together to further develop these ideas. Since that time MI has been widely disseminated, and is used in many areas of health care including smoking cessation, addictions treatment, dietary behavior change, increasing physical activity, compliance with medication, cardiac rehabilitation, diabetes treatment, physical therapy, the promotion of breast feeding, and others areas that have a strong lifestyle component. More recently, MI is being used in criminal justice, in leadership skills training, and to improve employer/employee relationships. In the early 1990s, a group of MI professionals formed an organization called the Motivational Interviewing Network of Trainers (MINT), which has grown into an international group of over 2,000 MI trainers (www.motivationalinterviewing.org).

A DEFINITION OF MI

Here is a technical definition of MI, from the 3rd edition of *Motivational Interviewing: Helping People Change* by Miller and Rollnick, 2013.

Motivational Interviewing is a collaborative, goal-oriented style of communication with particular attention to the language of change. It is designed to strengthen personal motivation for and commitment to a specific goal by eliciting and exploring the person's own reasons for change within an atmosphere of acceptance and compassion. (pg 29)

Before elaborating on the specifics of MI, let's highlight the important points of this definition.

- MI is *collaborative*. As clinicians, we see ourselves as *partners* with our clients as they proceed along the road to (possible) change.
- MI is *goal-oriented or directive*. The conversation has a particular goal for change. The client's goal may not be the same as the clinician's at first. As the relationship between client and clinician develops, these goals may or may not line up.
- MI is a *counseling style*. This refers to the basic emotional stance we take with our clients.
- Using MI, we pay special attention to the client's use of language in talking about change. Does the client's talk suggest that the client is focused on sustaining the current pattern of behavior, or does it indicate that change is possible?
- Instead of trying to *convince* the client that change is a good idea, the clinician is looking to enhance the client's personal motivation for and commitment to change. The decision about change is the client's.
- The clinician's role is one of *eliciting* or stimulating the client to articulate their own reasons for change, and helping them to explore those reasons in order to make decisions about change.
- In the interview there is an atmosphere of *compassion and acceptance*. This refers to the idea that the clinician works to understand the client's point of view and actively promotes the client's welfare. The clinician accepts the client's perspective and decision about whether or not to change and how that change might occur.

The rest of this chapter is devoted to an examination of these points in detail. As shown in Figure 1, the ideas can be expressed as a pyramid, with the **spirit** of MI as the base, the **processes** of MI as the next level up, the **listening skills**, and finally the technical skills or micro-skills and other **techniques of MI** and knowing how to respond to move the conversation with the client in the direction of positive change.

THE SPIRIT OF MOTIVATIONAL INTERVIEWING

The spirit of MI refers to the underlying premise and the clinician's general attitude when approaching the client. Each of the four *spirit points* is described here.

- **Collaboration or Partnership**

This refers to the idea that the clinician works together with the client to find answers to the problem at hand. This is in distinction to the "top-down" or "I have the answer and you don't, so I'll give it to you and you'll be all set" approach. The idea is that our clients have most of the answers they need and will find them together with the clinician. Miller and

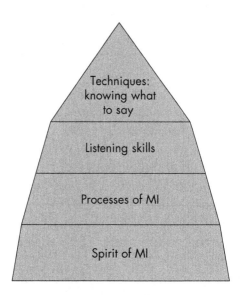

Figure 1. The Basic Concepts of Motivational Interviewing

Rollnick sum this up as the "profound respect for the other" (Miller and Rollnick 2013, 16). Another important idea is that Motivational Interviewing has a lot to do with what you *don't say*, in how you show restraint. It might be obvious to the clinician what the patient should do to improve his health, but *telling* him what to do doesn't usually work very well. The goal using MI is the help the client *find their own answers to the problem*.

- **Acceptance**

This means that I *accept* the patient for who they are, with no judgment. It also means that I accept their decision about whether or not to change the behavior in question. Another aspect of acceptance in MI is that we are interested in expressing *accurate empathy*. This is not sympathy and does not mean "I've had the same problem" or "poor you." It does mean that "I *get you*; I see you for who you are and I accept you."

It can be difficult for the clinician to accept a client's decision not to change, especially when the behavior in question is putting their health or that of others at risk. If the client decides *not to change* this behavior, we must accept that decision. The truth is that we can't make our patients do things, and not accepting their decisions actually makes things worse, by alienating them. Who wants to talk to someone who disapproves of you?

Accepting their decision may leave you feeling very uneasy and worried. If you're unhappy with the patient's decision, *you've got the problem, not the patient*. It is up to the clinician to deal with his or her own feelings about the client's decision.

Another important part of **acceptance** is affirming the client's autonomy. The clinician expresses respect for the other as a fully formed and functioning human being, with the ability and the right to make decisions for himself. We also want to look for what the other person does right, and affirm what we hear. The key is being able to see the glass as half full, and not half empty, and expressing that to the client. In any interaction in which we give advice, we make it very clear that it is up to the other person if, when, and how they will change. We rely on the client's own personal strengths, and acknowledge clearly that the client produces change, not the counselor.

- **Compassion**

Having compassion is to see the issues about the proposed change through the other's eyes. The goal is to actively promote the other person's welfare.

- **Evocation**

Using MI our goal is to *evoke* ideas, goals, and values from the patient, rather than telling them how things should work. This is the opposite of "installation therapy," which says "You're wrong, I've got the answers, I'll instill them in you, and you'll be all set." We want to encourage or stimulate the patient to find his own answers to the problem. Our role is to be a *guide*, not a director.

THE BASIC CONCEPTS OF MI

This section will address three basic concepts in MI: the *guiding style* used most often in MI, client *ambivalence*, and learning to listen for *change talk* from the client.

In talking with clients, we can use one of three basic styles: instructing, guiding and listening. Using MI we most often use a *guiding style*. A guide is saying "I can help you solve this for yourself." There is a place in the client/clinician relationship for instructing and listening, and one of the important skills in MI is in knowing which style to use in each instance. The goal here is to help the client find his or her own answer to the problem.

The second basic concept in MI is *ambivalence*. Most people faced with change are ambivalent, even if this change is something they really want, or even have longed for. Ambivalence means that we feel two ways about something. We may think we *should change*, or someone else thinks we should change, but *not be able to change*. An important aspect of MI is helping the client to resolve ambivalence, and so make a decision about whether or not to change.

People often say "Oh, I really hate change!", as though they hated change more than anyone else. Of course, some people dislike change more than others, but at the core, most of us are uncomfortable with change. Many of the changes we are asking clients to make are profound and stimulate the desire to avoid change. This happens even if they *think they should change.* To understand this, think of a time in your life when you were asked to change something about yourself, and you didn't do it. This may be something in the past or present, something you (or someone else) think you should change, something you have been thinking about changing, but haven't changed yet. Consider these two questions:

- Were you sure you *wanted* to change?
- Were you sure you were *able* to change?

You may find you were ambivalent, even though you may know it was in your best interest. Our clients feel the same way about the changes we are proposing for them.

It is important to understand that *wanting to change*, or wanting the eventual outcome of the changed behavior, is not the same as actually being able to change. The clinician must consider the context in which the person lives, and the constraints that may be present. For example, the teenager who wants to change his diet, but the foods needed to make these changes are simply not available in his or her environment. Or the person who would like to get more exercise, but really doesn't have time or resources. Another example is the client who thinks the Health At Every Size ideas are great, but can't let go of the desire to lose weight. In this last example, the client may not have the internal resources to shift her attitude away from a dieting mentality. The clinician can help her to see her own ambivalence about such change.

In MI we use a guiding style to help the client explore and resolve ambivalence, and ambivalence is seen as a good and normal occurrence. It means that the client is not saying "no, never," but "maybe." This means that the client is open to the possibility of change and to working through that ambivalence.

The third basic concept is *change talk*. When people are ambivalent about change, we may hear two distinct kinds of talk mixed together, often in the same sentence. *Change talk* refers to statements the client makes in favor of change, while *sustain talk* is any statement in favor of the status quo, or not changing. The client might say "I'd really like to start eating more mindfully, but I really like to eat whatever I want, whenever I want it. I really hate having limits on me." The language about wanting to eat mindfully is "change talk," while the reason not to is called "sustain talk." A crucial skill in MI is being able to hear, identify, and respond to both types of talk, and to reinforce in the direction of positive change. Change talk can be anything the client says that indicates something more than "I'm not going to change." There are two of types of change talk: *preparatory change talk* and *commitment talk.* The first type is heard when the client is in the process of deciding whether or not to change, while he or she is still ambivalent about the proposed change. As ambivalence is resolving or is resolved, we hear more commitment talk. This shift in the language of change talk is the signal to the clinician that ambivalence is resolving and the client may be ready for the planning process, which is discussed later in this chapter.

Change talk is heard in several categories, and being able to identify change talk is easiest when you are familiar with these categories. The preparatory change talk categories are *desire*, *ability*, *reason*, and *need*, and the commitment talk categories are *commitment*, *activation*, and *taking steps* (DARN-CAT). Figure 2 offers examples of the language the client might use in each of the categories of types of change talk. As the client moves through the process of resolving ambivalence, the *strength and frequency* of change talk increase. The strength refers to the client's use of language that indicates how close the client is to actually being ready to change. Here are some examples of different *strengths* of change talk.

- *Stopping dieting sounds good, but I can't give up the idea of losing weight.* Weak change talk.
- *I know that dieting is not the answer to my food problem.* Stronger change talk.
- *I am ready to experiment with eating mindfully.* Even stronger change talk.
- *I'm done with dieting and this week will try some of your non-diet ideas.* Commitment talk

Desire	I want... I wish... I hope that ___ will happen.
Ability	Positive, certain, assured that I can change... I might be able to... I know how to...
Reasons	I know it would be good for my health It would make it easier to...
Need	I have to... I ought to... I can't wait any longer
Commitment	I'm going to do it, My plan is to... My next step is.... It's time to take action

Figure 2. DARN-CAT Words and Phrases.

Change talk is an important concept in MI because we know that when the client is active in the conversation about change, making the "arguments" for change themselves, they are much more likely to actually make the changes under discussion. Miller and Rollnick put it succinctly, "If you are arguing for change, and your client is arguing against it, you've got it exactly backwards" (Miller and Rollnick 2013, 9).

The skill of being able to identify change talk is important because change-talk statements give the clinician indications of whether or not the client is moving ahead in the direction of positive change. They also give the clinician information about how to guide the client in the direction of positive behavior change. Remember that the goal in using MI is to help *clients convince themselves that they ought to change.*

Being able to hear and identify change talk are key listening skills in MI. Having heard *change talk* from your client, how do you know what to say next?

DEVELOPING THE SKILL OF KNOWING WHAT TO SAY: OARS

While listening skills are important in MI, knowing what to say in response is really what moves the conversation ahead in the direction of positive change. We think of these *micro-skills* by the acronym OARS, which refers to open-ended questions, affirmations, reflections, and summarizing.

Open-ended questions are those that cannot be answered by a "yes" or "no" or very short answer. When questions are open, we often learn more about our client, and are more likely to elicit change talk. For example, when asking about a client's consumption of certain foods, we could ask, "How many servings of fruit do you eat each day?" which is a closed question. If you ask instead, "Tell me about the fruit you eat," you are much more likely to hear about how eating fruit fits into the person's day and perhaps even how they feel about it. Working with a chronic dieter, you could ask "How many diets have you been on?" which is a closed question. A better question would be "Could you please tell me about your experience with diets in the past?" The second version is far more likely to elicit information from the client, including change talk.

As clinicians become more sophisticated in their MI skills, they ask more open than closed questions.

Affirmations are a positive statement about the client. It is something you have heard them say or know about them. There is almost always something good you can say about a person. The client who spends the first part of your session complaining and telling you all the things they haven't done can still be affirmed by thanking them for coming in to see you. You can express appreciation or admiration for the client, or an expression of hope, caring, or support. When the clinician helps clients to feel better about themselves, the client will feel more confident to make changes.

<u>Reflections</u> function to let the other person know you heard, and to confirm that you heard correctly. As seen in Figure 3, there are three possible places where communication can go wrong. Reflections can function to double check that you understood the other person's meaning clearly. There are two general types of reflections that can be used: simple or content reflections, and complex or meaning reflections. Simple reflections are a repeat or rephrase of what the client said. Complex reflections add the next sentence to the story, and may be a guess at what the client meant in terms of underlying emotion or meaning in their life. Here is an example.

> Client: *I know that this non-diet idea you're talking about would be good for me, and it sounds like a relief, but I really need to lose weight. Just look at me! I've never been so fat.*

> Simple/Content Reflection: *The non-diet ideas sound good, and your weight is a problem for you.*

> Complex/Meaning Reflection: *On one hand you find the non-diet ideas attractive, and you're worried that your weight will get out of hand if you quit dieting.*

The meaning reflection takes a guess at the underlying feeling this client is expressing.

If the guess is wrong, this can be awkward, and the client may feel offended. You can apologize and ask for clarification. It more often happens that your guess is exactly what the client is really feeling and your saying it brings that to light. That can be helpful even if disturbing for some clients.

In the example above, the meaning reflection is a *double-sided* reflection. It reflects the client's ambivalence and summarizes both sides of the story. Double-sided reflections can be very powerful. They bring together the client's ambivalence in a very clear and direct way and

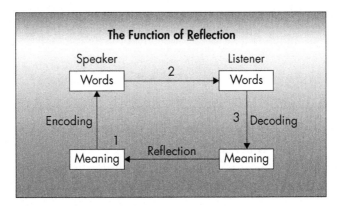

Figure 3. Numbers 1, 2, and 3 are places where communication can go wrong.

Figure 4. Sample Sentence Stems for Reflections

Sounds like ...
What I'm hearing is ...
So you're saying that ...
You're feeling like ...
This has been totally _____ for you
Almost as if ...
Like a. ...
Sounds as if you ...
For you, it's a matter of. ...
From your point of view, ...
I'm hearing that you ...
I'm really getting that you ...
I get the impression that you ...
You ...
You are ...
I would imagine you ...
Must be ...
I would think you ...
Through your eyes, ...
Your belief is that ...
Your concern is that ...
Your fear is that ...
It seems to you that ...
You're not terribly excited about ...
You're not much concerned about ...
The thing that bothers you is ...
The important thing as you see it is ...
I would bet that you ...
You must be ...

---

often people would rather avoid ambivalence because it is uncomfortable. Positive change involves moving through ambivalence.

As beginners in learning to use MI skills, many clinicians find it is easier to start with simple or content reflections. A higher-level skill in MI is learning to make complex reflections.

Figure 4 shows some ideas for "sentence stems" or words to use to begin reflective-listening statements. It takes practice to be skilled at forming reflections, but this skill can become intuitive, or automatic as you practice.

Summarizing is used in three ways in MI. A *collecting summary* is used to list the things that the client has said or the issues that have been discussed so far. This is an opportunity to reinforce the things that have been stated in favor of positive change.

> "So far you've expressed concern about your weight if you adopt some non-diet ideas, ways to keep healthy foods in your house, and your doctor telling you that your blood pressure is too high."

A *linking summary* is used to put together something just stated with something the client said earlier.

> "That sounds a little like what you said earlier about the sad feeling you get when you stop bingeing."

A *transitional summary* is used to pull together what has been said and what has happened and transition to a new task.

> "If it's OK with you, I'd like to talk with you about your blood sugar. Before we do that, let me summarize what we've talked about so far and see if I've missed anything important."

Note that in all three instances the clinician will emphasize the *change talk* the patient has stated.

As mentioned earlier, there is one more type of summary, a *double-sided summary*, which tells both sides of the story, and highlights the client's ambivalence. This is both a reflection and a summary.

> "On one hand you really like the way you've been eating, and your weight is getting out of hand and you're worried about your blood sugar and blood pressure. Did I get that right?"

The OARS skills are basic to developing and maintaining a relationship with the client. They also are key in eliciting change talk and guiding the client in the resolution of ambivalence and in making a decision about if, when, and how change will happen.

It is important to note at this point that the skills described are just that: skills that clinicians can develop. This is not something learned quickly, especially if you have been trained in the tradition medical, top-down model of interacting with clients. These skills take time and practice, and eventually begin to feel intuitive or automatic. This is really a set of *mental shifts* that the clinician makes: changes in attitude about your role in the relationship with your client. Many MI practitioners report that they continue to learn more about MI over time, sometimes over many years. There is much to explore and learn as the clinician broadens and deepens these skills. See the end of this chapter for more on learning MI skills.

THE FOUR PROCESSES THAT COMPRISE MI

Thus far we have discussed the definition of MI, its spirit, some basic concepts, and the OARS skills and techniques. Now we turn to the four basic and central interpersonal processes at work throughout our relationship with the client. The processes are **engaging, focusing, evoking,** and **planning.** They build on each other, as in Figure 5, and flow into each other at each stage of the relationship with the client.

Note that all of the ideas presented thus far in this chapter apply to the four processes. We continually apply the concepts of the spirit of MI: collaboration, acceptance, compassion, and eliciting. The clinician must listen carefully for change talk and ambivalence and use the OARS skills to elicit information and to guide the client.

Engaging refers to the ways in which you make a connection with the client by understanding the role of this issue in the client's life. It is more than simply being warm and open and a good listener, although these traits are a part of the engagement process. It means truly coming to understand the client's point of view about the proposed change. "I really *get you* and how this change is for you and what it might mean." This idea refers back to the spirit of MI, in which *accurate empathy* was described.

Engagement with the client really forms the basis of everything else that may occur in your relationship.

Focusing is the process of setting an agenda, deciding what the topic of conversation will be, and then what specific change, if any, will be addressed. The focus for the client and clinician may differ. For example, your client might come to you for help in losing weight. You may feel that weight is not really the issue, and that a non-diet approach to healing this client's difficult relationship with food is the best way to work together. In this case, as in many others, the process of focusing is a conversation and perhaps a negotiation rather than a foregone conclusion. In some cases, clients may have come to see you for reasons other than actually changing behavior; for instance, someone else wants them to do so, such as a physician, spouse, or parent. This might require other sorts of conversations to help the client clarify their own goals for change or no change. The focusing process involves harnessing the change conversation and helping the client decide what to change, based on their own goals and values. In the focusing process, we are navigating carefully between the client's autonomy

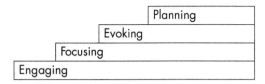

Figure 5. The Four Processes of Motivational Interviewing.

and the clinician's expertise. The initial focus of the conversation may change as the clinician and patient get to know each other.

At any time in our relationship with the client, it can be tempting to give advice or what you see as obvious or important solutions to the problem. Most health care providers are trained to give advice. After all, you have important expertise that you may feel is urgent to share. In MI this urge is called the *righting reflex*, in which you feel certain you have the answer to this client's problems, so why not tell them? When you give unasked-for advice, the client may feel defensive, dismissed, or downright angry. Think about how you might respond to being told what to do. Most of us don't really like it! Remember that the goal in using MI is to help the client find his or her *own answers to the problem.*

Evoking is encouraging the client to speak about the reasons for change and identify their own motivation for change. We are listening for *change talk*, which is the client talking about change, and not the clinician. Their reasons for or against change are what matters, and not ours. We are seeking to understand the patient's goals and values, and to highlight any discrepancy between those stated values and the client's behavior. One of the important skills in MI is using the guiding style, so that advice is given when appropriate, without telling the client what to do. The clinician's job in this process is to help the client to see discrepancies and make decisions about if, when, and how they will choose to change. This discrepancy is the *engine of change*. Often, once people state their goals and values and observe how their behavior does not fit, they can convince themselves that they should change.

Planning is the process of helping the client make a plan for action. It is not enough to stimulate change talk and move the client toward readiness to change. The clinician must also help the client, when ready, to form a specific and actionable plan for change. We know that people are more likely to change when they have a specific plan and voice that plan to another person (Miller and Rollnick 2013).

One trap clinicians often face at this point is the belief that "that MI stuff" is no longer useful and they can proceed to tell the client what to do. Nothing could be further from the truth. We continue to use MI skills and processes throughout our interactions with the client. Planning is a process of collaboration as is the rest of our relationship with the client. We add *negotiating* to the mix in the planning process. It is still important to watch for your *righting reflex*, that urge you may feel to "fix" things by providing what may seem to be an obvious solution to the problem.

	Tasks	In Practice
ELICIT	• Ask permission • Clarify information needs, gaps	• *May I...? or would you like to know about...?* • *What do you know about...?* • *What would you like to know about?* • *Is there any information I can help you with?*
PROVIDE	• Prioritize • Be clear • Support autonomy • Don't prescribe the person's response	• What does the person most want/need to know? • Avoid jargon; use everyday language • Offer small amounts with time to reflect • Acknowledge freedom to disagree or ignore • Present what you know without interpreting its meaning for the client
ELICIT	• Ask for the client's interpretation, understanding, or response	• Ask open questions • Reflect reactions that you see/hear • Allow time to process and respond to the information

Figure 6. Examples of Language in Elicit-Provide-Elicit.

How will you know when the client is ready for the planning process? You may hear an increase in the strength and frequency of change talk and less sustain talk or complaining about the problem. Questions about the process of change or actually taking steps to experiment with the change may be heard. The client might begin to envision what it would be like to make this change, and the clinician can ask the client to do so. All of these reflect the *resolution of ambivalence*. This resolution is really a process, so you might say that "ambivalence is resolved or *resolving*." The client is expressing stronger change talk; that is, *commitment, action, taking steps*. These are the last three types of change talk, described earlier in this chapter, specifically *commitment talk*, in the acronym DARN-CAT, which reflect readiness to change.

One way to "test the waters" regarding how ready the client is to make a plan is to make a collecting or *transitional* summary of what has been stated, followed by a *key question*. The clinician might include an element of sustain talk that the client has emphasized in the conversation. Whether or not to do this is a matter of clinical judgment.

Here is an example of a transitional or collecting summary, followed by a key question.

Let me summarize what you've said so far and see if I've missed anything important.	Collecting summary introduction
You're worried about your weight and your health and need something to be different. But, you are really fed up with dieting and find that it just increases your bingeing.	Collecting summary or Transitional summary
Being able to eat to soothe yourself is really important and you're not sure about giving this up.	Reflection of sustain talk
Where do we go from here?	Key Question

Once it is clear that the client is ready to participate in developing a change plan, there are three possible scenarios. Either the path and topic for change are very clear, or there are several clear paths to change, or there is no clear plan.

When the plan is clear, we can rely on the client to make specific goals, and the clinician's role may be to summarize, reinforce, and encourage clarification of those goals. The clinician can elicit *mobilizing change talk*; that is, the client making statements about what s/he will do next to follow through with the plan.

When there are several possibilities, the clinician's role is to guide the client in deciding which goal(s) they would like to tackle first. An example is the client with diabetes who is faced with changes that could be made in several areas of lifestyle such as diet, exercise, or testing blood sugar. The clinician's role is to enumerate these possible areas for change, and ask the client which they want to plan for. The process then includes confirming this goal, collaborating to make specific plans, and troubleshooting any potential difficulties.

When there is no clear set of options for change, the clinician's role is to guide the client in generating alternatives, options, or possible steps. The client's hunches or best guesses at what needs to be changed are very important in this instance. People really do have ideas about what will work best for them, and with some guidance, can come up with a plan that is their own.

Remember that our clients' ideas about what will work best for them, both in choosing the goal and in making plans to achieve it, are the most powerful. When people make a plan that is *their own*, they are much more likely to follow through.

In this spirit, we utilize the model of *elicit-provide-elicit* (E-P-E) in guiding our clients in making a plan for change. In all three of the above scenarios for goal setting, it is important to first ask the client what ideas they have for themselves. It may be that the client really doesn't know anything about the subject, or that they know quite a bit and have a plan in mind. Either way, we give the client the opportunity to state what they already know. This gives us the opportunity to correct any misinformation the client may have. The *provide* piece is where the clinician can give advice, *after obtaining permission*. Figure 6 gives examples of the tasks the clinician should accomplish and some clinical examples of *E-P-E*.

	No Change	Change
Benefits	**Sustain Talk** Good	**Change Talk** Pros
Costs	**Change Talk** Not-So-Good	**Sustain Talk** Cons

Figure 7. Decisional Matrix.

There are three ways to obtain permission to provide information or advice. Here are some examples of responses in each case.

1. The client asks for advice
   I have some thoughts on that subject, and I'm happy to share them. First I'd like to hear what you already know about_____.
2. You ask permission to give advice.
   Would it be OK if I made a suggestion about that?
3. You qualify your advice to emphasize autonomy.
   I have some ideas, I don't know if they will work for you; you'll be the best judge.

Asking permission before giving advice is simply respectful of the clients and their abilities as a complete human being. It is important to avoid the "expert trap" mentioned earlier. Asking permission indicates that you understand and acknowledge that the client has free will and can make their own decisions about change.

When providing information or advice, address only the pieces of information that the client most wants or needs to know. Offering advice in clear language and only one or two facts at a time is key. After a brief bit of information, *elicit* again, asking if it makes sense and what else they might like to know.

Clinician: So, you've decided to try out the "non-diet" ideas. What do you already know about these ideas? Elicit

Client: Well, I've read a little, and talked with a friend who runs her food that way. I know it has something to do with mindfulness, right?

Clinician: Yes, that's an important element of the concept. What would you like to know about it and how you could use this set of ideas? Provide-Elicit

Client: How do you know what and how much to eat? I've been dieting for so long, I really have no idea.

Clinician: I'd be happy to review the non-diet ideas with you and see what you think. Using a non-diet idea, we learn to respond to hunger and fullness signals from the body as a guide to when and how much to eat. The "what" is really up to you. I can help you get in tune with what you really want to eat. Does this make sense? Provide-Elicit

---

	The Way I'm Eating Now	Adopting a Non-Diet Approach
Benefits	• Rules of my diet are very clear • At least I know what I'm *supposed* to do • I really love bingeing when I can forget the guilt • Food is a great reward after a hard day	• I wouldn't have to diet anymore • I would feel less guilty • I might lose weight • Could eat what I really want • Would enjoy food more
Costs	• Been dieting all my life • Feel guilty most of the time • Hate my body for betraying me when I try not to eat • Worry about my health • Doctor yells at me for not losing weight • Feel out of control with food	• Where are the rules for how to do this? Diets make that clear • I'm afraid I won't be able to know intuitively what I want • I'm afraid I won't know when to stop eating when I'm full • I might have to give up the idea of losing weight • My doctor probably won't approve

Figure 8. Sample Completed Decisional Matrix.

The clinician in this example is using language that supports autonomy. Eliciting the client's ideas, affirming what she knows, and asking what she thinks about the information lets the client know she is free to do what she wishes with this information, and that the clinician is there to support her, rather than tell her what to do.

SOME HELPFUL TECHNIQUES USED IN MI

In this section two specific techniques in MI that can be helpful in moving the conversation forward are described.

The Decisional Matrix or *Decisional Balance* is a technique designed for the client and clinician to look at all sides of the questions regarding the change under consideration. This exercise works best with clients who have expressed at least some change talk. In the situation where the client is not considering change at any level, this approach does not make much sense.

This technique is most applicable in the focusing and evoking processes. It is designed to examine the "good" and the "not-so-good" aspects of the way things are right now, before change. Note that the language chosen is not "bad," but "not-so-good." We avoid negative language, since we are taking an objective look at all sides of the situation. We are also looking at the pros and cons of the ideas about change.

The exercise begins by asking the client for *permission* to ask some questions and help to complete the form at hand. Assuming permission is granted, we begin with the pros of change. *"If you were going to make this change, what would be good about it?"* As the client answers, the clinician jots them down in bullets as shown in Figure 6. We move from the top right, reasons to change, to the bottom left, costs of staying the same. The answers in these two boxes are *change talk*, while the answers in the other two boxes are *sustain talk*, or reasons not to change.

After the client has told you everything about each box, give a short summary of what you heard. After completing all four boxes, give a summary of everything you heard, expressing all sides of the story. This is best done as a *double-sided summary*. Figure 7 shows a simple version of the form used in this technique.

The clinician might say *"When we think about making changes, most of us don't really consider all sides in a complete way. Instead, we often do what we think we 'should' do, avoid doing things we don't feel like doing, or just feel confused or overwhelmed and give up thinking about it at all. Thinking through the pros and cons of both changing and not making a change is one way to help us make sure we have fully considered a possible change. This can help us to 'hang on' to our plan in times of stress or temptation."*

Figure 8 shows a sample of a completed Decisional Matrix. Here is an example of a double-sided summary the clinician might make for this client.

Let me see if I can summarize what you've told me so far. On one hand, you like the rules of the diets you follow, you sometimes love to binge, and food is a great reward for you. On the other hand, if you adopted the non-diet ideas instead of dieting, you wouldn't have to feel guilty, you could eat what you really want, and you could enjoy food more. Is there anything else?

In this case, the clinician is able to clearly state the ambivalence the client has expressed. This can be a very important turning point for some clients.

It is important to note that this entire exercise might be too much for some clients, or just might not be appropriate in your setting or with your own personality style. A simple pros and cons list can be equally effective:

- What would be good about change?
- What would make it hard for you to make these changes?

As you are moving through this process with your client, remember that the purpose is to examine all sides of the issue regarding whether or not the client will change behavior. We listen carefully to both *change talk* and *sustain talk*, but we reinforce in the direction of positive change. The skill here is being able to hear both types of language, and using OARS, knowing what to say in response.

Importance/Confidence Scaling

This technique is designed to evoke change talk, and to assess readiness to change. It is best used as the client is resolving ambivalence about change and approaching the planning process. You may also use this to check on whether or not the client is really ready for change. The client is asked to rate the *importance* of making the behavior change under discussion. The clinician could say:

> *Using a scale from one to ten, in which "1" is not at all important, and "10" is very important to you right now, how important is it for you right now to make this change?*

Assuming the client chooses a number higher than 1, this is followed up with the question:

> *Why are you at x and not at "1" (or a lower number)?*

The answer to the second question is almost always change talk, or reasons for change. The next question is

> *What would need to happen to increase your score a couple of points; that is, to make it more important?*

Here we are asking what would make this more important in your life.

The same questions can be asked about *confidence* to change. The answers to these questions are also change talk, and provide information to both the clinician and the client. For the client who says that importance is high, and confidence is low, the question to ask is

> *How can I help you feel more confident about this change?*

For the client who rates confidence high and importance low, the answer may be that this is not a good time to be pursuing this specific behavior change. The clinician could also further explore the idea of what would make this more important.

DEALING WITH DISCORD/RESISTANCE

Many clinicians wonder how to deal with the "resistant" client. It is more useful to think in terms of discord or something wrong in the relationship between the clinician and the client. *Sustain talk* is reasons not to change. This may sound like denial of the problem, such as,

- *I don't know what my doctor is so upset about. My blood sugar is not a problem.*
- *I don't see why everyone is so worried about my weight; I'm big boned and have always been this way.*

Signs of *discord* in the relationship include the client being defensive, blaming (the clinician or others), and minimizing the problem. Other signs of discord are the client becoming distracted, changing the subject, or interrupting.

- *You just don't understand how hard this is!*
- *How could you possibly know what my life is like? You've never been fat.*
- *Don't keep telling me I need to eat more vegetables. I have other priorities right now!*
- *My eating disorder isn't that bad. My roommate's is really bad.*
- *Why are all you health people so upset about my weight? I think you just don't get me and my life.*

The distinction between discord and sustain talk is that in sustain talk, the client is talking about themselves, not about your interactions. In either case, it points to an opportunity for the clinician to *do something differently.* The best responses to both sustain talk and discord are reflections, affirmations, or summaries. The goal is to let the client know you heard, and to verify that you heard it correctly. The clinician is also interested in letting the client hear what they have said in different words, which sometimes brings up different meanings. When people feel heard and acknowledged, anger and resentment tend to diminish, so communication can resume.

Here is an example of a conversation that demonstrates how to deal with discord and sustain talk.

Client: I'm just so sick of everyone talking and thinking about my weight! I'm eating healthy now, and just don't seem to be able to lose.	Sustain Talk, Discord
Clinician: It's hard for you to understand why you're eating healthy and still not losing weight. You're doing the best you possibly can.	Reflection, Affirmation
Client: Yes. ... but I suppose those afternoon candy bars aren't helping much.	Change Talk (weak)
Clinician: So perhaps there is some room for improvement. What do you think?	Reflection, Open Question
Client: I suppose so, but I really don't want to give those up. They really help get me through a hard afternoon at work.	Sustain Talk
Clinician: On one hand, it's worth it to you to get that comfort you need from the candy and not be perfect with your eating plan, but on the other hand you're seeing there might be some room for change.	Double-Sided Summary
Client: When you put it that way. ... I don't know. I guess I'll have to think about that.	
Clinician: Where do we go from here?	Open Question

In MI the metaphor is *dancing, not wrestling* with a client who expresses a lot of sustain talk or discord in their relationship with you. When we are wrestling, we are not collaborating, which is a key element of MI. An alternative is ballroom dancing; we can't be wrestling and dancing at the same time. In order to ballroom dance with a partner, you must be collaborating. Picture yourself gliding across the dance floor together, rather than wrestling. As a collaborator or partner, you have a much better chance of guiding the client in the direction of positive change.

WHY I LOVE USING AND TEACHING MI

Seventeen years ago I was introduced to the basic ideas of Motivational Interviewing. At the time, I was an outpatient and research dietitian at a large inner-city hospital. My job was to instruct patients on changes to their diet and exercise that would benefit them. Teaching patients what to do was what I was taught as a dietetic intern twenty-five years before, and thought was the only way of communicating with patients. After several years of doing this, I found that *almost no one had done what I told them to do.* This was quite discouraging. I felt that I needed a different, better approach. I ran across MI at a conference, where a colleague and I were on the same panel. I was presenting on a non-diet approach, and he spoke about MI. I felt so drawn to these ideas, and quickly realized they were a better, more productive way to go about helping people change.

Over the next few years, I found a teacher, another clinician who agreed to mentor me in the process of my learning how to use MI as a clinician. I attended many different MI trainings around the country, to learn how other trainers expressed these ideas and trained people in MI. I felt so energized and excited about MI that I really wanted to share it with others professionals. I found that I was a lot less tired and felt involved and happy about my work again. Using MI, many clinicians feel less tired because we are no longer responsible for whether or not our clients decide to change. We certainly may have feelings about their decisions, but if their decision is not to change, we accept that. What a relief!

In 2006, I was trained by the Motivational Interviewing Network of Trainers (MINT) in how to *teach MI to others.* This is a very different set of skills than using MI as a clinician. I have been privileged to provide training in MI to a wide variety of organizations and conferences around the US since then. It is particularly exciting to learn something new myself in nearly every training session I conduct. There is always something new in MI, a new way of looking at some of the ideas, or a refinement of the way in which I have been teaching it. My trainees are often my best teachers!

I still use MI as a clinician in my private practice treating eating disorders and chronic weight management issues. I find that it really works to help my clients decide if, when, and how they will change their behavior with food and physical activity.

How to Learn Motivational Interviewing

Over the past 30 years there has been much research on how people learn the ideas of MI and how to implement them in practice. Here are some ideas, in no particular order.

1. Attend a workshop.
   A live, hands-on workshop with a professional MI trainer is the best way to learn MI. If the trainer is a member of MINT, you can be sure they have been trained to very high standards and you can expect a quality workshop. Your training should ideally include

practice sessions, in small groups and in pairs. A short lecture is better than nothing, but don't expect to be able to use the MI skills. People need several days, or the equivalent, of direct training to achieve minimum competence in MI.

2. Read and learn.

    There are many excellent books on MI, which are included in the bibliography at the end of this book. You will also find articles and other materials that can help advance your skills.

3. Practice and listen.

    Listen to professionally produced video tapes of MI being used by other professionals. Practice the MI skills with your clients, patients, and colleagues.

4. Get feedback and supervision in MI.

    The best way to advance your MI skills is to have direct coaching with an MI trainer. This can take the form of telephone or in-person coaching, either one on one or in small groups. You can submit audio or video tapes of yourself with a client or someone role playing a client, have it rated, and receive written and verbal feedback. Remember that an expert trainer in MI will always *model the methods* with you by looking for what you do right, and reinforcing *you in the direction of positive change.*

People vary in the ways in which they learn best. Some have the best experiences listening to discussion, some learn best viewing video clips and critiquing them in a group, and still others do best with hands-on practice. Such practice can happen in small groups or pairs at a training session, or one on one with a coach.

How you learn MI is up to you, and may be the product of limitations in resources such as time and money. Remember that attending a lecture and reading about MI will not make you an expert. The best you can expect from those experiences is to have an *understanding* of the basis of MI, and perhaps of the spirit. Learning the skills described in this chapter takes training, patience, and lots of practice. You will be rewarded with proficiency in a very powerful and compassionate way of relating to your clients and patients.

References

1. Miller, WM and Rollnick, S. *Motivational Interviewing: Helping People Change.* New York: Guilford Press, 2013.

2. Miller, WM, "Motivational Interviewing with Problem Drinkers." *Behavioural Psychotherapy* 11, no. 02 (April 1983): 147–172.

3. Miller, WM and Rollnick, S. "Motivational Interviewing: Helping People Change," DVD set. The Change Companies, www.changecompanies.net, 2013.

INTRODUCTION TO PART TWO, MORE ON EACH TOPIC

This section provides the scientific basis for Health At Every Size, as well as discussions of the scientific literature relating to the value of weight loss in improving health. It also explores the use of an HAES, non-diet perspective for special populations including individuals and families with eating disorders, children, and athletes. This is followed by an examination of the weight centered approach used to training dietetics professionals, and the arguments in favor of changing this philosophy to a health-centered, HAES approach. The last chapter in Part Two explores ways in which the principles of HAES can be taught to health care professionals.

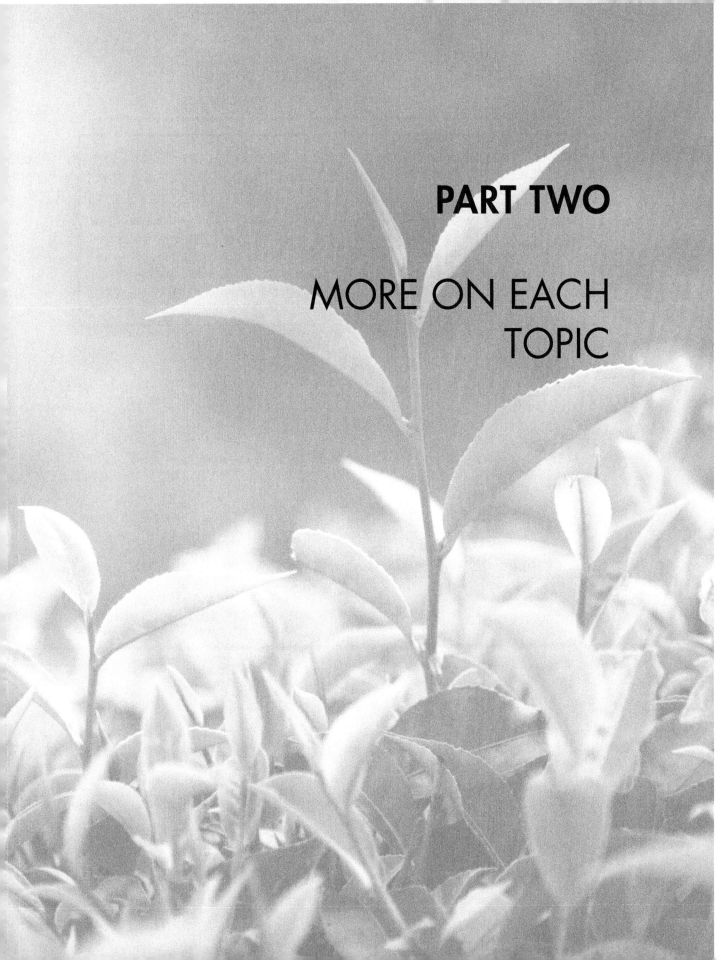

PART TWO

MORE ON EACH
TOPIC

SPOTLIGHT

The first chapter in this section, by Paul Ernsberger, compares the Health At Every Size model to current medical approaches to the treatment of chronic disease. Ernsberger makes the central argument that HAES is at its core conservative in the medical sense, while a weight-centered medical approach is radical. HAES focuses on avoiding harmful and ineffective treatments, while using the full armamentarium of modern medicine that has been validated in controlled trials.

Chapter Four

Biomedical Rationale for a Wellness Approach to Obesity

Paul Ernsberger

Health At Every Size is a practical approach to maximizing the health of larger individuals. The current paradigm for health care for large bodies is to focus on weight reduction, based on the assumption that reducing body mass will reverse each and every presenting health concern. The current paradigm is not supported by clinical trial evidence, despite claims to the contrary. Clinical trial data for weight loss treatments, other than one trial of surgery,[1] show only short-term results in the first one to two years. Because current remedies for obesity have little long-term effectiveness, no controlled clinical trial has demonstrated improved longevity after weight loss. One trial tracked mortality following weight loss surgery.[2] Mortality increased in the first two years relative to the comparison group that was placed on a very low calorie diet, then crossed over after 8 years and seemed to show a benefit, but by this point after surgery, few of the original patients were being followed up.[2] In contrast to the stark example of a single trial with an ambiguous outcome, literally hundreds of clinical trials that include thousands of obese subjects have repeatedly proven that drug therapy for diabetes, hypertension, and high cholesterol extend life and improve health. Clinical drug trials for lipid lowering and cardiovascular drugs have, by default if not by design, followed a Health At Every Size model because outcomes were focused on clinical lab values and health outcomes, not on changes in body weight despite the fact that a majority of the subjects in these drugs trials were obese. Thus, clinical drug trials represent a large body of evidence that support the treatment of obese persons with conventional drug therapy to improve health and extend life. Furthermore, as medical science has advanced, the cardiovascular risks associated with high body mass index have declined progressively since the 1970's, as shown by successive cohorts in the NHANES study.[3]

In contrast, while a focus on weight loss might theoretically be effective in improving health outcomes, because there is no method to reliably and permanently reverse obesity, the long-term impact on health and longevity of weight loss are not known. We cannot assume that persons who have been thin all their lives are physically identical to formerly obese persons who are now thin, and in fact studies show there are biochemical differences between the always-thin and formerly fat.[4,5] As others in this volume have shown (refer to chapter 6 by Dharini M. Bhammar and Glenn A. Gaesser and chapter 7 by Brandon J. Sawyer, Siddhartha S. Angadi and Glenn A. Gaesser), beneficial effects of exercise and healthy eating do not depend on weight loss but are a direct result of lifestyle changes. Therefore, the proven benefits of drug therapy, exercise, and an optimized diet composition support a redirection of therapeutic goals from weight loss to health gain.

Conservative medicine is defined in the Oxford Dictionary as "intended to control rather than eliminate a condition, with existing tissue preserved as far as possible." The opposite of conservative medical care is aggressive or radical treatment. The classic distinction is between surgery and medication. Surgical treatment is aggressive, and radical surgery is the most aggressive intervention. Prescription medicine is more conservative, and almost always has fewer side effects and lower costs. A conservative approach to prescribing medicine will focus on drugs with the fewest side effects and greatest effectiveness.

Possibly the greatest recent triumph of conservative medicine has come in the cardiovascular arena. Many clinical trials have studied cardiac patients and pitted surgical intervention against conservative treatments, such as a cocktail of medications combined with cardiac rehabilitation to promote moderate graded physical activity. Most recent trials show that conservative treatment, mainly with drugs by mouth, is just as effective in preventing heart attacks and death as surgery in all but the most dire emergencies.[6] Over time, fewer cardiac patients are sent for open heart surgery and more are sent for angioplasty or for the most conservative option, which is medication alone.

The key weapons against heart disease today are the statin drugs. Clinical trials have shown again and again that the incidence of death, heart attack, and stroke decline following statin treatment.[7] In the recent JUPITER double-blind trial of rosuvastatin (Crestor) in over 17,000 subjects, the risk of death and the risk of heart attack were reduced equally effectively in those with a BMI over 30 kg/m^2 as in those who were leaner.[7] A combined analysis of eight double-blind trials of statins, including JUPITER, confirmed in a pool of 38,000 subjects that obese and non-obese subjects benefit equally.[8]

The life-prolonging benefits in these controlled trials are calculated on an intention-to-treat basis. In other words, you were included in the statin group if you got a prescription for statins, whether you actually took them or not. Several trials have compared people who were prescribed statins and took them versus those who got the prescriptions and never filled them or never refilled their prescriptions. Remarkably, the death rate for people who failed to take their medication was three times higher.[9] Even after adjusting for differences in medical history and risk factors, merely neglecting to refill your statin prescription doubled the risk of death.

Unfortunately, over half of all people prescribed statins will fail to take them, and the rate rises with time. The most common reason given is the side effect of muscle pain. However, in double-blind trials, an equally high rate of complaints of muscle pain arises in the placebo group.[8] This suggests that a negative placebo effect, or nocebo effect, may lead to the perception of muscle pain. There is some evidence that treatment with the nutrient CoQ10 can lessen side effects of statins, which is logical because statins impair the ability of the cells to synthesize CoQ10.[10]

Many patients and even physicians view statins as an alternative to diet and exercise, i.e., "Should I eat right and exercise or take the easy way out and just pop a statin pill?" On the contrary, the evidence shows that statins work synergistically to improve health in obese persons, even in obese Type 2 diabetics.[11]

Thus, numerous high-quality studies conducted in large groups of people consistently show that statin drugs lower the risk of disease and death in obese people. Besides heart attack and stroke, statins may prevent other diseases including gastrointestinal disorders,[12] colon cancer,[13] autoimmune diseases,[14] and asthma.[15] One thing statins do not do is cause weight loss. No study has ever shown a persistent change in body weight from statin treatment. All of the health benefits of statin therapy in obese patients are accomplished without any loss of body fat whatsoever. Therefore, statin treatment should be considered to be an evidence-based treatment consistent with the Health At Every Size model.

A conservative treatment with an even greater impact on the health and life expectancy than statins is antihypertensive medications. The use of medications to lower blood pressure is believed to be the primary innovation that has led to dramatic declines in the death rate from stroke and heart attack in developed nations around the world since 1950. These declines in cardiovascular disease have notably occurred at the same time as rising rates of obesity from 1980 to 2000.[16] Nearly all of the controlled clinical trials of antihypertensive drugs have included obese subjects, usually as a majority of their test subjects. These trials consistently show that obese people are protected from stroke and heart attack when they treat their high blood pressure with safe and effective medications, and they benefit as much as or more than lean persons.[17] Even very obese persons with a BMI over 40 show excellent benefits from antihypertensive drugs, although the drug of choice may be different for obese and lean hypertensives.[18] None of the clinical trials with blood pressure–lowering drugs show any loss of weight in obese persons. Thus, antihypertensive medications are another evidence-based treatment promoting health regardless of size.

An aggressive medical approach to the obese patient will start with extremely low-calorie "crash" diets and proceed to stimulant drugs such as phentermine and others in the amphetamine class. These stimulant diet medications can increase blood pressure and heart rate, can be strongly habit forming, and can have psychiatric side effects.[19] Another category of diet drugs includes Orlistat, which blocks absorption of dietary fat, but its effectiveness is limited by side effects such as oily stool and anal leakage. Orlistat can also lead to depletion of fat-soluble vitamins.[20] Weight loss clinics run by bariatric physicians use a number of drugs "off label," meaning they are used for weight loss although not approved by the FDA for this purpose.[21] Popular off-label drugs for weight loss include high-dose thyroid hormone and a variety of drugs for other conditions that have a side effect of nausea. For example, the antiepileptic drug topiramate is given to obese patients in bariatric clinics because the resulting nausea can lead to a small weight loss, even though the drug has a number of potentially serious side effects including memory loss and confusion.[22] The FDA has recently approved a combination tablet containing topiramate and phentermine, even though weight loss is minimal and side effects are considerable.[23, 24] Topiramate is a sedative and apparently reduces the insomnia and agitation that can come from long-term stimulant use. This is the same rationale that was used for the notorious fen-phen combination of phentermine with another sedating drug, fenfluramine, which together had side effects of pulmonary hypertension and cardiac complications.

Even more aggressive than weight loss medications are surgical procedures. Weight loss surgeries fall along a spectrum of increasing risks of complications and increasing effectiveness in terms of weight loss. Gastric bypass is the most dangerous and results in the most weight loss.[25–28] The more of the intestinal tract that is bypassed, the greater the risk of malnutrition-related complications. The biliopancreatic bypass, which bypasses much of the small intestine, carries all of the risks of gastric bypass surgery but can also result in kwashiorkor, a disease of malnutrition formerly limited to African famine victims but now occurring in people in the US. Gastric banding reduces the risk of malnutrition relative to the bypass operations, but also results in less weight loss and more rapid weight regain. Gastric banding carries other risks, however, especially erosion of the stomach under the band, which becomes necrotic from lack of blood supply. Vomiting is especially frequent with the band, but also occurs after all of the gastric weight loss operations because the capacity of the stomach is reduced to two ounces or less. Any meal or beverage greater than this volume may be ejected, sometimes forcefully. Chronic vomiting carries the risk of B-vitamin deficiencies such as those seen with severe alcohol abuse. Electrolyte disturbances can result in strokes and cardiac arrest, similar to bulimia. Vomiting can be triggered by certain foods. High-protein foods are common triggers, even after treatment with meat tenderizer and mincing into fine pieces. High-fiber vegetables and foods with concentrated sugars may also be difficult to tolerate.

Contrasting with highly aggressive and risky interventions with weight loss drugs and surgery, a Health At Every Size approach favors low-risk or risk-free interventions. Medically, this is the essence of a conservative approach. The recent history of medicine records the progression from aggressive to conservative treatments as technology advances. For example, surgery used to be the standard treatment for ulcers and hospital wards were filled with people recovering form ulcer surgery. The development of cimetidine in 1976 led to the almost complete elimination of ulcer surgery.[29] Cimetidine was the first drug to achieve a billion dollars a year in sales and led to a Nobel Prize being awarded to its discoverer, Sir James Black. Further advances have led to the treatment of acid reflux, or heartburn, forestalling the development of ulcers. In another example, surgery used to be common treatment for chronic back pain. Clinical trials showed that physical therapy is more effective than surgery, and this far more conservative approach to treatment now predominates.[30] Weight loss surgery is a major anomaly in this historical trend for medical progress, and has become a common surgery done in the United States.

One remedy for diseases and conditions associated with a high body weight is a wellness approach focused on healthy lifestyle, positive attitude to health and self-care, and a disregarding of predetermined weight standards in favor of preventing further weight gain and reducing risk factors. Medical conditions common in obese patients, including hypertension, Type 2 diabetes, hyperlipidemia, and sleep apnea, are dealt with directly and aggressively rather than relying on weight loss as the primary treatment. This new approach is supported by the highest-quality controlled clinical trials and should improve the physical and mental well-being of obese patients. An important role of HAES practitioners is to encourage adherence to conservative medical therapies such as medications and physical rehabilitation.

References

1. M. Neovius et al., "Health Care Use During 20 Years Following Bariatric Surgery," *Journal of the American Medical Association* 308, no. 11 (2012): 1132–1141.

2. L. Sjostrom et al., "Effects of Bariatric Surgery on Mortality in Swedish Obese Subjects," *N. Engl. J Med.* 357, no. 8 (2007): 741–752.

3. K. M. Flegal et al., "Cause-Specific Excess Deaths Associated with Underweight, Overweight, and Obesity," *Journal of the American Medical Association* 298, no. 17 (2007): 2028–2037.

4. R. L. Leibel and J. Hirsch, "Diminished Energy Requirements in Reduced-Obese Patients," *Metabolism: Clinical and Experimental* 33 (1984): 164–170.

5. A. Tremblay et al., "Metabolic Fitness in Active Reduced-Obese Individuals," *Obes.Res.* 7, no. 6 (1999): 556–563.

6. S. Pursnani et al., "Percutaneous Coronary Intervention versus Optimal Medical Therapy in Stable Coronary Artery Disease: A Systematic Review and Meta-Analysis of Randomized Clinical Trials," *Circ.Cardiovasc.Interv.* 5, no. 4 (2012): 476–490.

7. P. M. Ridker et al., "Cardiovascular Benefits and Diabetes Risks of Statin Therapy in Primary Prevention: An Analysis from the JUPITER Trial," *Lancet* 380, no. 9841 (2012): 565–571.

8. S. M. Boekholdt et al., "Association of LDL Cholesterol, Non-HDL Cholesterol, and Apolipoprotein B Levels with Risk of Cardiovascular Events Among Patients Treated with Statins: A Meta-Analysis," *Journal of the American Medical Association* 307, no. 12 (2012): 1302–1309.

9. J. Allonen et al., "Mortality Rate Increases Steeply with Nonadherence to Statin Therapy in Patients with Acute Coronary Syndrome," *Clin. Cardiol.* 35, no. 11 (2012): E22–E27.

10. E. Mas and T. A. Mori, "Coenzyme Q(10) and Statin Myalgia: What Is the Evidence?" *Curr. Atheroscler. Rep.* 12, no. 6 (2010): 407–413.

11. R. C. Meex et al., "The Use of Statins Potentiates the Insulin-Sensitizing Effect of Exercise Training in Obese Males with and Without Type 2 Diabetes," *Clin. Sci.(Lond)* 119, no. 7 (2010): 293–301.

12. M. Cortes-Bergoderi, A. M. Pineda, and O. Santana, "The Pleiotropic Effects and Therapeutic Potential of the Hydroxy-Methyl-Glutaryl-CoA Reductase Inhibitors in Gastrointestinal Tract Disorders: A Comprehensive Review," *J. Gastrointestin. Liver Dis.* 22, no. 2 (2013): 199–204.

13. P. Lochhead and A. T. Chan, "Statins and Colorectal Cancer," *Clin. Gastroenterol. Hepatol.* 11, no. 2 (2013): 109–118.

14. C. Lopez-Pedrera et al., "To Cardiovascular Disease and Beyond: New Therapeutic Perspectives of Statins in Autoimmune Diseases and Cancer," *Curr. Drug Targets.* 13, no. 6 (2012): 829–841.

15. R. Miyata et al., "Statins Reduce Ambient Particulate Matter-Induced Lung Inflammation by Promoting the Clearance of Particulate Matter, < 10 µm from Lung Tissues," *Chest* 143, no. 2 (2013): 452–460.

16. P. Ernsberger and R. J. Koletsky, "Biomedical Rationale for a Wellness Approach to Obesity: An Alternative to a Focus on Weight Loss," *Journal of Social Issues* 55, no. 2 (1999): 221–259.

17. M. A. Weber et al., "Effects of Body Size and Hypertension Treatments on Cardiovascular Event Rates: Subanalysis of the ACCOMPLISH Randomised Controlled Trial," *Lancet* 381, no. 9866 (2013): 537–545.

18. J. Jordan et al., "Antihypertensive Treatment in Patients With Class 3 Obesity," *Ther.Adv.Endocrinol. Metab* 3, no. 3 (2012): 93–98.

19. L. L. Ioannides-Demos et al., "Safety of Drug Therapies Used for Weight Loss and Treatment of Obesity," *Drug Safety* 29, no. 4 (2006): 277–302.

20. A. T. Melia, S. G. Koss Twardy, and J. Zhi, "The Effect of Orlistat, an Inhibitor of Dietary Fat Absorption, on the Absorption of Vitamins A and E in Healthy Volunteers," *J. Clin. Pharmacol.* 36, no. 7 (1996): 647–653.

21. P. Ernsberger and P. Haskew, "Health Implications of Obesity: An Alternative View," *Journal of Obesity and Weight Regulation* 6 (1987): 55–137.

22. C. K. Kramer et al., "Efficacy and Safety of Topiramate on Weight Loss: A Meta-Analysis of Randomized Controlled Trials," *Obes. Rev.* 12, no. 5 (2011): e338–e347.

23. W. R. Hiatt, A. Thomas, and A. B. Goldfine, "What Cost Weight Loss?" *Circulation* 125, no. 9 (2012): 1171–1177.

24. M. S. Lauer, "Lemons for Obesity," *Annals of Internal Medicine* 157, no. 2 (2012): 139–140.

25. P. Ernsberger, "Complications of the Surgical Treatment of Obesity," *American Journal of Psychiatry* 144 (1987): 833–834.

26. T. Al Fahad et al., "Very Early Onset of Wernicke's Encephalopathy After Gastric Bypass," *Obes. Surg.* 16, no. 5 (2006): 671–672.

27. B. M. Koffman et al., "Neurologic Complications After Surgery for Obesity," *Muscle Nerve* 33, no. 2 (2006): 166–176.

28. S. S. Malinowski, "Nutritional and Metabolic Complications of Bariatric Surgery," *Am. J Med Sci.* 331, no. 4 (2006): 219–225.

29. D. T. Hansell et al., "Maintenance Cimetidine Instead of Surgery for Duodenal Ulcer: The First Decade," *Gut* 30, no. 6 (1989): 786–789.

30. M. B. Lequin et al., "Surgery versus Prolonged Conservative Treatment for Sciatica: 5-Year Results of a Randomised Controlled Trial," *BMJ Open.* 3, no. 5 (2013).

SPOTLIGHT

The next chapter, by Linda Bacon and Lucy Aphramor, elaborates further on the difficulties with the traditional medical model of focusing on weight loss as the solution to many health problems. The authors examine a number of assumptions typically made in the research literature on overweight and obesity. They critique the conclusions made about the need for weight loss for health, and state that there is no evidence to support the idea that, for most people, weight loss will improve health and longevity, and therefore should be pursued from a medical point of view.

Chapter Five

Weight Science: Evaluating the Evidence for a Paradigm Shift

Linda Bacon and Lucy Aphramor

ASSUMPTIONS UNDERLYING THE CONVENTIONAL (WEIGHT-FOCUSED)PARADIGM

Dieting and other weight loss behaviors are popular in the general population and widely encouraged in public health policy and health care practice as a solution for the "problem" of obesity. There is increasing concern about the endemic misrepresentation of evidence in these weight management policies.[1, 2] Researchers have demonstrated ways in which bias and convention interfere with robust scientific reasoning such that obesity research seems to "enjoy special immunity from accepted standards in clinical practice and publishing ethics".[1-3] This section discusses the assumptions that underlie the current weight-focused paradigm, presenting evidence that contests their scientific merit and challenges the value of promoting weight management as a public health measure.

Assumption: Adiposity poses significant mortality risk.

Evidence: Except at statistical extremes, body mass index (BMI)—or amount of body fat—only weakly predicts longevity.[4] Most epidemiological studies find that people who are overweight or moderately obese live at least as long as normal weight people, and often

Linda Bacon and Lucy Aphramor, "Assumptions Underlying the Conventional Paradigm of Health," *Nutrition Journal*, vol. 10, no. 9, pp. 4–13. Copyright © 2011 by Linda Bacon and Lucy Aphramor, (CC BY 2.0) at: http://www.nutritionj.com/content/10/1/9.

longer.[4–7] Analysis of the National Health and Nutrition Examination Surveys I, II, and III, which followed the largest nationally representative cohort of United States adults, determined that greatest longevity was in the overweight category. As per the report, published in the *Journal of the American Medical Association* and reviewed and approved by the Centers for Disease Control and Prevention and the National Cancer Institute, "[this] finding is consistent with other results reported in the literature."[4] Indeed, the most comprehensive review of the research pooled data for over 350,000 subjects from 26 studies and found overweight to be associated with greater longevity than normal weight.[8] More recently, Janssen analyzed data in the elderly (among whom more than 70% of all deaths occur)—also from 26 published studies—and similarly found no evidence of excess mortality associated with overweight.[9] The Americans' Changing Lives study came to a similar conclusion, indicating that "when socioeconomic and other risk factors are controlled for, obesity is not a significant risk factor for mortality; and … for those 55 or older, both overweight and obesity confer a significant decreased risk of mortality."[10] The most recent analysis, published in the *New England Journal of Medicine*, concluded that overweight was associated with increased risk, but only arrived at this conclusion after restricting the analysis by excluding 78% of the deaths.[11] They also used a reference category much narrower than the entire "normal weight" category used by most other studies, which also contributed to making the relative risk for overweight higher.

There is a robust pattern in the epidemiological literature that has been named the "obesity paradox"[12, 13]: obesity is associated with longer survival in many diseases. For example, obese persons with type 2 diabetes,[14] hypertension,[15, 16] cardiovascular disease,[13, 17] and chronic kidney disease[18] all have greater longevity than thinner people with these conditions.[19–21] Also, obese people who have had heart attacks, coronary bypass,[22] angioplasty,[23] or hemodialysis[24] live longer than thinner people with these histories.[21] In addition, obese senior citizens live longer than thinner senior citizens.[25]

It is also interesting to note that life expectancy increased dramatically during the same time period in which weight rose (from 70.8 years in 1970 to 77.8 years in 2005).[26] Both the World Health Organization and the Social Security Administration project life expectancy will continue to rise in coming decades.[27, 28]

Assumption: Adiposity poses significant morbidity risk.

Evidence: While it is well established that obesity is *associated* with increased risk for many diseases, causation is less well-established. Epidemiological studies rarely acknowledge factors like fitness, activity, nutrient intake, weight cycling or socioeconomic status when considering connections between weight and disease. Yet all play a role in determining health risk. When studies *do* control for these factors, increased risk of disease disappears or is significantly reduced.[29] (This is less true at statistical extremes.) It is likely that these other factors increase disease risk at the same time they increase the risk of weight gain.

Consider weight cycling as an example. Attempts to lose weight typically result in weight cycling, and such attempts are more common among obese individuals.[30] Weight cycling results in increased inflammation, which in turn is known to increase risk for many obesity-associated diseases.[31] Other potential mechanisms by which weight cycling contributes to morbidity include hypertension, insulin resistance and dyslipidemia.[32] Research also indicates that weight fluctuation is associated with poorer cardiovascular outcomes and increased mortality risk.[32–36] Weight cycling can account for all of the excess mortality associated with obesity in both the Framingham Heart Study[37] and the National Health and Nutrition Examination Survey (NHANES).[38] It may be, therefore, that the association between weight and health risk can be better attributed to weight cycling than adiposity itself.[31]

As another example, consider type 2 diabetes, the disease most highly associated with weight and fat distribution. There is increasing evidence that poverty and marginalization are more strongly associated with type 2 diabetes than conventionally-accepted risk factors such as weight, diet or activity habits.[39–42] A large Canadian report produced in 2010, for example, found that low income was strongly associated with diabetes even when BMI (and physical activity) was accounted for.[42] Also, much evidence suggests that insulin resistance is a product of an underlying metabolic disturbance that predisposes the individual to increased fat storage due to compensatory insulin secretion.[29, 43–47] In other words, obesity may be an early symptom of diabetes as opposed to its primary underlying cause.

Hypertension provides another example of a condition highly associated with weight; research suggests that it is two to three times more common among obese people than lean people.[48] To what extent hypertension is caused by adiposity, however, is unclear. That BMI correlates more strongly with blood pressure than percent body fat[49] indicates that the association between BMI and blood pressure results from higher lean mass as opposed to fat mass. Also, the association may have more to do with the weight cycling that results from trying to control weight than the actual weight itself.[20, 50, 51] One study conducted with obese individuals determined that weight cycling was strongly positively associated with incident hypertension.[51] Another study showed that obese women who had dieted had high blood pressure, while those who had never been on a diet had normal blood pressure.[35] Rat studies also show that obese rats that have weight cycled have very high blood pressures compared to obese rats that have not weight cycled.[52, 53] This finding could also explain the weak association between obesity and hypertension in cultures where dieting is uncommon.[20, 54]

Additionally, it is well documented that obese people with hypertension live significantly longer than thinner people with hypertension[15, 55–57] and have a lower risk of heart attack, stroke, or early death.[17] Rather than identifying health risk, as it does in thinner people, hypertension in heavier people may simply be a requirement for pumping blood through their larger bodies.[58]

It is also interesting to note that the prevalence of hypertension dropped by half between 1960 and 2000, a time when average weight sharply increased, declining much more steeply among those deemed overweight and obese than among thinner individuals.[59] Incidence of cardiovascular disease also plummeted during this time period and many common diseases now emerge at older ages and are less severe.[59] (The notable exception is diabetes, which showed a small, non-significant increase during this time period.[59]) While the decreased morbidity can at least in part be attributed to improvements in medical care, the point remains that we are simply not seeing the catastrophic disease consequences predicted to result from the "obesity epidemic."

Assumption: Weight loss will prolong life.

Evidence: Most prospective observational studies suggest that weight loss *increases* the risk of premature death among obese individuals, even when the weight loss is intentional and the studies are well controlled with regard to known confounding factors, including hazardous behavior and underlying diseases.[60–65] Recent review of NHANES, for example, a nationally representative sample of ethnically diverse people over the age of fifty, shows that mortality *increased* among those who lost weight.[66]

While many short-term weight loss intervention studies do indicate improvements in health measures, because the weight loss is always accompanied by a change in behavior, it is not known whether or to what extent the improvements can be attributed to the weight loss itself. Liposuction studies that control for behavior change may provide more accurate information about the effects of weight loss itself. One study which explicitly monitored that there were no changes in diet and activity for 10–12 weeks post abdominal liposuction determined that participants lost 10.5 kgs but saw no improvements in obesity-associated metabolic abnormalities, including blood pressure, triglycerides, cholesterol, or insulin sensitivity.[67]

Evidence also challenges the assumption that weight loss is associated with improvement in long-term glycemic control, as reflected in HbA1c values.[68, 69] One review of controlled weight-loss studies for people with type 2 diabetes showed that initial improvements were followed by a deterioration back to starting values six to eighteen months after treatment, *even when the weight loss was maintained.*[70]

Furthermore, health benefits associated with weight loss rarely show a dose response (in other words, people who lose small amounts of weight generally get as much health benefit from the intervention as those who lose larger amounts). In studies on type 2 diabetes, the improvement in glycemic control is seen within days, before significant weight or fat is lost.

These data suggest that the behavior change as opposed to the weight loss itself may play a greater role in health improvement.

Assumption: Anyone who is determined can lose weight and keep it off through appropriate diet and exercise.

Evidence: Long-term follow-up studies document that the majority of individuals regain virtually all of the weight that was lost during treatment, regardless of whether they maintain their diet or exercise program.[2, 71] Consider the Women's Health Initiative, the largest and longest randomized, controlled dietary intervention clinical trial, designed to test the current recommendations. More than 20,000 women maintained a low-fat diet, reportedly reducing their calorie intake by an average of 360 calories per day. After almost eight years on this diet, there was almost no change in weight from starting point (a loss of 0.1 kg), and average waist circumference, which is a measure of abdominal fat, had *increased* (0.3 cm).[72]

A panel of experts convened by the National Institutes of Health determined that "one third to two thirds of the weight is regained within one year [after weight loss], and almost all is regained within five years."[73] More recent review finds one-third to two-thirds of dieters regain more weight than was lost on their diets; "In sum," the authors report, "there is little support for the notion that diets lead to lasting weight loss or health benefits."[2] Other reviews demonstrate the unreliability of conventional claims of sustained weight loss.[74, 75] There is a paucity of long term data regarding surgical studies, but emerging data indicates gradual post-surgery weight regain as well.[76, 77] Weight loss peaks about one year postoperative, after which gradual weight regain is the norm.

Assumption: The pursuit of weight loss is a practical and positive goal.

Evidence: As discussed earlier, weight cycling is the most common result of engaging in conventional dieting practices and is known to increase morbidity and mortality risk. Research identifies many other contraindications to the pursuit of weight loss. For example, dieting is known to reduce bone mass, increasing risk for osteoporosis;[78–81] this is true even in an obese population, though obesity is typically associated with reduced risk for osteoporosis.[78] Research also suggests that dieting is associated with increased chronic psychological stress and cortisol production, two factors known to increase disease risk.[82] Also, there is emerging evidence that persistent organic pollutants (POPs), which bioaccumulate in adipose tissue and are released during its breakdown, can increase risk of various chronic diseases including type 2 diabetes,[83, 84] cardiovascular disease[85] and rheumatoid arthritis;[86] two studies document that people who have lost weight have higher concentration of POPs in their blood.[87, 88] One review of the diabetes literature indicates "that obese persons that (sic) do not have elevated POPs are not at elevated risk of diabetes, suggesting that the POPs rather than the obesity per se is responsible for the association."[84]

Positing the value of weight loss also supports widespread anxiety about weight.[89, 90] Evidence from the eating disorder literature indicates an emphasis on weight control can promote eating disordered behaviors.[91] Prospective studies show that body dissatisfaction is associated with binge eating and other eating disordered behaviors, lower levels of physical

Table 1. Cost of Using BMI as a Proxy for Health[a]

		Abnormal cariometabolic profile	Normal cardiometabolic profile	TOTAL
Untreated	"Normal weight (BMI = 18.5–24.9)	23.5% (16.3 million people)[b]	76.5% (53.0 million people)	100% (69.3 million people)
Treated	"Overweight" (BMI = 25.0–29.9)	48.7% (34.1 million people)	51.3% (35.9 million people)[c]	100% (70.0 million people)
	"Obese" (BMI ≥ 30.0)	68.3% (42.0 million people)	31.7% (19.5 million people)[c]	100% (61.5 million people)
TOTAL		46% 92.4 million people	54% 108.4 million people	100% 200.8 million people

[a]Based on study by Widman et al.

[b]False negative: 16.3 million of 92.4 million (17.6%) who have abnormal cardiometabolic profile are overlooked

[c]False positive: 55.4 million of 131.5 million (42%) are identified as ill who are not

Bacon and Aphramor *Nutrition Journal* 2011 10:9 doi: 10.1186/1475-2891-10-9

activity and increased weight gain over time.[92, 93] Many studies also show that dieting is a strong predictor of future weight gain.[34, 94–99]

Another unintended consequence of the weight loss imperative is an increase in stigmatization and discrimination against fat individuals. Discrimination based on weight now equals or exceeds that based on race or gender.[100] Extensive research indicates that stigmatizing fat demotivates, rather than encourages, health behavior change.[101] Adults who face weight stigmatization and discrimination report consuming increased quantities of food,[102–105] avoiding exercise,[104, 106–108] and postponing or avoiding medical care (for fear of experiencing stigmatization).[109] Stigmatization and bias on the part of health care practitioners is well-documented, resulting in lower quality care.[110, 111]

Assumption: The only way for overweight and obese people to improve health is to lose weight.

Evidence: That weight loss will improve health over the long-term for obese people is, in fact, an untested hypothesis. One reason the hypothesis is untested is because no methods have proven to reduce weight long-term for a significant number of people. Also, while normal weight people have lower disease incidence than obese individuals, it is unknown if weight loss in individuals already obese reduces disease risk to the same level as that observed in those who were never obese.[60, 62]

As indicated by research conducted by one of the authors and many other investigators, most health indicators can be improved through changing health behaviors, regardless of whether weight is lost.[112] For example, lifestyle changes can reduce blood pressure, largely or completely independent of changes in body weight.[112–115] The same can be said for blood lipids.[112, 115–117] Improvements in insulin sensitivity and blood lipids as a result of aerobic exercise training have been documented even in individuals who *gained* body fat during the intervention.[117, 118]

Assumption: Obesity-related costs place a large burden on the economy, and this can be corrected by focused attention to obesity treatment and prevention.

Evidence: The health cost attributed to obesity in the United States is currently estimated to be $147 billion annually[119] and this cost estimate has been used to justify efforts at obesity treatment and prevention. Although this estimate has been granted credence by health experts, the word "estimate" is important to note: as the authors state, most of the cost changes are not "statistically different from zero." Also, the estimate fails to account for many potentially confounding variables, among them physical activity, nutrient intake, history of weight cycling, degree of discrimination, access to (quality) medical care, etc. All are independently correlated with both weight and health and could play a role in explaining the costs associated with having a BMI over 30. Nor does it account for costs associated with unintended consequences of positing the value of a weight focus, which may include eating disorders, diet attempts, weight cycling, reduced self-esteem, depression, and discrimination.

Because BMI is considered a risk factor for many diseases, obese persons are automatically relegated to greater testing and treatment, which means that positing BMI as a risk factor results in increased costs, regardless of whether BMI itself is problematic. Yet using BMI as a proxy for health may be more costly than addressing health directly. Consider, for example, the findings of a study which examined the "healthy obese" and the "unhealthy normal weight" populations.[120] The study identified six different risk factors for cardiometabolic health and included subjects in the "unhealthy" group if they had two or more risk factors, making it a more stringent threshold of health than that used in categorizing metabolic syndrome or diabetes. The study found a substantial proportion of the overweight and obese population, at every age, who were healthy and a substantial proportion of the "normal weight" group who were unhealthy. Psychologist Deb Burgard examined the costs of overlooking the normal weight people who need treatment and over-treating the obese people who do not (personal communication, March 2010). She found that BMI profiling overlooks 16.3 million "normal weight" individuals who are not healthy and identifies 55.4 million overweight and obese people who are not ill as being in need of treatment (see Table 1). When the total population is considered, this means that 36 percent of the population is mis-identified when BMI is used as a proxy for health.

The weight bias inherent in BMI profiling may actually result in higher costs and sicker people. As an example, consider a 2009 study published in the American Journal of Public Health.[121] The authors compared people of similar age, gender, education level, and rates of diabetes and hypertension, and examined how often they reported feeling sick over a 30-day period. Results indicated that body image had a much bigger impact on health than body size. In other words, two equally fat women would have very different health outcomes, depending on how they felt about their bodies. Likewise, two women with similar body insecurities would have similar health outcomes, even if one were fat and the other thin. These results suggest that the stigma associated with being fat is a major contributor to obesity-associated disease. BMI and health are only weakly related in cultures where obesity is not stigmatized, such as in the South Pacific.[20, 122]

References

1. Bacon, L., *Health at Every Size: The Surprising Truth About Your Weight (Second Edition)*. 2010, Dallas: BenBella Books.

2. Mann, T., et al., *Medicare's Search for Effective Obesity Treatments: Diets Are Not the Answer.* American Psychologist, 2007. 62(3): p. 220–33.

3. Aphramor, L., *Validity of claims made in weight management research: a narrative review of dietetic articles.* Nutr J, 2010. 9: p. 30.

4. Flegal, K.M., et al., *Excess deaths associated with underweight, overweight, and obesity.* Journal of the American Medical Association, 2005. 293(15): p. 1861–7.

5. Durazo-Arvizu, R., et al., *Mortality and optimal body mass index in a sample of the US population.* American Journal of Epidemiology, 1998. 147: p. 739–749.

6. Troiano, R., et al., *The relationship between body weight and mortality: A quantitative analysis of combined information from existing studies.* International Journal of Obesity and Related Metabolic Disorders, 1996. 20: p. 63–75.

7. Flegal, K., et al., Supplement: Response to "Can Fat Be Fit", in *Scientific American*. 2008. p. 5–6.

8. McGee, D.L., Body mass index and mortality: a meta-analysis based on person-level data from twenty-six observational studies. *Annals of Epidemiology*, 2005. 15(2): p. 87–97.

9. Janssen, I. and A.E. Mark, Elevated body mass index and mortality risk in the elderly. *Obes Rev*, 2007. 8(1): p. 41–59.

10. Lantz, P.M., et al., Socioeconomic and behavioral risk factors for mortality in a national 19-year prospective study of U.S. adults. *Soc Sci Med*, 2010. 70(10): p. 1558–66.

11. Berrington de Gonzalez, A., et al., Body-mass index and mortality among 1.46 million white adults. *N Engl J Med,* 2010. 363(23): p. 2211–9.

12. Childers, D. and D. Allison, The 'obesity paradox': a parsimonious explanation for relations among obesity, mortality rate and aging? *Int J Obes (Lond)*, 2010. 34(8): p. 1231–8.

13. Morse, S., R. Gulati, and E. Reisin, The obesity paradox and cardiovascular disease. *Curr Hypertens Rep,* 2010. 12(2): p. 120–6.

14. Ross, C., R.D. Langer, and E. Barrett-Connor, Given diabetes, is fat better than thin? *Diabetes Care,* 1997. 20(4): p. 650–2.

15. Barrett-Connor, E. and K. Khaw, Is hypertension more benign when associated with obesity? *Circulation,* 1985. 72: p. 53–60.

16. Barrett-Connor, E.L., Obesity, atherosclerosis and coronary artery disease. *Annals of Internal Medicine,* 1985. 103: p. 1010–1019.

17. Kang, X., et al., Impact of body mass index on cardiac mortality in patients with known or suspected coronary artery disease undergoing myocardial perfusion single-photon emission computed tomography. *Journal of the American College of Cardiology,* 2006. 47(7): p. 1418–26.

18. Beddhu, S., The body mass index paradox and an obesity, inflammation, and atherosclerosis syndrome in chronic kidney disease. *Seminars in Dialysis,* 2004. 17(3): p. 229–32.

19. Ernsberger, P. and P. Haskew, Health implications of obesity: An alternative view. *Journal of Obesity and Weight Regulation,* 1987. 9(2): p. 39–40.

20. Ernsberger, P. and R.J. Koletsky, Biomedical rationale for a wellness approach to obesity: An alternative to a focus on weight loss. *Journal of Social Issues,* 1999. 55(2): p. 221–260.

21. Lavie, C.J., R.V. Milani, and H.O. Ventura, Obesity, heart disease, and favorable prognosis--truth or paradox? *American Journal of Medicine,* 2007. 120(10): p. 825–6.

22. Gruberg, L., et al., Impact of body mass index on the outcome of patients with multivessel disease randomized to either coronary artery bypass grafting or stenting in the ARTS trial: The obesity paradox II? *Am J Cardiol,* 2005. 95(4): p. 439–44.

23. Lavie, C.J., et al., Body composition and prognosis in chronic systolic heart failure: the obesity paradox. *American Journal of Cardiology,* 2003. 91(7): p. 891–4.

24. Schmidt, D.S. and A.K. Salahudeen, Obesity-survival paradox-still a controversy? *Semin Dial,* 2007. 20(6): p. 486–92.

25. Kulminski, A.M., et al., Body mass index and nine-year mortality in disabled and nondisabled older U.S. individuals. *J Am Geriatr Soc,* 2008. 56(1): p. 105–10.

26. National Center for Health Statistics, *Health, United States, 2007. With Chartbook on Trends in the Health of Americans.* 2007, Hyattsville, MD.

27. Mathers, C. and D. Loncar, Projections of Global Mortality and Burden of Disease from 2002 to 2030. *PLoS Med,* 2006. 3(11): p. 2011–2029.

28. Social Security Administration, *Periodic Life Table.* 2007 (updated 7/9/07).

29. Campos, P., et al., The epidemiology of overweight and obesity: public health crisis or moral panic? *International Journal of Epidemiology,* 2005. 35(1): p. 55–60.

30. Kruger, J., et al., Attempting to lose weight: specific practices among U.S. adults. *Am J Prev Med,* 2004. 26(5): p. 402–6.

31. Strohacker, K. and B. McFarlin, Influence of obesity, physical inactivity, and weight cycling on chronic inflammation. *Frontiers in Bioscience*, 2010. E2: p. 98–104.

32. Montani, J.P., et al., Weight cycling during growth and beyond as a risk factor for later cardiovascular diseases: the 'repeated overshoot' theory. *Int J Obes (Lond)*, 2006. 30 Suppl 4: p. S58–66.

33. Olson, M.B., et al., Weight cycling and high-density lipoprotein cholesterol in women: evidence of an adverse effect: a report from the NHLBI-sponsored WISE study. Women's Ischemia Syndrome Evaluation Study Group. *J Am Coll Cardiol*, 2000. 36(5): p. 1565–71.

34. French, S.A., et al., Predictors of weight change over two years among a population of working adults: The Healthy Worker Project. *International Journal of Obesity*, 1994. 18: p. 145–154.

35. Guagnano, M.T., et al., Weight fluctuations could increase blood pressure in android obese women. *Clinical Sciences (London)*, 1999. 96(6): p. 677–80.

36. Rzehak, P., et al., Weight change, weight cycling and mortality in the ERFORT Male Cohort Study. *Eur J Epidemiol*, 2007. 22(10): p. 665–73.

37. Lissner, L., et al., Variability of body weight and health outcomes in the Framingham population. *New England Journal of Medicine*, 1991. 324: p. 1839–1844.

38. Diaz, V.A., A.G. Mainous, 3rd, and C.J. Everett, The association between weight fluctuation and mortality: results from a population-based cohort study. *Journal of Community Health*, 2005. 30(3): p. 153–65.

39. McDermott, R., Ethics, Epidemiology, and the Thrifty Gene: Biological Determinism as a Health Hazard. *Social Science & Medicine*, 1998. 47(9): p. 1189–1195.

40. Brunner, E. and M. Marmot, Social Organization, Stress, and Health, in *Social Determinants of Health, 2nd ed.*, M. Marmot, Wilkinson, R.G, Editor. 2006, Oxford University Press: New York. p. 17–43.

41. Wamala, S., J. Lynch, and M. Horsten, Education and the Metabolic Syndrome in Women. *Diabetes Care,* 1999. 22(12): p. 1999–2003.

42. Raphael, D., et al., *Type 2 Diabetes: Poverty, Priorities and Policy. The Social Determinants of the Incidence and Management of Type 2 Diabetes.* 2010, Toronto: York University School of Health Policy and Management and School of Nursing.

43. Charles, M.A., et al., Development of impaired glucose tolerance with or without weight gain. *Diabetes Care*, 1993. 16(4): p. 593–6.

44. Odeleye, O.E., et al., Fasting hyperinsulinemia is a predictor of increased body weight gain and obesity in Pima Indian children. *Diabetes,* 1997. 46(8): p. 1341–5.

45. Sigal, R.J., et al., Acute postchallenge hyperinsulinemia predicts weight gain: a prospective study. *Diabetes,* 1997. 46(6): p. 1025–9.

46. Yost, T.J., D.R. Jensen, and R.H. Eckel, Weight regain following sustained weight reduction is predicted by relative insulin sensitivity. *Obes Res*, 1995. 3(6): p. 583–7.

47. Halberg, N., et al., Effect of intermittent fasting and refeeding on insulin action in healthy men. *J Appl Physiol.*, 2005. 99(6): p. 2128–36.

48. Akram, D.S., et al., *Obesity: Preventing and managing the global epidemic. Report of a WHO consultation on obesity.* 1997, Geneva, Switzerland: World Health Organization.

49. Weinsier, R.L., et al., The relative contribution of body fat and fat pattern to blood pressure level. *Hypertension*, 1985. 7(4): p. 578–85.

50. Ernsberger, P. and D.O. Nelson, Effects of fasting and refeeding on blood pressure are determined by nutritional state, not by body weight change. *American Journal of Hypertension*, 1988: p. 153S–157S.

51. Schulz, M., et al., Associations of short-term weight changes and weight cycling with incidence of essential hypertension in the EPIC-Potsdam Study. *Journal of Human Hypertension*, 2005. 19(1): p. 61–7.

52. Ernsberger, P., et al., Consequences of weight cycling in obese spontaneously hypertensive rats. *American Journal of Physiology*, 1996. 270: p. R864–R872.

53. Ernsberger, P., et al., Refeeding hypertension in obese spontaneously hypertensive rats. *Hypertension*, 1994. 24: p. 699–705.

54. Chernin, K., *The Obsession: Reflections on the tyranny of slenderness.* 1981, New York: Harper & Row.

55. Cambien, F., et al., Is the relationship between blood pressure and cardiovascular risk dependent on body mass index? *American Journal of Epidemiology*, 1985. 122: p. 434–42.

56. Weinsier, R., et al., Body fat: Its relationship to coronary heart disease, blood pressure, lipids, and other risk factors measured in a large male population. *American Journal of Medicine*, 1976. 61: p. 815–24.

57. Uretsky, S., et al., Obesity paradox in patients with hypertension and coronary artery disease. *American Journal of Medicine*, 2007. 120(10): p. 863–70.

58. Messerli, F.H., Cardiovascular adaptations to obesity and arterial hypertension: detrimental or beneficial? *Int J Cardiol*, 1983. 3(1): p. 94–7.

59. Gregg, E.W., et al., Secular trends in cardiovascular disease risk factors according to body mass index in US adults. *Journal of the American Medical Association*, 2005. 293(15): p. 1868–74.

60. Williamson, D.F., et al., Prospective study of intentional weight loss and mortality in never-smoking overweight U.S. white women aged 40–64 years. *American Journal of Epidemiology*, 1995. 141: p. 1128–1141.

61. Williamson, D.F., et al., Prospective study of intentional weight loss and mortality in overweight white men aged 40–64 years. *American Journal of Epidemiology*, 1999. 149(6): p. 491–503.

62. Andres, R., D.C. Muller, and J.D. Sorkin, Long-term effects of change in body weight on all-cause mortality. A review. *Annals of Internal Medicine,* 1993. 119: p. 737–743.

63. Yaari, S. and U. Goldbourt, Voluntary and involuntary weight loss: associations with long term mortality in 9,228 middle-aged and elderly men. *American Journal of Epidemiology*, 1998. 148: p. 546–55.

64. Sørensen, T., et al., Intention to lose weight, weight changes, and 18-y mortality in overweight individuals without co-morbidities. *PLoS Med,* 2005. 2: p. E171.

65. Simonsen, M.K., et al., Intentional weight loss and mortality among initially healthy men and women. *Nutr Rev,* 2008. 66(7): p. 375–86.

66. Ingram, D.D. and M.E. Mussolino, Weight loss from maximum body weight and mortality: the Third National Health and Nutrition Examination Survey Linked Mortality File. *International Journal of Obesity,* 2010. 34(6): p. 1044–1050.

67. Klein, S., et al., Absence of an effect of liposuction on insulin action and risk factors for coronary heart disease. *N Engl J Med,* 2004. 350(25): p. 2549–57.

68. Manning, R.M., et al., The comparison of four weight reduction strategies aimed at overweight patients with diabetes mellitus: four-year follow-up. *Diabet Med,* 1998. 15(6): p. 497–502.

69. Wing, R.R. and K. Anglin, Effectiveness of a behavioral weight control program for blacks and whites with NIDDM. *Diabetes Care,* 1996. 19(5): p. 409–13.

70. Ciliska, D., et al., A review of weight loss interventions for obese people with non-insulin dependent diabetes mellitus. *Canadian Journal of Diabetes Care,* 1995. 19: p. 10–15.

71. Miller, W.C., How effective are traditional dietary and exercise interventions for weight loss? *Medicine and Science in Sports and Exercise,* 1999. 31(8): p. 1129–1134.

72. Howard, B.V., et al., Low-fat dietary pattern and weight change over 7 years: the Women's Health Initiative Dietary Modification Trial. *Journal of the American Medical Association,* 2006. 295(1): p. 39–49.

73. National Institutes of Health (NIH), Methods for voluntary weight loss and control (Technology Assessment Conference Panel). *Annals of Internal Medicine,* 1992. 116(11): p. 942–949.

74. Aphramor, L., Is A Weight-Centred Health Framework Salutogenic? Some Thoughts on Unhinging Certain Dietary Ideologies. *Social Theory and Health,* 2005. 3(4): p. 315–340.

75. Aphramor, L., Weight management as a cardioprotective intervention raises issues for nutritional scientists regarding clinical ethics. *Proc Nut Soc,* 2009. 67: p. E401.

76. Sjostrom, L., et al., Lifestyle, diabetes, and cardiovascular risk factors 10 years after bariatric surgery. *New England Journal of Medicine,* 2004. 351(26): p. 2683–93.

77. Christou, N.V., D. Look, and L.D. Maclean, Weight gain after short- and long-limb gastric bypass in patients followed for longer than 10 years. *Ann Surg,* 2006. 244(5): p. 734–40.

78. Bacon, L., et al., Low bone mass in premenopausal chronic dieting obese women. *European Journal of Clinical Nutrition,* 2004. 58(6): p. 966–71.

79. Van Loan, M.D. and N.L. Keim, Influence of cognitive eating restraint on total-body measurements of bone mineral density and bone mineral content in premenopausal women 18–45 y: a cross-sectional study. *American Journal of Clinical Nutrition,* 2000. 72: p. 837–843.

80. Van Loan, M.D., et al., Effect of drive for thinness during adolescence on adult bone mass. *Journal of Bone and Mineral Research,* 2000. 15(Suppl 1): p. S412.

81. Barr, S.I., J.C. Prior, and Y.M. Vigna, Restrained eating and ovulatory disturbances: Possible implications for bone health. *American Journal of Clinical Nutrition*, 1994. 59: p. 92–97.

82. Tomiyama, A.J., et al., Low calorie dieting increases cortisol. *Psychosom Med*, 2010. 72(4): p. 357–64.

83. Lee, D.H., et al., A strong dose-response relation between serum concentrations of persistent organic pollutants and diabetes: results from the National Health and Examination Survey 1999–2002. *Diabetes Care*, 2006. 29(7): p. 1638–44.

84. Carpenter, D.O., Environmental contaminants as risk factors for developing diabetes. *Reviews on Environmental Health*, 2008. 23(1): p. 59–74.

85. Ha, M.H., D.H. Lee, and D.R. Jacobs, Association between serum concentrations of persistent organic pollutants and self-reported cardiovascular disease prevalence: results from the National Health and Nutrition Examination Survey, 1999–2002. *Environmental Health Perspectives*, 2007. 115(8): p. 1204–9.

86. Lee, D.H., M. Steffes, and D.R. Jacobs, Positive associations of serum concentration of polychlorinated biphenyls or organochlorine pesticides with self-reported arthritis, especially rheumatoid type, in women. *Environmental Health Perspectives,* 2007. 115(6): p. 883–8.

87. Chevrier, J., et al., Body weight loss increases plasma and adipose tissue concentrations of potentially toxic pollutants in obese individuals. *International Journal of Obesity and Related Metabolic Disorders*, 2000. 24(10): p. 1272–8.

88. Lim, J.S., et al., Inverse associations between long-term weight change and serum concentrations of persistent organic pollutants. *Int J Obes (Lond)*, 2010 (E pub ahead of print).

89. Davison, K.K., C.N. Markey, and L.L. Birch, A longitudinal examination of patterns in girls' weight concerns and body dissatisfaction from ages 5 to 9 years. *Int J Eat Disord*, 2003. 33(3): p. 320–32.

90. Holm, S., Obesity interventions and ethics. *Obes Rev, 2007.* 8 Suppl 1: p. 207–10.

91. Daníelsdóttir, S., D. Burgard, and W. Oliver-Pyatt, *AED Guidelines for Childhood Obesity Prevention Programs.* 2009, Academy of Eating Disorders.

92. Neumark-Sztainer, D., et al., Prevention of body dissatisfaction and disordered eating: What next? *Eat Disord*, 2006. 14(4): p. 265–85.

93. van den Berg, P. and D. Neumark-Sztainer, Fat 'n happy 5 years later: is it bad for overweight girls to like their bodies? *Journal of Adolescent Health*, 2007. 41(4): p. 415–7.

94. Stice, E., et al., Naturalistic weight-reduction efforts prospectively predict growth in relative weight and onset of obesity among female adolescents. *Journal of Consulting and Clinical Psychology,* 1999. 67: p. 967–974.

95. Coakley, E.H., et al., Predictors of weight change in men: Results from the Health Professionals Follow-Up Study. *International Journal of Obesity and Related Metabolic Disorders*, 1998. 22: p. 89–96.

96. Bild, D.E., et al., Correlates and predictors of weight loss in young adults: The CARDIA study. *International Journal of Obesity and Related Metabolic Disorders*, 1996. 20(1): p. 47–55.

97. Korkeila, M., et al., Weight-loss attempts and risk of major weight gain. *American Journal of Clinical Nutrition*, 1999. 70: p. 965–973.

98. Neumark-Sztainer, D., et al., Obesity, disordered eating, and eating disorders in a longitudinal study of adolescents: how do dieters fare 5 years later? *J Am Diet Assoc*, 2006. 106(4): p. 559–68.

99. Field, A.E., et al., Relation between dieting and weight change among preadolescents and adolescents. *Pediatrics*, 2003. 112(4): p. 900–6.

100. Puhl, R.M., T. Andreyeva, and K.D. Brownell, Perceptions of weight discrimination: prevalence and comparison to race and gender discrimination in America. *Int J Obes (Lond)*, 2008. 32: p. 992–1000.

101. Brownell, K., et al., *Weight bias: Nature, consequences, and remedies*. 2005, New York: Guilford.

102. Puhl, R.M. and K.D. Brownell, Confronting and coping with weight stigma: an investigation of overweight and obese adults. *Obesity* (Silver Spring), 2006. 14(10): p. 1802–15.

103. Haines, J., et al., Weight teasing and disordered eating behaviors in adolescents: longitudinal findings from Project EAT (Eating Among Teens). *Pediatrics,* 2006. 117(2): p. e209–15.

104. Neumark-Sztainer, D., et al., Weight-teasing among adolescents: correlations with weight status and disordered eating behaviors. *Int J Obes Relat Metab Disord*, 2002. 26(1): p. 123–31.

105. Puhl, R.M., C.A. Moss-Racusin, and M.B. Schwartz, Internalization of weight bias: Implications for binge eating and emotional well-being. *Obesity* (Silver Spring), 2007. 15(1): p. 19–23.

106. Faith, M.S., et al., Weight criticism during physical activity, coping skills, and reported physical activity in children. *Pediatrics*, 2002. 110(2 Pt 1): p. e23.

107. Storch, E.A., et al., Peer victimization, psychosocial adjustment, and physical activity in overweight and at-risk-for-overweight youth. *J Pediatr Psychol*, 2007. 32(1): p. 80–9.

108. Vartanian, L.R. and J.G. Shaprow, Effects of weight stigma on exercise motivation and behavior: a preliminary investigation among college-aged females. *J Health Psychol*, 2008. 13(1): p. 131–8.

109. Amy, N., et al., Barriers to routine gynecological cancer screening for White and African-American obese women. *International Journal of Obesity and Related Metabolic Disorders*, 2006. 30(1): p. 147–155.

110. Puhl, R. and K. Brownell, Bias, discrimination and obesity. *Obesity Research*, 2001. 9(12): p. 788–805.

111. Puhl, R.M. and C.A. Heuer, The stigma of obesity: a review and update. *Obesity* (Silver Spring), 2009. 17(5): p. 941–64.

112. Bacon, L., et al., Size acceptance and intuitive eating improve health for obese, female chronic dieters. *Journal of the American Dietetic Association*, 2005. 105: p. 929–36.

113. Fagard, R.H., Physical activity in the prevention and treatment of hypertension in the obese. *Med Sci Sports Exerc*, 1999. 31(11 Suppl): p. S624–30.

114. Appel, L.J., et al., A clinical trial of the effects of dietary patterns on blood pressure. *New England Journal of Medicine*, 1997. 33: p. 1117–1124.

115. Gaesser, G.A., Exercise for prevention and treatment of cardiovascular disease, type 2 diabetes, and metabolic syndrome. *Curr Diab Rep*, 2007. 7(1): p. 14–9.

116. Kraus, W.E., et al., Effects of the amount and intensity of exercise on plasma lipoproteins. *N Engl J Med,* 2002. 347(19): p. 1483–92.

117. Lamarche, B., et al., Is body fat loss a determinant factor in the improvement of carbohydrate and lipid metabolism following aerobic exercise training in obese women? *Metabolism,* 1992. 41: p. 1249–1256.

118. Bjorntorp, P., et al., The effect of physical training on insulin production in obesity. *Metabolism,* 1970. 19: p. 631–638.

119. Finkelstein, E.A., et al., Annual medical spending attributable to obesity: payer-and service-specific estimates. *Health Aff* (Millwood), 2009. 28(5): p. w822–31.

120. Wildman, R.P., et al., The obese without cardiometabolic risk factor clustering and the normal weight with cardiometabolic risk factor clustering: prevalence and correlates of 2 phenotypes among the US population (NHANES 1999–2004). *Arch Intern Med,* 2008. 168(15): p. 1617–24.

121. Muennig, P., et al., I Think Therefore I Am: Perceived Ideal Weight as a Determinant of Health. *American Journal of Public Health*, 2008. March.

122. Beaglehole, R., et al., Death in the South Pacific. *N Z Med J, 1980.* 91(660): p. 375–8.

SPOTLIGHT

The next chapter, by Dharini Bhammar and Glenn Gaesser, explores the topic of "weight cycling," in which people lose and regain weight repeatedly in an effort to be healthier. They present evidence to support the idea that weight cycling may in fact be more damaging to health than being consistently overweight or obese.

Chapter Six

Health Risks Associated With Weight Cycling

Dharini M. Bhammar and Glenn A. Gaesser

Losing weight is a preoccupation among many Americans. According to the Behavioral Risk Factor Surveillance System surveys, approximately 46% of women and 33% of men attempt weight loss each year.[1] An even greater percentage of women (64.9%) and men (62.9%) considered overweight or obese by body mass index (BMI: weight (kg)/height (m²)) criteria attempt weight loss.[2] However, permanent weight-loss maintenance is rare, as dieting has a very high long-term failure rate.[3] Multiple attempts at weight loss can lead to a life of weight cycling, where individuals go through repeated gains and losses of weight over time. The prevalence of weight cycling has been reported to range between 18% and 34% for men[4] and between 20% and 55% for women.[5] Weight cycling may carry significant health risks, including increased cancer risk[6–9] and higher mortality rates.[10–22] Weight cycling has also been linked to gall bladder disease[4,5] and increased bone fracture risk[23,24] that may increase mortality risk in older men and women.[25] These risks do not appear to have deterred efforts to lose weight, and despite the poor long-term success rates for weight-loss maintenance, caloric restriction remains a cornerstone for treatment of weight-related health conditions. The purpose of this chapter is to briefly review the research on the health risks associated with weight cycling.

WEIGHT CYCLING AND LONGEVITY

Although the term "weight cycling" is commonly used in research and lay publications, there is no universally accepted definition of weight cycling. In prospective observational studies, researchers have used statistical methods to define weight cycling (e.g., interpersonal standard deviation or coefficient of variation of body weight over time), or by merely counting the number of weight-cycling episodes combined with the magnitude of weight loss/gain in each cycle over time. Weight cycling could be attributable to unintentional weight changes as well as to the quite common experience of purposeful weight loss followed by inevitable regain of weight. In view of the prevalence of weight-loss attempts in the United States, it seems likely that weight cycling to a large extent reflects intentional attempts to lose weight. Involuntary weight losses are relatively uncommon. For example, in cancer the spontaneous loss of weight is a late symptom and often signals a terminal course.

Since 1989, a number of studies have reported a significantly increased mortality risk associated with weight cycling.[10-22] The increased mortality risk has been observed in men[10-13,15,22] and women,[11,14] in both sexes combined[16,17] and in older populations.[18-21] By contrast, some studies have not consistently found higher mortality risk associated with weight cycling.[22,26-32] It should be noted, however, that several of these studies did report higher mortality risk associated with weight cycling,[22,26,30] but the increased risk of weight cycling was not entirely independent of other factors, such as starting level of body weight and weight loss.

The reasons for the discrepancies in the literature are not entirely clear. As mentioned above, there is no standard definition of weight cycling. Additionally, much of the data are obtained by self-report, and it is not always clear whether weight loss was intentional or not. However, several of the studies in which body weight was actually measured over time, and thus did not rely on self-report, revealed significantly higher mortality rates associated with weight cycling. For example, 32-year follow-up data from the Framingham Heart Study indicated that weight cycling (defined as the coefficient of variation derived from eight measurements of body weight that were taken during the first 14 years and self-report weight at 25 years) was associated with a 65% to 93% increased risk of all-cause mortality and a 55% to 78% increase in coronary heart disease mortality in both men and women, even after adjusting for BMI, weight change, smoking, physical activity, serum cholesterol, systolic blood pressure, and glucose tolerance.[11] Additionally, mortality data for four years following the last weight measurement were not used in the analysis in order to eliminate variability in body weight that may have been attributable to antecedent disease, such as late stage cancer.

Two years after the results of the Framingham Heart Study were published, data from the multiple risk factor intervention trial (MRFIT) also demonstrated that weight cycling was associated with increased mortality risk.[15] Annual measures of body weight were taken for 6 to 7 years for men ages 35 to 57. Intrapersonal standard deviation (ISD) and weight change categories were used as measures of weight cycling. Based on the quartile of ISD for weight, the relative risk for all-cause and cardiovascular disease mortality increased steadily from the first through the fourth quartile and this was statistically significant even after adjustment for confounding variables (e.g., diastolic BP, diuretic use, serum cholesterol, initial level of physical activity, BMI, and reported number of alcoholic drinks). Weight cycling, regardless of whether the men had lost or gained weight by the end of the cycle, was also significantly associated with higher all-cause and cardiovascular disease mortality rates, with lowest mortality in the weight-stable group.

More recently, data on men and women from the National Health and Nutrition Examination Surveys (NHANES)[16] and on men in the Erfort Male Cohort Study (ERFORT)[12] showed that weight cycling, defined as the sum of variations in BMI compared to average BMI, was associated with higher mortality risk. In the NHANES analyses, weight cycling was determined from five weight measurements assessed between 1971 and 1987, with mortality follow-up through 1992. Weight cycling was associated with an 86% higher risk of cardiovascular mortality and an 83% higher risk of all-cause mortality. These risks were observed even when participants who were incapacitated or in poor health at the last weight assessment period in 1987 were excluded from the analysis. Thus it is likely that the risks of weight cycling reported in the NHANES study were in apparently healthy men and women, especially because of the thorough examination of each subject by physicians. In the ERFORT study, weight cycling was assessed via direct measurements of body weight at four time points between 1973 and 1990. In these middle-aged men, weight cycling—even when controlling for pre-existing cardiovascular disease or diabetes, smoking, and socioeconomic status—was associated with an 86% higher all-cause mortality risk during follow-up until 2003.

Even more recently, the Cardiovascular Health Study examined the association between weight cycling and all-cause mortality in adults ages > 65 years.[21] Seven weight measurements were taken annually between 1992 and 1999, and subjects were followed up on through 2006. Subjects were considered to be weight cycling if they had both lost and gained greater than or equal to 5% of their body weight over time. After adjusting for many common comorbidities and overall health status, the authors found that weight cycling was associated with a 20% higher all-cause mortality rate. Weight instability, assessed by the coefficient of variation in body weight over the seven measurement periods, was associated with a 66% increase mortality risk.

In contrast to these findings, a number of studies have claimed to have found no increased mortality risk associated with weight cycling.[22,26–31] In three of these studies,[22,26,29] body weights were actually measured. In the Chicago Western Electric Company Study, men with the highest degree of weight variability had higher risk of all-cause and cardiovascular disease mortality, but the authors nonetheless concluded that weight variability may not increase mortality risk independently of the overall slope of weight loss or weight gain.[26] Field et al.[27] conducted a prospective study of 44,822 women in the Nurses' Health Study cohort and they classified women who reported that they had intentionally lost at least 20 pounds at least 3 times as severe weight cyclers (8% of the cohort) and those who had lost at least 10 pounds at least 3 times as mild weight cyclers (18.8% of the cohort). They found no significant increase in all-cause or cardiovascular disease mortality in women who were mild or severe weight cyclers after controlling for

BMI at age 18, physical activity, smoking, hormone replacement therapy, alcohol intake, and net weight change from age 18 years. However, this study did not include the entire cohort of the Nurses' Health Study and appears to be an undefined subset of the original subjects.

Recent results from the Cancer Prevention Study II Nutrition Cohort also found no significant link between weight cycling and mortality.[32] In this study, however, weight cycling was assessed entirely by questionnaire, and did not quantify the exact amount of weight lost or gained. Interestingly, women who reported 1–4 cycles of losing and regaining 10 or more pounds, and men who reported either 1–4 or 5–9 weight cycles of losing and regaining 10 or more pounds, had slightly reduced (7%) all-cause mortality risks. These findings are similar to those in the Nurses' Health Study cohort, which found that women who intentionally lost at least 10 pounds at least three times had a 17% lower risk of all-cause mortality.[27] This was not observed in women classified as severe cyclers (intentional weight loss of at least 20 pounds at least three times), nor was it observed for cardiovascular disease mortality. These are the only two studies that have found a slightly reduced risk of all-cause mortality associated with weight cycling. It must be noted that the results were not uniformly observed in all subsets within these cohorts, and that weight cycling was assessed entirely by questionnaires. Also, these studies used a model of weight cycling that assumed that its ill effects were permanent and cumulative over the lifespan. This does conform to the model advanced by laboratory data, which shows transient effects that are not cumulative.

In summation, although a number of studies do not show an increased mortality risk associated with weight cycling, the fact that at least a dozen studies published since 1989 have shown elevated mortality risk associated with weight cycling, suggests that chronic weight fluctuation may not be benign. However, many of these studies relied on self-report of weight history. Another major limitation of these epidemiological studies is that they are observational, and cannot by themselves establish cause and effect.

Despite these limitations, there is a fairly substantial body of literature that provides insight into the possible mechanisms by which weight cycling could compromise health, thus increasing mortality rates compared to weight-stable persons. In the next section we describe the research that supports the link between weight cycling and adverse cardiovascular and metabolic outcomes.

WEIGHT CYCLING AND RISK FACTORS FOR CARDIOVASCULAR DISEASE

A number of studies have examined the effects of weight cycling on cardiovascular disease risk factors and related health outcomes. Blood pressure is one cardiovascular risk factor that may be adversely affected by weight cycling. Among 258 obese healthy women ages 25–64, weight cycling was significantly associated with hypertension.[33] Weight cycling was established on the basis of at least five weight losses in the previous five years due to dieting with a weight loss of at least 10 pounds per cycle. A weight-cycling index was also calculated as the difference between the highest and lowest adult lifetime BMI of each subject. The risk of hypertension was 4.1 times higher in subjects with a positive history of weight cycling. The weight-cycling index and the sum of weight regained were also correlated with risk of hypertension. Another study by the same research team reported that blood pressure of 96 obese women with a history of weight cycling (147 ± 12/90 ± 8 mmHg) was significantly greater than that of 96 equally obese women with no history of weight cycling (125 ± 14/79 ± 8 mmHg).[34] These results are consistent the findings of the European Prospective Investigation in Cancer and Nutrition-Potsdam Study that also found that weight cycling in men and women was associated with increased risk of hypertension.[35]

A direct cause-effect of weight fluctuation on increasing blood pressure was demonstrated in a small study of lean Japanese women.[36] In this study, women first lost ~4 kg via caloric restriction over a period of 30 days. They regained their weight during a subsequent 14-day period of *ad libitum* diet. After a second 30-day weight-loss period in which they again lost ~4 kg via caloric restriction, they regained weight during an *ad libitum* diet period once again, and were assessed 106 days later. Although body weight had returned to baseline levels, both systolic and diastolic blood pressures were significantly elevated by 8–10 mmHg at the end of the study compared to baseline values. Systolic blood pressure alone had increased by ~25 mmHg during the 106 days between the end of the second weight-loss period (where systolic blood pressure had decreased) and the end of study. This is the only intervention study to directly assess the impact of controlled, intentional weight cycling on blood pressure in women around the time of the weight fluctuation rather than looking retrospectively at the distant past

Blood lipids may also be adversely affected by weight cycling. In the Women's Ischemia Syndrome Evaluation (WISE) study, among 485 women with coronary risk factors who were undergoing coronary angiography for evaluation of suspected myocardial ischemia, weight cycling, defined as a weight loss ≥ 10 pounds at least 3 times, was associated with reduced high-density lipoprotein cholesterol (HDL-C) as compared to non-weight cyclers.[37] The reduction in HDL-C was directly related to the amount of weight cycled, with women who lost at least 50 pounds per cycle having HDL-C 27% lower than non-cyclers (41 mg/dl vs. 56 mg/dl). In contrast to these findings, several studies have reported no adverse effects of weight cycling on cardiovascular risk factors.[38–40]

Weight cycling also may increase risk of the metabolic syndrome. Among middle-aged French men and women, those in the highest one third of the group of weight fluctuation had a 2.06-fold increase in risk of metabolic syndrome compared to the most weight-stable tertile.[41] Odds ratios for increased blood pressure, low HDL-C, and increased waist circumference were also significantly higher for the third of the group of weight fluctuation compared to the first. Similarly, among middle-aged Japanese men, weight cycling was significantly and positively associated with the prevalence of metabolic syndrome components (hypertriglyceridemia, high fasting glucose, and obesity).[42]

An elevated blood pressure and worsened blood lipid profile associated with weight cycling may increase risk of vascular disease. In fact, weight cycling has been reported to be associated with impaired coronary artery endothelial function. Among 18 postmenopausal women with at least one risk factor for cardiovascular disease, weight cycling (defined as the number of weight swings per year with a gain/loss of at least 10 pounds) was found to be a strong predictor of lower resting ($r = 0.53$) and endothelium-dependent ($r = 0.76$) myocardial blood flow assessed by dynamic N-13 positron emission tomography.[43]

In the Iowa Women's Health Study,[44,45] weight cycling due to both intentional and unintentional weight loss was associated with increased prevalence of heart attack, other heart diseases or angina, high blood pressure, diabetes mellitus, liver disease, and arthritis. Large weight cycles (defined as a loss and regain of at least 10% of body weight) were also associated with an 89% higher risk of myocardial infarction and a 71% higher risk of stroke.[45] Although a higher risk of diabetes mellitus was associated with weight cycling in this study, there is no consistent finding regarding weight cycling and diabetes risk.[46–49] Weight cycling has been reported to be associated with increased risk of developing hyperinsulinemia,[50] but this has not been a consistent finding.[51]

Weight cycling may increase levels of C-reactive protein[52] and compromise immune function.[53] Among 114 healthy, overweight, sedentary, postmenopausal women, increasing frequency of intentional weight loss of at least 10 pounds or more was associated with lower natural killer cell activity.[53] Weight cycling also has been reported to be associated with reduced telomere length in 647 women ages 35–74 participating in the National Institute of Environmental Health Sciences Sister Study.[54] Short telomeres have been associated with increased risk of cardiovascular disease and certain cancers.[54]

INTERPRETATION OF THE INCONSISTENT FINDINGS AND CONCLUDING REMARKS

Overall, the data on health risks of weight cycling are mixed. Many studies have reported increased health risks, including higher mortality rates, associated with weight cycling.[10–22] In contrast, a number of studies have reported no adverse health risks among weight cyclers.[22,26–31] One problem with interpretation of the data is that there is no universally accepted definition of weight cycling. In some cases, relatively small weight fluctuations were treated as weight cycles. Another major limitation of virtually all studies of weight cycling is that they are mostly snapshots that do not capture the time course of changes in body weight or health markers that may change during periods of weight change.[55] The blood pressure or level of a particular blood lipid, for example, may be only transiently elevated during a period of weight regain after an episode of caloric restriction.[36] Patients are typically lost to follow up during the time when they are regaining weight after successful weight loss. Blood pressure, or markers of metabolic or cardiovascular function, may have returned to normal at the time researchers obtained measurements.

As proposed by Montani et al., the "overshoots" above normal values during weight regain may place a strain on the cardiovascular system, which, if repeated over time with subsequent weight cycles, could trigger higher cardiovascular morbidity.[55] Thus, long-term instability of cardiovascular disease risk factors that result from chronic weight fluctuation could contribute to the atherosclerotic process.[56] The fact that no studies have shown chronic and severe weight cycling to be associated with reduced risk of chronic disease suggests that the weight loss that *is* achieved (however transient) does not provide sustained health benefits.

Thus recommendations for perpetually unsuccessful dieters to just keep trying to lose weight seem ill-advised, and potentially harmful. A non-weight-loss-centered approach has substantial published research support.[57] Many so-called weight-related health problems can be improved by exercise and a healthy, non-energy-restrictive diet independently of weight loss. Shifting the focus of behavior change away from weight loss and toward a health-at-every-size approach may produce better outcomes without the pitfalls associated with caloric restriction.

References

1. Bish CL, Blanck HM, Serdula MK, Marcus M, Kohl HW, and Khan LK. 2005. "Diet and Physical Activity Behaviors Among Americans Trying to Lose Weight: 2000 Behavioral Risk Factor Surveillance System." *Obes Res,* 13(3):596–607.

2. Andreyeva T, Long MW, Henderson KE, and Grode GM. 2010. "Trying to Lose Weight: Diet Strategies Among Americans with Overweight or Obesity in 1996 and 2003." *J Am Diet Assoc.,* 110(4):535–542.

3. Aphramor L. 2010. "Validity of Claims Made in Weight Management Research: A Narrative Review of Dietetic Articles." *Nutr J.,* 9:30.

4. Tsai CJ, Leitzmann MF, Willett WC, and Giovannucci EL. 2006. "Weight Cycling and Risk of Gallstone Disease in Men." *Arch Intern Med.,* 166(21):2369–2374.

5. Syngal S, Coakley EH, Willett WC, Byers T, Williamson DF, and Colditz GA. 1999. "Long-Term Weight Patterns and Risk for Cholecystectomy in Women." *Ann Intern Med.,* 130:471–477.

6. Trentham-Dietz A, Nichols H, Hampton J, and Newcomb P. 2006. "Weight Change and Risk of Endometrial Cancer." *Int J Epidemiol.,* 35(1):151–158.

7. Luo J, Margolis KL, Adami HO, Lopez AM, Lessin L, and Ye W. 2007. "Body Size, Weight Cycling, and Risk of Renal Cell Carcinoma Among Postmenopausal Women: The Women's Health Initiative (United States)." *Am J Epidemiol.,* 166(7):752–759.

8. Lindblad P, Wolk A, Bergstrom R, Persson I, and Adami HO. 1994. "The Role of Obesity and Weight Fluctuations in the Etiology of Renal-Cell Cancer: A Population-Based Case-Control Study." *Cancer Epidemiol Biomarkers Prev.,* 3(8):631–639.

9. Bird CL, Frankl HD, Lee ER, and Haile RW. 1998. "Obesity, Weight Gain, Large Weight Changes, and Adenomatous Polyps of the Left Colon and Rectum." *Am J Epidemiol.,* 147(7):670–680.

10. Hamm P, Shekelle RB, and Stamler J. 1989. "Large fluctuations in Body Weight During Young Adulthood and Twenty-Five Year Risk of Coronary Death in Men." *Am J Epidemiol.*, 129(2):312–318.

11. Lissner L, Odell PM, D'Agostino RB, et al. 1991. "Variability of Body Weight and Health Outcomes in the Framingham Population." *N Engl J Med.*, 324(26):1839–1844.

12. Rzehak P, Meisinger C, Woelke G, Brasche S, Strube G, and Heinrich J. 2007. "Weight Change, Weight Cycling and Mortality in the ERFORT Male Cohort Study." *Eur J Epidemiol.*, 22(10):665–673.

13. Peters ETJ, Seidell JC, Menotti A, et al. 1995. "Changes in Body-Weight in Relation to Mortality in 6441 European Middle-Aged Men: The 7 Countries Study." *Int J Obes.*, 19(12):862–868.

14. Folsom A, French S, Zheng W, Baxter J, and Jeffery R. 1996. "Weight Variability and Mortality: The Iowa Women's Health Study." *Int J Obes Relat Metab Disord.*, 20(8):704–709.

15. Blair SN, Shaten J, Brownell K, Collins G, and Lissner L. 1993. "Body Weight Change, All-Cause Mortality, and Cause-Specific Mortality in the Multiple Risk Factor Intervention Trial." *Ann Intern Med.*, 119(7 Pt 2):749–757.

16. Diaz VA, Mainous AG, and Everett CJ. 2005. "The Association Between Weight Fluctuation and Mortality: Results from a Population-Based Cohort Study." *J Community Health.*, 30(3):153–165.

17. Hanson RL, Jacobsson LTH, McCance DR, et al. 1996. "Weight Fluctuation, Mortality and Vascular Disease in Pima Indians." *Int J Obes.*, 20(5):463–471.

18. Reynolds MW, Fredman L, Langenberg P, and Magaziner J. 1999. "Weight, Weight Change, and Mortality in a Random Sample of Older Community-Dwelling Women." *J Am Geriatr Soc.*, 47(12):1409–1414.

19. Zoppini G, Verlato G, Targher G, Bonora E, Trombetta M, and Muggeo M. 2008. "Variability of Body Weight, Pulse Pressure and Glycaemia Strongly Predict Total Mortality in Elderly Type 2 Diabetic Patients. The Verona Diabetes Study." *Diabetes Metab Res.*, 24(8):624–628.

20. Nguyen ND, Center JR, Eisman JA, and Nguyen TV. 2007. "Bone Loss, Weight Loss, and Weight Fluctuation Predict Mortality Risk in Elderly Men and Women." *J Bone Miner Res.*, 22(8):1147–1154.

21. Arnold AM, Newman AB, Cushman M, Ding J, and Kritchevsky S. 2010. "Body Weight Dynamics and Their Association with Physical Function and Mortality in Older Adults: The Cardiovascular Health Study." *J Gerontol A Biol Sci Med Sci.*, 65(1):63–70.

22. Iribarren C, Sharp DS, Burchfiel CM, and Petrovitch H. 1995. "Association of Weight-Loss and Weight Fluctuation with Mortality Among Japanese-American Men." *N Engl J Med.*, 333(11):686–692.

23. Fogelholm M, Sievanen H, Heinonen A, et al. 1997. "Association Between Weight Cycling History and Bone Mineral Density in Premenopausal Women." *Osteoporosis Int.*, 7(4):354–358.

24. Søgaard AJ, Meyer HE, Tonstad S, Håheim LL, and Holme I. 2008. "Weight Cycling and Risk of Forearm Fractures: A 28-Year Follow-Up of Men in the Oslo Study." *Am J Epidemiol.*, 167(8):1005–1013.

25. Bliuc D, Nguyen ND, Milch VE, Nguyen TV, Eisman JA, and Center JR. 2009. "Mortality Risk Associated with Low-Trauma Osteoporotic Fracture and Subsequent Fracture in Men and Women." *JAMA*, 301(5):513–521.

26. Dyer AR, Stamler J, and Greenland P. 2000. "Associations of Weight Change and Weight Variability with Cardiovascular and All-Cause Mortality in the Chicago Western Electric Company Study." *Am J Epidemiol.*, 152(4):324–333.

27. Field AE, Malspeis S, and Willett WC. 2009. "Weight Cycling and Mortality Among Middle-Aged or Older Women." *Arch Intern Med.*, 169(9):881–886.

28. Stevens J and Lissner L. 1990. "Body Weight Variability and Mortality in the Charleston Heart Study." *Int J Obes.*, 14(4):385–386.

29. Lissner L, Andres R, Muller D, and Shimokata H. 1990. "Body Weight Variability in Men: Metabolic Rate, Health and Longevity." *Int J Obes.*, 14(4):373–383.

30. Wannamethee SG, Shaper AG, and Walker M. 2002. "Weight Change, Weight Fluctuation, and Mortality." *Arch Intern Med.*, 162(22):2575–2580.

31. Taing KY, Ardern CI, and Kuk JL. 2012. "Effect of the Timing of Weight Cycling During Adulthood on Mortality Risk in Overweight and Obese Postmenopausal Women." *Obesity.*, 20(2):407–413.

32. Stevens VL, Jacobs EJ, Sun J, et al. 2012. "Weight Cycling and Mortality in a Large Prospective US Study." *Am J Epidemiol.*, 175(8):785–792.

33. Guagnano MT, Ballone E, Pace-Palitti V, et al. 2000. "Risk Factors for Hypertension in Obese Women: The Role of Weight Cycling." *Eur J Clin Nutr.*, 54(4):356–360.

34. Guagnano MT, Pace-Palitti V, Carrabs C, Merlitti D, and Sensi S. 1999. "Weight Fluctuations Could Increase Blood Pressure in Android Obese Women." *Clin Sci.*, 96(6):677–680.

35. Schulz M, Liese A, Boeing H, Cunningham J, Moore C, and Kroke A. 2004. "Associations of Short-Term Weight Changes and Weight Cycling with Incidence of Essential Hypertension in the EPIC-Potsdam Study." *J Hum Hypertens.*, 19(1):61–67.

36. Kajioka T, Tsuzuku S, Shimokata H, and Sato Y. 2002. "Effects of Intentional Weight Cycling on Non-Obese Young Women." *Metabolism-Clinical and Experimental.*, 51(2):149–154.

37. Olson MB, Kelsey SF, Bittner V, et al. 2000. "Weight Cycling and High-Density Lipoprotein Cholesterol in Women: Evidence of an Adverse Effect—A Report from the NHLBI-Sponsored WISE Study." *J Am Coll Cardiol.*, 36(5):1565–1571.

38. Taylor CB, Jatulis DE, Fortmann SP, and Kraemer HC. 1995. "Weight Variability Effects—A Prospective Analysis from the Stanford 5-City Project." *Am J Epidemiol.*, 141(5):461–465.

39. Petersmarck KA, Teitelbaum HS, Bond JT, Bianchi L, Hoerr SM, and Sowers MF. 1999. "The Effect of Weight Cycling on Blood Lipids and Blood Pressure in the Multiple Risk Factor Intervention Trial Special Intervention Group." *Int J Obes.*, 23(12):1246–1255.

40. Lee J, Kawakubo K, Kobayashi Y, Mori K, Kasihara H, and Tamura M. 2001. "Effects of Ten Year Body Weight Variability on Cardiovascular Risk Factors in Japanese Middle-Aged Men and Women." *Int J Obes Relat Metab Disord.*, 25(7):1063–1067.

41. Vergnaud A, Bertrais S, Oppert J, et al. 2008. "Weight Fluctuations and Risk for Metabolic Syndrome in an Adult Cohort." *Int J Obes.*, 32(2):315–321.

42. Zhang H, Tamakoshi K, Yatsuya H, et al. 2005. "Long-Term Body Weight Fluctuation Is Associated with Metabolic Syndrome Independent of Current Body Mass Index Among Japanese Men." *Circ J.*, 69(1):13–18.

43. Martin JW, Briesmiester K, Bargardi A, Muzik O, Mosca L, and Duvernoy CS. 2005. "Weight Changes and Obesity Predict Impaired Resting and Endothelium-Dependent Myocardial Blood Flow in Postmenopausal Women." *Clin Cardiol.*, 28(1):13–18.

44. French SA, Folsom AR, Jeffery RW, Zheng W, Mink PJ, and Baxter JE. 1997. "Weight Variability and Incident Disease in Older Women: The Iowa Women's Health Study." *Int J Obes.*, 21(3):217–223.

45. French SA, Jeffery RW, Folsom AR, Williamson DF, and Byers T. 1995. "Relation of Weight Variability and Intentionality of Weight Loss to Disease History and Health-Related Variables in a Population-Based Sample of Women Aged 55–69 Years." *Am J Epidemiol.*, 142(12):1306–1314.

46. Field AE, Manson JE, Laird N, Williamson DF, Willett WC, and Colditz GA. 2004. "Weight Cycling and the Risk of Developing Type 2 Diabetes Among Adult Women in the United States." *Obes Res.*, 12(2):267–274.

47. Graci S, Izzo G, Savino S, et al. 2004. "Weight Cycling and Cardiovascular Risk Factors in Obesity." *Int J Obes.*, 28(1):65–71.

48. Waring ME, Eaton CB, Lasater TM, and Lapane KL. 2010. "Incident Diabetes in Relation to Weight Patterns During Middle Age." *Am J Epidemiol.*, 171(5):550–556.

49. Kataja-Tuomola M, Sundell J, Männistö S, et al. 2010. "Short-Term Weight Change and Fluctuation as Risk Factors for Type 2 Diabetes in Finnish Male Smokers." *Eur J Epidemiol.*, 25(5):333–339.

50. Yatsuya H, Tamakoshi K, Yoshida T, et al. 2003. "Association Between Weight Fluctuation and Fasting Insulin Concentration in Japanese Men." *Int J Obes.*, 27(4):478–483.

51. Weyer C, Hanson K, Bogardus C, and Pratley R. 2000. "Long-Term Changes in Insulin Action and Insulin Secretion Associated with Gain, Loss, Regain and Maintenance of Body Weight." *Diabetologia.*, 43(1):36–46.

52. Tamakoshi K, Yatsuya H, Kondo T, et al. 2003. "Long-Term Body Weight Variability Is Associated with Elevated C-Reactive Protein Independent of Current Body Mass Index Among Japanese Men." *Int J Obes.*, 27(9):1059–1065.

53. Shade ED, Ulrich CM, Wener MH, et al. 2004. "Frequent Intentional Weight Loss Is Associated with Lower Natural Killer Cell Cytotoxicity in Postmenopausal Women: Possible Long-Term Immune Effects." *J Am Diet Assoc.*, 104(6):903–912.

54. Kim S, Parks CG, DeRoo LA, et al. 2009. "Obesity and Weight Gain in Adulthood and Telomere Length." *Cancer Epidemiology Biomarkers & Prevention.*, 18(3):816–820.

55. Montani J-P, Viecelli AK, Prevot A, and Dulloo AG. 2006. "Weight Cycling During Growth and Beyond as a Risk Factor for Later Cardiovascular Diseases: The 'Repeated Overshoot' Theory." *Int J Obes.*, 30:S58–S66.

56. Christen A, Efstathiadou Z, Laspa E, Johnston DG, and Godsland IF. 2007. "Rate of Change and Instability in Body Mass Index, Insulin Resistance, and Lipid Metabolism as Predictors of Atherosclerotic Vascular Disease." *J Clin Endocrinol Metab.*, 92(10):3780–3787.

57. Bacon L and Aphramor L. 2011. "Weight Science: Evaluating the Evidence for a Paradigm Shift." *Nutr J.*, 10(9):1–13.

SPOTLIGHT

The next chapter, by Brandon Sawyer, Siddartha Angadi, and Glenn Gaesser, explores the idea that significant improvements in health can be achieved without any weight loss at all. The authors present data from many studies which reveal that weight loss itself may not be the cause of improvements in health indicators and measures of risk of chronic illness. This flies in the face of the conventional wisdom that for overweight or obese people, weight loss is the best and really the only solution to improving health.

Chapter Seven

Health Benefits of Physical Activity and Diet are Independent of Weight Loss

Brandon J. Sawyer, Siddhartha S. Angadi and Glenn A. Gaesser

INTRODUCTION

Weight loss is routinely recommended for treating health conditions attributed to obesity, such as comorbidities associated with cardiovascular disease (CVD) and type 2 diabetes (T2D). A weight loss of ~10% of initial body weight has been recommended as an initial target goal,[1] although this goal is seldom achieved via lifestyle interventions.[2] Furthermore, studies of long-term weight-loss maintenance indicate high recidivism rates.[3] This failure to maintain weight loss creates a pattern of chronic weight fluctuation, or yo-yo dieting, that can have negative impact on health (refer to chapter on weight cycling).

Consequently, lifestyle interventions focused more on behaviors (e.g., exercise and diet), rather than on weight loss, have been advocated.[4,5] Many obesity-related health conditions can be ameliorated by changes in physical activity and diet, independent of weight loss, thus avoiding the pitfalls of weight cycling.[4,5] The remainder of this chapter will highlight research findings that demonstrate the health benefits of physical activity and dietary changes independent of weight loss. The information should help health professionals provide a scientifically sound rationale for supporting healthy behaviors rather than achieving weight loss in treating so-called obesity-related health conditions.

REDUCTION IN TYPE 2 DIABETES RISK

Two very high-profile lifestyle interventions that induced significant weight loss have been reported to reduce incidence of T2D, the Finnish Diabetes Prevention Program[6] and the Diabetes Prevention Program.[7] Weight loss, however, was just one outcome of these studies, and may not have been the most important factor explaining the reduction in T2D. Two more recent lifestyle intervention programs revealed significant reductions in T2D incidence with either no weight loss[8] or with only very minor weight loss.[9] In the PREDIMED trial, a Mediterranean diet supplemented with either virgin olive oil or nuts reduced T2D incidence by 52% over 4 years, compared to a control, low-fat diet group.[8] In the 3-year Study of Lifestyle Intervention and Impaired glucose tolerance Maastricht (SLIM),[9] the lifestyle intervention group experienced a 58% reduction in T2D incidence despite a mean weight loss of only 1.08 kg. A mean weight loss of only ~1 kg over a 3-year period should hardly be viewed as substantial. Yet the reductions in T2D incidence in these two studies are comparable to those observed in other large-scale studies[6,7] where significant weight loss occurred. Thus lifestyle interventions may be effective in reducing T2D in at-risk populations even when body weight remains largely unchanged.

GLUCOSE METABOLISM AND INSULIN ACTION

The reductions in T2D risk are attributable in large part to the beneficial effects of physical activity and diet on glucose metabolism and insulin action. For example, aerobic exercise training, independent of changes in body weight, induces significant improvements in markers of glucose metabolism in overweight and obese individuals with either no, or minimal, change (e.g., <2%) in body weight or body fat.[10–19] In fact exercise training may enhance insulin sensitivity even in the face of increasing adiposity after training.[20] These findings may be explained in part by the fact that just a single bout of exercise can improve insulin sensitivity,[17,21] an effect that may last for several days after the exercise session.[17]

Long-term blood glucose control can be assessed by measuring glycated hemoglobin (HbA_{1c}). A meta-analysis of 27 exercise training studies in patients with T2D lasting up to one year revealed that exercise training decreased HbA_{1c} by ~0.8%.[10] The authors noted that this effect is in the same range as observed with dietary, drug, and insulin treatments. Weight loss appeared to have little to do with the improvement in glycemic control because the improvement in HbA_{1c} with aerobic exercise training alone (−0.7%) was about the same as that observed for combined aerobic and resistance exercise training (−0.8%), even though weight loss was much greater for the combined training (−5.1%) than for aerobic exercise training alone (−1.5%). A large randomized clinical trial of 251 adults with T2D demonstrated that both aerobic and resistance training reduced HbA_{1c} by ~0.4%–0.5%, but improvements were greatest for combined aerobic and resistance training (0.9%).[19] Although combined training reduced HbA_{1c} by twice as much as either mode alone, changes in body weight (2.6 kg) and fat mass (1.6–1.9 kg) were modest and were the same for all groups.

Both aerobic and resistance exercise training are also effective for improving insulin sensitivity. Six months of either aerobic or resistance training in overweight and obese men increased glucose disposal by 20% to 25%.[22] The fact that body fat mass was reduced by 2.1 kg after aerobic exercise training but was unchanged after resistance exercise training (actually a nonsignificant increase of 0.7 kg) demonstrates that the improvement in insulin sensitivity after exercise training was not dependent on loss of body fat.

Dietary interventions that focus on improving diet quality also enhance glucose metabolism and insulin action, in the absence of clinically significant weight loss.[12,23] Among adults with T2D or impaired fasting glucose, a 12-week dietary intervention that centered on replacing refined rice with whole grains and increasing vegetable intake resulted in significant improvements in fasting glucose and insulin sensitivity, despite body mass index (BMI) decreasing by just 0.2 units.[12] Similarly, in overweight and obese men and women at risk for T2D, following a Mediterranean diet for 3 months reduced fasting glucose and insulin, and improved insulin sensitivity, despite no statistically significant changes in body weight or waist circumference.[23] Additionally, after 4 years of follow-up in these individuals, the Mediterranean diet reduced incidence of T2D by 52%, despite no reduction in body weight.[8]

BLOOD PRESSURE

In addition to the improvements in metabolic control, discussed above, exercise training reduces resting and ambulatory blood pressures, with blood pressure improvements largely independent of weight loss.[10,24,25] Among 168 overweight men and women with stage I hypertension, a 6-week program of brisk walking reduced 24-hour ambulatory systolic (143.1 to 135.5 mmHg) and diastolic (91.1 to 84.8 mmHg) blood pressures.[25] The program had no effect on body weight. A meta-analysis of 72 exercise intervention trials found that training induced significant reductions in resting and ambulatory blood pressure on the order of 3–4 mmHg, with the reduction in blood pressure being more pronounced among hypertensive individuals (~5–7 mmHg).[11] It is noteworthy that these improvements occurred despite average reductions in body weight of 1.2 kg, and percent body fat of 1.4%. Furthermore, correlations between changes in BMI and both systolic blood pressure (r = 0.09) and diastolic blood pressure (r = 0.07) are extremely low,[24] demonstrating that reductions in body weight explain less than 1% of the changes in blood pressure with exercise training. In other studies where a correlation between weight loss and blood pressure reduction does exist, compliance may be a confounding factor. That is, persons who exercise the most in a given cohort will be the ones to lose weight, gain the most fitness, and have the greatest improvements in blood pressure. It does not necessarily follow that the weight loss is the cause of the blood pressure drop.

Diet quality also affects blood pressure independently of weight loss.[13,15,26,27] This is best illustrated by the Dietary Approaches to Stop Hypertension (DASH) trial.[27] Specifically designed to assess the effect of diet composition on blood pressure while maintaining a constant body weight, the DASH diet reduced both systolic (−5.5 mmHg) and diastolic (−3.0 mmHg) blood pressures. The results were more impressive among 133 men and women with hypertension. Simply eating more fruits and vegetables and consuming dairy foods low in saturated fat was sufficient to reduce systolic blood pressure by an average of 11.4 mmHg and diastolic blood pressure by an average of 5.5 mmHg within two weeks.[27] The mechanism for the fall in blood pressure during the DASH and Mediterranean diets is thought to be simultaneous increases in monounsaturated fat, fiber, potassium, magnesium and calcium intakes with decreases in sodium and saturated fat intakes. These dietary changes apparently have synergistic health benefits.

LIPIDS AND LIPOPROTEINS

Exercise training generally has favorable effects on lipids and lipoproteins, even in the face of unchanged body weight[10,11,14,18,29] or clinically insignificant weight loss (<2%).[30] A meta-analysis (72 studies) indicated a small but statistically significant effect of aerobic exercise on elevation of high-density lipoprotein cholesterol (HDL-C) and a trend (P = 0.07) for a reduction in serum triglycerides.[11] In these studies, the overall changes in body mass (~1.2 kg) and body fat (<2.0%) were rather small. In Asian Indians with T2D, Misra et al.[14] reported that 12 weeks of resistance exercise training reduced total cholesterol (8.5%), triglycerides (19.6%), and very-low-density lipoprotein cholesterol (VLDL-C) (32.1%), with no changes in BMI or total body fat. Among overweight, sedentary, and dyslipidemic men and women, 8 months of exercise training varying in amount and intensity (the equivalent of either walking 10–12 miles per week or jogging 10–20 miles per week) improved 11 different lipid and lipoprotein variables in the absence of clinically significant weight loss (≤1.52 kg).[30] In both overweight/obese adults with and without T2D, an 8-week program of aerobic exercise significantly reduced total (~8$–13%) and low-density lipoprotein cholesterol (LDL-C) (~13%–19%), and increased HDL-C/total cholesterol (~10%–17%), but did not significantly alter body weight or fat mass.[29]

Dietary interventions also show that blood lipid profiles can be improved independently of weight loss.[12,13,31] In patients with T2D, the addition of 26 g/day of soluble and insoluble fiber to the American Diabetes Association diet for 6 weeks reduced total cholesterol (−14 mg/dl), triglycerides (−21mg/dl), and VLDL-C (−5 mg/dl), with no changes in body weight.[31] Replacing refined rice with whole grains and increasing vegetable intake for 12 weeks reduced triglycerides, total and LDL-C, and increased HDL-C in T2D with only a modest (0.4 kg) decrease in body weight.[12]

ENDOTHELIAL FUNCTION

One of the first steps in atherosclerosis is endothelial dysfunction. Consequently, endothelial-dependent dilation of blood vessels (typically assessed noninvasively by ultrasound imaging of arterial responses to increases in blood flow, or invasively by arterial infusion of acetylcholine) has been reported to be a strong and independent predictor of cardiovascular morbidity and mortality.[33] Both aerobic and resistance exercise training, in the absence of weight loss, can improve endothelial function.[34,35] In men and women with the metabolic syndrome, 12 weeks of aerobic interval training, resistance exercise training, or combined training increased endothelial function by in all groups, despite no change in body weight.[35] In obese adults with T2D, four weeks of aerobic training and a hypocaloric diet reduced body weight by 6.1% (6 kg), but had no effect on coronary vasodilation.[34] After an additional 5 months of exercise training, during which time dietary restrictions were relaxed, body weight had increased by 3.1 kg. Despite regaining approximately 50% of the weight lost after the initial 4-week period that included a hypocaloric diet, coronary blood flow in response to either acetylcholine or adenosine had increased by 127% and 58.7%, respectively. That significant improvements in coronary endothelial function could be achieved in the face of a weight gain of 3.1 kg, suggests that exercise training may be more important than weight loss per se for improving vascular health.

Improving diet quality has also been shown to positively affect vascular health independently of weight loss.[36–38] Three months of close adherence to a Mediterranean diet improved endothelial function by 50% in abdominally obese adults.[36] Although the participants lost a modest amount of weight (2.7 kg; 2.9% of initial body weight), this probably was not the critical factor for improving vascular health because a comparison diet group lost a similar amount of weight (2.1 kg; 2.2% of initial body weight) yet experienced no change in endothelial function. Supplementation of an *ad libitum* diet with walnuts (56 g/day) for 8 weeks improved endothelial function by 25.6% in obese men and women with T2D despite no changes in body weight.[37] These studies suggest that improved diet quality, rather than minor weight loss, is primarily responsible for improvements in vascular health that accompany dietary interventions. A low-carbohydrate diet, for example, has been reported to induce weight loss but impairs endothelial function.[38] In overweight or obese men and women, one year of a low-carbohydrate diet reduced body weight by 14.9 kg (15.8% of initial body weight), yet impaired endothelial function by 35%.[38]

HEMOSTASIS

Overweight and obese individuals typically have impaired ability to control blood clotting in artery walls, in part due to insufficient release of the anti-coagulant tissue plasminogen activator (t-PA) and excess levels of plasminogen activator inhibitor (PAI-1) released from far cells. Regular exercise, in the absence of weight loss, may reverse defects in blood coagulation. Three months of aerobic exercise training in overweight and obese adults improved t-PA release by 55%, to levels not different from normal weight controls.[39] The exercise program did not reduce body weight, body fat, or waist circumference, which illustrates that the impaired blood clotting control was linked to the sedentary lifestyle and not the excess body weight.[39] Dietary modifications that result in little, if any, weight loss have also been shown to improve blood clotting factors in diseased populations.[16,26] In a sample of 49 asymptomatic subjects at high risk for CVD, three months of a Mediterranean diet with added nuts, high in monounsaturated fatty acids, polyunsaturated fatty acids, and various bioactive dietary compounds, increased tissue factor pathway inhibitor (TFPI) by 39%, despite no changes in body weight.[26] TFPI is known to decrease blood clotting and reduce restenosis of arteries.

Plasminogen activator inhibitor-1 (PAI-1), which inhibits the dissolution of blood clots, has been shown to be increased in obese populations.[40] Ten weeks of a low-glycemic diet reduced PAI-1 by 15% in overweight females, despite minimal weight loss of only 1.9 kg.[16] The fact that PAI-1 activity was not changed in women who consumed a high-glycemic diet, despite similar weight loss (–1.3 kg), suggests that the improvement was attributable to diet quality rather than weight loss itself. However, substantially greater diet-induced weight loss (8%–10%) has been shown to reduce PAI-1 by 31 to 38%.[40] This suggests that weight loss itself may play a role in reducing PAI-1. This conforms to the fact that PAI-1 is produced by adipocytes. Exercise can reduce the production of PAI-1 by adipocytes, but shrinking adipocytes is likely to have an additional effect. It is important to note that the addition of exercise to a hypocaloric diet produced a 71% reduction in PAI-1,[40] suggesting roles for both exercise and weight loss.

INFLAMMATION

Low-grade inflammation is an established characteristic of CVD and T2D[41] and is detected by elevations in numerous pro-inflammatory biomarkers including C-reactive protein (CRP) and various cytokines, or by lower levels of anti-inflammatory biomarkers. Although weight loss has been reported to affect inflammatory molecules, it is clear that inflammatory status can be improved with exercise and/or diet in the absence of weight loss.[15,18,23,42–45] In a study of men and women with T2D, 12 months of either aerobic or combined aerobic and resistance exercise training significantly reduced pro-inflammatory biomarkers and increased anti-inflammatory biomarkers.[18] Body weight was not reduced in either group, indicating that exercise training, om the absence of weight loss, has a full anti-inflammatory effect.[18]

The weight-loss-independent effect of exercise training on reducing inflammation is best exemplified by a study of 235 patients with coronary heart disease (CHD) before and after cardiac rehabilitation.[42] Patients who lost weight (6 pounds; 3% of initial body weight) reduced CRP by 31%; patients who *gained* weight (6 pounds; 3% of initial body weight) also reduced CRP, by 42%. Additionally, Lambert et al.[43] reported that significant weight loss (7.5 kg) via diet had no effect on markers of muscle inflammation, whereas exercise training in the absence of weight loss reduced pro-inflammatory markers by 37%–50%. Thus weight loss itself does not appear to be the cause of the reduction in low-grade inflammation observed after lifestyle interventions involving exercise and diet.

Non-calorically restricted dietary interventions can also improve inflammatory status.[15,23,44,45] In overweight and obese adults at high risk for CVD, three months of a Mediterranean diet supplemented with either virgin olive oil (1 liter/week) or nuts (30 g/day) significantly reduced pro-inflammatory markers.[15,23] Body fat was not reduced during this dietary intervention. Similarly, dietary interventions that replaced typical Western protein products that are high in saturated fats (i.e., red meat) with other protein-rich foods (e.g., soy[45], almonds[44]) have reported decreases in pro-inflammatory markers in the absence of weight loss.

CONCLUSION

The published research described in this chapter clearly shows that exercise and non-calorically restricted dietary interventions can lead to marked improvements in the cardiometabolic risk profiles of men and women considered overweight and obese by current body mass index criteria, in the absence of clinically significant weight loss. Many of the studies revealed that significant improvements in health can be achieved without any weight loss at all, thus undermining the conventional wisdom about the importance of weight loss as a cornerstone of obesity treatment. Because caloric restriction suffers from a high failure rate, and chronic weight cycling is associated with increased health risks, a non-weight-loss-centered focus on improving health is warranted. Men and women should be encouraged to focus on the achievable lifestyle goals of improving diet quality and increasing physical activity regardless of changes in body weight.

References

1. National Institutes of Health. 1998. *Clinical Guidelines on the Identification, Evaluation, and Treatment of Overweight and Obesity in Adults*. 98–4083.

2. Norris SL, Zhang XP, Avenell A, et al. 2004. "Long-Term Effectiveness of Lifestyle and Behavioral Weight Loss Interventions in Adults with Type 2 Diabetes: A Meta-Analysis." *Am J Med.*, 117(10):762–774.

3. Anderson JW, Konz EC, Frederich RC, and Wood CL. 2001. "Long-Term Weight-Loss Maintenance: A Meta-Analysis of US Studies." *Am J Clin Nutr.*, 74(5):579–584.

4. Gaesser GA, Angadi SS, and Sawyer BJ. 2011. "Exercise and Diet, Independent of Weight Loss, Improve Cardiometabolic Risk Profile in Overweight and Obese Individuals." *Physician Sportsmed.*, 39(2):87–97.

5. Tuomilehto J, Lindstrom J, Eriksson JG, et al. 2001. "Prevention of Type 2 Diabetes Mellitus by Changes in Lifestyle Among Subjects with Impaired Glucose Tolerance." *N Engl J Med.*, 344(18):1343–1350.

6. Knowler WC, Barrett-Connor E, Fowler SE, et al. 2002. "Reduction in the Incidence of Type 2 Diabetes with Lifestyle Intervention or Metformin." *N Engl J Med.*, 346(6):393–403.

7. Salas-Salvado J, Bullo M, Babio N, et al. 2011. "Reduction in the Incidence of Type 2 Diabetes with the Mediterranean Diet: Results of the PREDIMED-Reus Nutrition Intervention Randomized Trial." *Diabetes Care*, 34(1):14–19.

8. Roumen C, Corpeleijn E, Feskens EJM, Mensink M, Saris WHM, and Blaak EE. 2008. "Impact of 3-Year Lifestyle Intervention on Postprandial Glucose Metabolism: The SLIM Study." *Diabetic Med.*, 25(5):597–605.

9. Snowling NJ and Hopkins WG. 2006. "Effects of Different Modes of Exercise Training on Glucose Control and Risk Factors for Complications in Type 2 Diabetic Patients—A Meta-Analysis." *Diabetes Care*, 29(11):2518–2527.

10. Cornelissen VA and Fagard RH. 2005. "Effects of Endurance Training on Blood Pressure, Blood Pressure-Regulating Mechanisms, and Cardiovascular Risk Factors." *Hypertension*, 46(4):667–675.

11. Chung HK, Chae JS, Hyun YJ, et al. 2009. "Influence of Adiponectin Gene Polymorphisms on Adiponectin Level and Insulin Resistance Index in Response to Dietary Intervention in Overweight-Obese Patients with Impaired Fasting Glucose or Newly Diagnosed Type 2 Diabetes." *Diabetes Care*, 32(4):552–558.

12. Estruch R, Martinez-Gonzalez MA, Corella D, et al. 2006. "Effects of a Mediterranean-Style Diet on Cardiovascular Risk Factors—A Randomized Trial." *Ann Intern Med.*, 145(1):1–11.

13. Misra A, Alappan NK, Vikram NK, et al. 2008. "Effect of Supervised Progressive Resistance-Exercise Training Protocol on Insulin Sensitivity, Glycemia, Lipids, and Body Composition in Asian Indians with Type 2 Diabetes." *Diabetes Care*, 31(7):1282–1287.

14. Mena MP, Sacanella E, Vazquez-Agell M, et al. 2009. "Inhibition of Circulating Immune Cell Activation: A Molecular Antiinflammatory Effect of the Mediterranean Diet." *Am J Clin Nutr.*, 89(1):248.

15. Jensen L, Sloth B, Krog-Mikkelsen I, et al. 2008. "A Low-Glycemic-Index Diet Reduces Plasma Plasminogen Activator Inhibitor-1 Activity, But Not Tissue Inhibitor of Proteinases-1 or Plasminogen Activator Inhibitor-1 Protein, in Overweight Women." *Am J Clin Nutr.*, 87(1):97.

16. DiPietro L, Dziura J, Yeckel CW, and Neufer PD. 2006. "Exercise and Improved Insulin Sensitivity in Older Women: Evidence of the Enduring Benefits of Higher Intensity Training." *J Appl Physiol.*, 100(1):142–149.

17. Balducci S, Zanuso S, Nicolucci A, et al. 2010. "Effect of an Intensive Exercise Intervention Strategy on Modifiable Cardiovascular Risk Factors in Subjects with Type 2 Diabetes Mellitus—A Randomized Controlled Trial: The Italian Diabetes and Exercise Study (IDES)." *Arch Intern Med.*, 170(20):1794–1803.

18. Sigal RJ, Kenny GP, Boule NG, et al. 2007. "Effects of Aerobic Training, Resistance Training, or Both on Glycemic Control in Type 2 Diabetes—A Randomized Trial." *Ann Intern Med.*, 147(6):357–369.

19. Björntorp P, de Jounge K, Sjöström L, and Sullivan L. 1970. "The Effect of Physical Training on Insulin Production in Obesity." *Metab Clin Exp.*, 19(8):631–638.

20. Thompson PD, Crouse SF, Goodpaster B, Kelley D, Moyna N, and Pescatello L. 2001. "The Acute versus the Chronic Response to Exercise." *Med Sci Sports Exerc.*, 33(6):S438–S445.

21. Ferrara CM, Goldberg AP, Ortmeyer HK, and Ryan AS. 2006. "Effects of Aerobic and Resistive Exercise Training on Glucose Disposal and Skeletal Muscle Metabolism in Older Men." *Journals of Gerontology Series A: Biological Sciences and Medical Sciences*, 61(5):480–487.

22. Estruch R, Martinez-Gonzalez MA, Corella D, et al. 2006. "Effects of a Mediterranean-Style Diet on Cardiovascular Risk Factors: A Randomized Trial." *Ann Intern Med.*, 145(1):1–11.

23. Fagard RH. 1999. "Physical Activity in the Prevention and Treatment of Hypertension in the Obese." *Med Sci Sports Exerc.*, 31(11):S624–S630.

24. Pinto A, Di Raimondo D, Tuttolomondo A, Fernandez P, Arna V, and Licata G. 2006. "Twenty-Four Hour Ambulatory Blood Pressure Monitoring to Evaluate Effects on Blood Pressure of Physical Activity in Hypertensive Patients." *Clinical Journal of Sport Medicine*, 16(3):238–243.

25. Llorente-Cortés V, Estruch R, Mena MP, et al. 2010. "Effect of Mediterranean Diet on the Expression of Pro-Atherogenic Genes in a Population at High Cardiovascular Risk." *Atherosclerosis*, 208(2):442–450.

26. Appel LJ, Moore TJ, Obarzanek E, et al. 1997. "A Clinical Trial of the Effects of Dietary Patterns on Blood Pressure." *N Engl J Med*, 336(16):1117–1124.

27. De Filippis E, Cusi K, Ocampo G, et al. 2006. "Exercise-Induced Improvement in Vasodilatory Function Accompanies Increased Insulin Sensitivity in Obesity and Type 2 Diabetes Mellitus." *Journal of Clinical Endocrinology & Metabolism*, 91(12):4903–4910.

28. Kraus WE, Houmard JA, Duscha BD, et al. 2002. "Effects of the Amount and Intensity of Exercise on Plasma Lipoproteins." *N Engl J Med.*, 347(19):1483–1492.

29. Chandalia M, Garg A, Lutjohann D, von Bergmann K, Grundy SM, and Brinkley LJ. 2000. "Beneficial Effects of High Dietary Fiber Intake in Patients with Type 2 Diabetes Mellitus." *N Engl J Med.*, 342(19):1392–1398.

30. Widlansky ME, Gokce N, Keaney JF, and Vita JA. 2003. "The Clinical Implications of Endothelial Dysfunction." *J Am Coll Cardiol.*, 42(7):1149–1160.

31. Sixt S, Beer S, Blüher M, et al. 2010. "Long- But Not Short-Term Multifactorial Intervention with Focus on Exercise Training Improves Coronary Endothelial Dysfunction in Diabetes Mellitus Type 2 and Coronary Artery Disease." *Eur Heart J.*, 31(1):112–119.

32. Stensvold D, Tjonna AE, Skaug E, et al. 2010. "Strength Training versus Aerobic Interval Training to Modify Risk Factors of Metabolic Syndrome." *J Appl Physiol.*, 108(4):804–810.

33. Rallidis LS, Lekakis J, Kolomvotsou A, et al. 2009. "Close Adherence to a Mediterranean Diet Improves Endothelial Function in Subjects with Abdominal Obesity." *Am J Clin Nutr.*, 90(2):263–268.

34. Ma Y, Njike VY, Millet J, et al. 2010. "Effects of Walnut Consumption on Endothelial Function in Type 2 Diabetic Subjects—A Randomized Controlled Crossover Trial." *Diabetes Care*, 33(2):227–232.

35. Wycherley TP, Brinkworth GD, Keogh JB, Noakes M, Buckley JD, and Clifton PM. 2010. "Long-Term Effects of Weight Loss with a Very Low Carbohydrate and Low Fat Diet on Vascular Function in Overweight and Obese Patients." *J Intern Med.*, 267(5):452–461.

36. Van Guilder GP, Hoetzer GL, Smith DT, et al. 2005. "Endothelial t-PA Release Is Impaired in Overweight and Obese Adults But Can Be Improved with Regular Aerobic Exercise." *American Journal of Physiology—Endocrinology and Metabolism*, 289(5):E807.

37. Murakami T, Horigome H, Tanaka K, et al. 2007. "Impact of Weight Reduction on Production of Platelet-Derived Microparticles and Fibrinolytic Parameters in Obesity." *Thromb Res.*, 119(1):45–53.

38. Haffner SM. 2006. "The Metabolic Syndrome: Inflammation, Diabetes Mellitus, and Cardiovascular Disease." *Am J Cardiol.*, 97(2):3–11.

39. Milani RV, Lavie CJ, and Mehra MR. 2004. "Reduction in C-Reactive Protein Through Cardiac Rehabilitation and Exercise Training." *J Am Coll Cardiol.*, 43(6):1056–1061.

40. Lambert CP, Wright NR, Finck BN, and Villareal DT. 2008. "Exercise But Not Diet-Induced Weight Loss Decreases Skeletal Muscle Inflammatory Gene Expression in Frail Obese Elderly Persons." *J Appl Physiol.*, 105(2):473–478.

41. Rajaram S, Connell KM, and Sabate J. 2010. "Effect of Almond-Enriched High-Monounsaturated Fat Diet on Selected Markers of Inflammation: A Randomised, Controlled, Crossover Study." *Br J Nutr.*, 103(6):907–912.

42. Azadbakht L, Kimiagar M, Mehrabi Y, Esmaillzadeh A, Hu FB, and Willett WC. 2007. "Soy Consumption, Markers of Inflammation, and Endothelial Function." *Diabetes Care*, 30(4):967.

SPOTLIGHT

The following chapter by Janet Treasure and Pamela McDonald discusses the use of Motivational Interviewing with patients with eating disorders, as well as their families. The authors review the scientific literature on the treatment of eating disorders using MI and related treatment approaches. They then discuss the practicalities of using such approaches and offer examples of how to use them.

Chapter Eight

Eating Disorders and Motivational Interviewing

Pamela McDonald and Janet Treasure

Anorexia nervosa (AN), bulimia nervosa (BN), eating disorders not otherwise specified (EDNOS), and binge eating disorder (BED) are prevalent disorders affecting mainly young women[1] that typically follow a chronic course with major psychiatric and medical co-morbidities.[2,3] Anorexia nervosa has the highest mortality of any psychiatric disorder, with the risk of death three times higher than that of depression, schizophrenia, or alcoholism.[4] Individuals with eating disorders are notoriously ambivalent about recovery and treatment refusal; drop-out and relapse are common occurrences.[5] As a result of these difficulties, motivational therapies are increasingly being incorporated into treatment models, such as cognitive behavioral therapy[6] and working with family members to enhance motivation for change in their loved ones.[7]

Motivational Interviewing (MI) was originally developed for the treatment of substance abuse and is an approach designed to increase clients' willingness to engage in future intensive treatment.[8] It has since been adapted and used to help people with a wide range of psychological problems,[9] including eating disorders.[1] The goal of MI is to help the client recognize their problem, build commitment to therapy, and reach a decision to change their behavior. MI is client-centered and the therapist's role is to enhance their client's motivation for change by exploring and resolving their ambivalence about recovery.[10] The MI model has been increasingly utilized in the field of eating disorders, building on existing assessment and treatment procedures. Some modifications to the standard MI model, however, are required depending on the eating disorder subtype. MI is often combined with structured biological and psychological feedback from clinical assessments. This combination of MI and individual feedback is called Motivational Enhancement Therapy (MET).[11,12]

People with eating disorders are frequently dependent on their families either because of their age or because of the severity of their illness. In the United Kingdom, the National Institute for Health and Clinical Excellence (NICE)[13] guidelines recommend that most people with AN be managed on an outpatient basis, a policy that places primary responsibility on family members. Eating disorder symptoms and the associated high medical risk have profound social ramifications, especially within the family. Caregivers often report lacking the skills and resources required to care for their loved ones.[14,15] Consequently, the manner in which the family attempts to reduce the symptoms often inadvertently plays a role in maintaining or aggravating the problem.[16] MI has also proved a useful tool in working with the family of people with eating disorders. It has helped to model more adaptive communication skills that both address symptom management and help families themselves change attitudes and behaviors that can maintain the disorder.

THEORETICAL BASE

In the United Kingdom, the MRC guidelines for developing and evaluating complex interventions[17] states that implications for development and evaluation of a complex intervention should include: a) a good theoretical understanding of how an intervention causes change so that any weak links in the causal chain can be identified/strengthened; b) lack of impact may reflect methodological/design faults rather than genuine ineffectiveness; c) identifying a single primary outcome may not make the best use of the data; and d) strict fidelity to a protocol may be inappropriate, adaptation may be required. These points are particularly pertinent when it comes to the implementation of MI in eating disorders.

MI arose from intuitive clinical practice rather than any particular theoretical model. It emerged, in part, as an alternative to the directive and even confrontational style of substance use counseling commonly used throughout the 1980s.[18] Many of its principles and techniques are rooted in the client-centered approach of Rogers and Carkauff, although MI is perhaps more goal driven and unidirectional than classic Rogerian client-centered therapy.[19-22] Despite MI's largely atheoretical origins,[23] in recent years, an increasing number of MI researchers and practitioners have begun to use self-determination theory (SDT) as a defacto model for understanding how and why MI works.[24,25] The differences in the nature of the two approaches in that SDT is a macro-theory of human motivation that began with basic laboratory research and has gradually been applied to health care. In contrast, MI is a bottom-up approach to health-behavior change,[26] an approach that is largely atheoretical and was based on intuition, trial and error, and clinical observations when treating addicted patients within the counseling venue. In fact, there is a similar interpersonal perspective to working with people within MI and SDT and the intervention techniques used within these two approaches have much in common.[23] Both approaches can be thought of as person-centered; non-judgmental and supportive, both provide information that is responsive to patient needs, both buttress patients' attempts to come into deeper contact with their inner experiences and motivations, and both place heavy emphasis on patients' autonomy while at the same time work to promote patients taking responsibility in a healthy way.[23]

EFFECTIVENESS OF MI IN EATING DISORDERS

In a systematic review, the aim of which was to examine the effectiveness of interventions that include the principles and techniques of MI and its adaptations in the treatment of eating disorders,[27] studies showed more promising results in *readiness to change* than a reduction in symptoms. Consequently, it may well be that MI is a behavior change process designed to be helpful when an individual is not ready to instigate change; in other words, it may be more useful with proximal rather than distal outcomes. According to Miller, if people are already in "action" mode, then the skill is to step back from motivational interviewing to a more action-based, cognitive-based therapeutic approach.[8] MI, then, may be more effective as an introduction or a preliminary phase before any of the interim behavior change processes that may be needed in order to produce symptom change. An MI approach, for example, may be helpful to instigate several behavior change activities that are used within cognitive behavioral therapy (CBT), e.g., food diaries, structured eating, exposure, behavioral experiment, surveys, etc.

Studies of MI being utilized in the field of eating disorders show a lack of homogeneity that makes it difficult to effectively assess the use of MI in eating disorders. In the recent systematic review, for example, samples were predominantly small, which may suggest lack of power in several studies. There were also considerable variations in intervention timeline, frequency and duration of actual MI/MET sessions, illness diagnosis, duration of illness, and age of patient (Macdonald et al. 2012, under review). The main problematic area encountered was focused on the variation in design and methodology. This has also been a challenge in other studies.[28,29] In a systematic review of motivational interviewing in physical health care settings, for example, Knight et al.[29] voiced their concerns that the internal content validity of studies in their review remains worryingly low. It appears that the field would benefit from more randomized clinical trials (RCTs) with larger samples as well as studies that present a clearer description of the process implemented, in terms of MI techniques, along with a more transparent depiction of the training, monitoring, and supervision procedures administered.

Despite the difficulties in making comparative conclusions between studies that utilize MI in eating disorders, there are promising results that do indicate the potential for using MI in this arena. These is particularly evident when working in the stage that signifies a *readiness for change.*[30–33,10] A key challenge for MI practitioners is deciding when and how to transition from building motivation to more action-oriented counseling within a patient-centered framework.[23] With this thought in mind, the next section will examine working with the MI model, first with the sufferer and then with the carer.

MI WITH THE SUFFERER

The literature shows a current theme of anorexics' reluctance to change.[34] One prominent framework for conceptualizing and assessing motivation and readiness for change is the transtheoretical model,[35] the key assumptions of which are that people move through a predictable sequence of stages from precontemplation to contemplation, preparation, action, and finally maintenance. Studies in adults with anorexia nervosa found that about half of those presenting for treatment were either in precontemplation or contemplation (no desire to change or highly ambivalent).[36,37] The mismatch in the desire for change between the person with the illness and those around them, coupled with the sense of urgency of intervention resulting from the person's compromised medical state, makes the process of engaging people with AN into treatment a challenging task.[1]

A treatment was developed on an evidence-based model of how anorexia is maintained.[38] Although a full description of the model is beyond the scope of this chapter, in summary, the cognitive-interpersonal approach (the Maudsley model of anorexia nervosa) proposes that the core psychopathology of AN is a need for the avoidance of intense negative emotions in people who have anxious/avoidant and perfectionist/rigid personality traits and who develop beliefs about the positive function of the anorexia in their life (pro-anorexia beliefs). These beliefs help them manage difficult emotions and the relationships that arouse them. A further maintenance factor is the response of others, which is characterized by concern and worry or criticism and hostility. If the benefits of AN go unrecognized in therapy, increased resistance to change can occur.[1]

MI combined with the cognitive interpersonal model has been regarded as very useful in helping clients question those valued functions of the illness. Treatment is conducted in the MI spirit, using a collaborative and empathic stance throughout.[8] Expressing empathy, developing discrepancy, rolling with resistance, and supporting self-efficacy are combined with reflective listening and open questioning to help elicit and reinforce change and commitment talk in helping resolve the ambivalence commonly found in eating disorders. There is, however, one important difference in that a classical application of MI accepts the client's autonomy to accept or reject treatment at any stage as an integral part of the MI spirit. However, in the treatment of AN, the client is not always an autonomous agent. For example, In the United Kingdom the Mental Health Act can be invoked to hospitalize and feed against their will some patients who have life-threatening AN. Nevertheless, even within these boundaries, it is still possible to use a motivational approach that offers an element of choice, particularly if non-negotiable matters are presented in an empathic "one-down position" that points out how both patient and practitioner are bound by societal rules.

Within SDT, recommendations must be given after eliciting and acknowledging client perspectives, non-coercively and in an autonomy-supportive way. When provided in this manner, the recommendation is more likely to be experienced by the patient as being informational, as opposed to coercive, and thus supports the patient in making the decision himself or herself. More recent formulations of MI have allowed for medical practitioners to make recommendations. The Elicit-Provide-Elicit style, for example, first *elicits* the person's understanding and need for information, then *provides* new information in a neutral manner, followed by *eliciting* what this information might mean for the client.[8] Often a key challenge for clinicians is determining when and how to move from building motivation to planning a course of action in a style that is MI-consistent.[23] Presently in the field of eating disorders, these components have been unified by using MI as a precursor to more action-oriented therapies, such as CBT.[39–41] Less work has been done on truly integrating the two approaches. In particular, there is a need to develop autonomy-supportive variants of CBT and other action-oriented approaches that are conceptually consistent with MI, not just stitched together.[23] Resnicow and McMaster's three-component model of MI is an attempt to bridge this gap. This model includes three core tasks: *Exploring*, *Guiding*, and *Choosing*, this model is an adaptation of models previously proposed by Miller and Rollnick.[42] Each task or phase is characterized by different counseling objectives and usually applies specific skills and techniques.

The following, then, is a clinical illustration of MI being used with an eating disorder sufferer in the precontemplation phase. We have noted the important techniques of MI in this example.

Therapist:	Thanks for coming today, Rose, I know how uncomfortable these meetings are for you. *[empathy]*
Rose:	It's not that. I just do not see the point in my being here… it's a waste of everybody's time.
Therapist:	So there's some heavy pressure from your family to come to these sessions. That must be pretty frustrating for you. I'd be interested in hearing more about your feelings on this. *[complex reflection + open question]*

Rose:	(deep sigh) Well mum cries all the time, dad shouts—that's their default positions. … *"You're wasting away," "Why don't you just eat?," "You're a shadow of your former self," "You've lost your spark"* and on and on and on—you get the picture?
Therapist:	Yup, that must be hard for you, especially when you feel that the attention is unwarranted. *[complex reflection]*
Rose:	It is… it really plays with my head. *Silence…* I mean it's not that the concern is *entirely* unwarranted. I mean I do have a lot of pressure from school and stuff on at the moment and I don't feel as great as I did, say, last year. …
Therapist:	That's interesting… part of you feels that your parents are over-reacting yet you also notice that you *have* been feeling a bit more stressed and anxious than usual. *[developing discrepancy]*
Rose:	I guess… yeah sometimes. …
Therapist:	That must be a bit puzzling for you—may even add to your anxiety. *pause…* How do you feel about spending the next half hour just talking about this pressure you're experiencing at the moment? *[complex reflection + open question]*
Rose:	Guess I'd be OK with that… may even help a bit… because the *last* thing I need right now is them banging on and making me even more hyped up. …

In the above scenario, the therapist uses double-sided reflections to help the client explore discrepancy. The therapist rolls with any resistance while using reflections and open questions to examine the client's perspective on a deeper level. At this stage, the therapist's goal will be to establish a connection with the sufferer.

MI WITH THE CARER

People with eating disorders are usually dependent on their families either because of their age or severity of their illness. However, carers often report lacking the skills and resources required to care for their loved ones.[14] Eating disorder symptoms and the associated high medical risk have profound social ramifications, especially within the family and the reactions and behaviors of family members often inadvertently reinforce ED symptoms.[43]

The outcome of many psychiatric conditions is influenced by the response of close others,[38] an aspect that is reflected in the concept of expressed emotion (EE), which indicates the amount of positive and negative comments (criticism, hostility, and emotional overinvolvement) expressed by relatives of psychiatric patients toward them. Several studies have found that EE affects adherence either to treatment and/or outcome in AN.[44–48] Carers can also find themselves accommodating and enabling ED behaviors by removing or covering up negative consequences of the illness in a bid to keep the peace. A clear benefit derived from research into EE is the development of family interventions. Skills-training interventions for carers have shown a reduction in expressed emotion and accommodating and enabling behaviors.[49–51, 47]

Most people have behaviors that they know are unhelpful or situations where they would like to see some change. Many people also experience a certain degree of ambivalence as to whether or not they want or, indeed, would be able to change those situations or behaviors. MI has proved a useful tool in skills-training programs to work with families in modeling communication skills that both address symptom management as well as helping families change those attitudes and behaviors that serve to maintain the disorder. Motivational interviewing can be an effective intervention for reducing maladaptive interpersonal responses to the symptoms within the family as a way of improving communication and reducing expressed emotion, anxiety, and burden. The therapist uses MI to work with the family in reflecting upon changing any maladaptive responses to the illness. Carers are also encouraged to themselves use basic MI skills with their loved one to communicate more effectively in a bid to instigate change.[1] The following excerpt illustrates clinical application of MI when working with a carer:

Therapist:	So from you've been telling me, Sue, things are pretty rough at home at the moment with lots of tears and conflict. *[complex reflection]* That must be pretty tough on all of you, particularly when you're trying so hard to be supportive. *[expressing empathy + affirmation]*
Carer:	It's awful, the weight is dropping off her and she's still insisting that there's nothing wrong. I spend my time in tears, Pete deals with it by yelling and meanwhile Rose grows more and more distant. We desperately want to help her but we don't know how to. …
Therapist:	So you and Pete recognize that there's a problem here but you're having difficulty knowing the best way to respond to it. *[complex reflection]*

Carer: Yeah... I know that perhaps we're not dealing with it the right way but then at the same time I feel kinda ticked off—I mean it's not like we're the ones who should be examining our behavior. ...

Therapist: So a bag of mixed emotions then. *[simple reflection]* On the one hand, you feel that perhaps the way you respond to the symptoms may be adding to the stress, yet you feel that it's Rose who really should be changing her behavior. Meanwhile there's lots of confusion and bewilderment. *[developing discrepancy]* What would be most helpful to you right now? *[open question]*

Carer: For you to tell us what to do for the best... or how to make her eat (laugh).

Therapist: (smiling) Unfortunately there's no magic pill for an eating disorder, nor can I tell you what to do for the best. Every family has their own unique needs. However, many carers I have worked with appreciate information and support interventions on how best to respond to the illness. I have some information you may find very useful and relevant in regards to your own needs. How would you feel if I gave you this to take away with you today then next appointment we can discuss some of this and plan the next step forward? *[giving information + open question]*

Carer: I guess it would be a start. ...

In the above excerpt the therapist uses the *elicit-provide-elicit* (EPE) information exchange to elicit the carer's needs, thus emphasizing the carer's active involvement in the recovery process. The second part of the EPE cycle involves providing information in a manageable chunk. If the carer has been asked whether or not they would welcome information, this permits therapist to elaborate opening the door for further discussion in future sessions.

CONCLUSION

There is evidence to suggest that MI is a useful intervention when working with both sufferers and their carers. Nevertheless, RCTs must be designed that provide a more thorough description of the methods used. This would not only make replication easier but would also allow researchers to distinguish between variations in the interventions being offered and examine the extent to which MI is being administered. It is important for researchers and clinicians to understand the range of effects and how they vary among recipients of the intervention, i.e., comparing effects between individuals in the various stages of change and the causes of that variation. Analyzing the results of those RCTs that utilize a control "treatment as usual" group would address this issue, allowing for further investigation of the intervention's active ingredients and how they exert their effects. Only by building a cumulative understanding of the influences of MI and its variants can we then design effective interventions tailored specifically to the field of eating disorders.

References

1. Treasure, J. and Schmidt, U. 2008. "Motivational Interviewing in the Management of Eating Disorders." In H.Arkowitz, H. A. Westra, W. R. Miller, and S. Rollnick (Eds.), *Motivational Interviewing in the Treatment of Psychological Problems* (pp. 194–224). New York: The Guildford Press.

2. Fairburn, C. G. and Brownell, K. D. 2001. *Eating Disorders and Obesity: A Comprehensive Handbook (2nd ed.).* New York: Guildford Press.

3. Zipfel, S. L. B. and Herzog, W. 2003. "Medical Complications in Eating Disorders and Obesity." In J. Treasure, U. Schmidt, and E. F. van Furth (Eds.), *Handbook of Eating Disorders: Theory, Treatment and Research. (2nd ed.)* Chichester, UK: Wiley.

4. Harris, E. C. and Barrowclough, B. 1998. "Excess Mortality of Mental Disorder." *British Journal of Psychiatry, 173,* 11–53.

5. Kahn, C. and Pike, K. M. 2001. "In Search of Predictors of Dropout from Inpatient Treatment for Anorexia Nervosa." *International Journal of Eating Disorders, 30,* 237–244.

6. Fairburn, C. G. 2008. *Cognitive Behavior Therapy and Eating Disorders.* New York: Guildford Press.

7. Treasure, J., Sepulveda, A. R., Whitaker, W., Todd, G., Lopez, C., and Whitney, J. 2007. "Collaborative Care Between Professionals and Non-Professionals in the Management of Eating Disorders: A Description of Workshops Focussed on Interpersonal Maintaining Factors." *European Eating Disorders Review, 15,* 24–34.

8. Miller, W. R. and Rollnick, S. 2002. *Motivational Interviewing: Preparing People for Change, 2nd Edition.* New York: Guildford.

9. Arkowitz, H., Westra, H. A., Miller, W. R., and Rollnick, S. 2008. *Motivational Interviewing in the Treatment of Psychological Problems.* New York: The Guildford Press.

10. Geller, J., Brown, G. K., and Srikameswaran, S. 2011. "The Efficacy of a Brief Motivational Intervention for Individuals with Eating Disorders: A Randomized Control Trial." *International Journal of Eating Disorders, 44,* 497–505.

11. Miller, W. R., Zweben, A., DiClemente, C., and Rychtarik, R. G. 1992. *Motivational Enhancement Therapy Manual: A Clinical Research Guide for Therapists Treating Individuals with Alcohol Abuse and Dependence.* Rockville, MD: National Institute on Alcohol Abuse and Alcoholism.

12. Treasure, J. and Ward, A. 1997. "A Practical Guide to the Use of Motivational Interviewing in Anorexia Nervosa." *European Eating Disorders Review, 5,* 102–114.

13. National Institute for Clinical Excellence 2004. *National Clinical Practice Guideline. Eating Disorders. Core Interventions in the Treatment and Management of Anorexia Nervosa, Bulimia Nervosa, and Related Eating Disorders.* London.

14. Haigh, R. and Treasure, J. 2003. "Investigating the Needs of Carers in the Area of Eating Disorders: Development of the Carers' Needs Assessment Measure (CaNAM)." *European Eating Disorders Review, 11*, 125–141.

15. Treasure, J., Murphy, T., Szmukler, T., Todd, G., Gavan, K., and Joyce, J. 2001. "The Experience of Caregiving for Severe Mental Illness: A Comparison Between Anorexia Nervosa and Psychosis." *Social Psychiatry and Psychiatric Epidemiology., 36*, 343–347.

16. Treasure, J., Sepulveda, A. R., Macdonald, P., Whitaker, W., Lopez, C., and Zabala, M. 2008b. "Interpersonal Maintaining Factors in Eating Disorders: Skill Sharing Interventions for Carers." *International Journal of Child and Adolescent Health, 1*, 331–338.

17. Medical Research Council 2008. *Developing and Evaluating Complex Interventions: New Guidance* www.mrc. ac.uk/complexinterventionsguidance.

18. Miller, W. R. and Rose, G. S. 2009. "Towards a Theory of Motivational Interviewing." *American Psychologist, 64*, 527–537.

19. Carkhuff, R., Anthony, W. A., Cannon, J., Pierce, R., and Zigon, F. 1979. *The Skills of Helping: An Introduction to Counseling Skills.* Amherst, MA: Human Resource Development Press.

20. Carkhuff, R. 1993. *The Art of Helping. (7th ed.).* Amherst, MA: Human Resource Development Press.

21. Miller, W. B. and Rollnick, S. 2009. "Ten Things That Motivational Interviewing Is Not." *Behavioural and Cognitive Psychotherapy, 37*, 129–140.

22. Rogers, C. R. 1986. "Carl Rogers on the Development of the Person-Centered Approach." *Person Centered Review, 1*, 257–289.

23. Resnicow, K. and McMaster, F. 2012. "Motivational Interviewing: Moving from Why to How with Autonomy Support." *International Journal of Behavioral Nutrition and Physical Activity, 9*, 19.

24. Markland, D., Ryan, R. M., Tobin, V. J., and Rollnick, S. 2005. "Motivational Interviewing and Self-Determination Theory." *Journal of Social and Clinical Psychology, 24*, 811–831.

25. Vansteenkiste, M. and Sheldon, K. M. 2006. "There's Nothing More Practical Than a Good Theory: Integrating Motivational Interviewing and Self-Determination Theory." *British Journal of Clinical Psychology, 45*, 63–82.

26. Miller, W. R. and Rollnick, S. 2012. "Meeting in the Middle: Motivational Interviewing and Self-Determination Theory." *International Journal of Behavioral Nutrition and Physical Activity, 9*, 25.

27. Macdonald, P., Hibbs, R., Corfield, F., & Treasure, J. (2012). The use of motivational interviewing in eating disorders: a systematic review. *Psychiatry Res, 200*, 1–11.

28. Dunn, C., Deroo, L., and Rivara, F. P. 2001. "The Use of Brief Interventions Adapted from Motivational Interviewing Across Behavioral Domains: A Systematic Review." *Addictions, 96*, 1725–1742.

29. Knight, K. M., Mcgowan, L., Dickens, C., and Bundy, C. 2006. "A Systematic Review of Motivational Interviewing in Physical Health Care Settings." *British Journal of Health Psychology, 11*, 319–332.

30. Cassin, S. E., von Ranson, K. M., Heng, K., Brar, J., and Wojtowicz, A. E. 2008. "Adapted Motivational Interviewing for Women with Binge Eating Disorder: A Randomized Controlled Trial." *Psychology of Addictive Behaviors, 22*, 417–425.

31. Dean, H. Y., Touyz, S. W., Rieger, E., and Thornton, C. E. 2008. "Group Motivational Enhancement Therapy as an Adjunct to Inpatient Treatment for Eating Disorders: A Preliminary Study." *European Eating Disorders Review, 16,* 256–267.

32. Dunn, E. C., Neighbors, C., and Larimer, M. E. 2006. "Motivational enhancement therapy and Self-Help Treatment for Binge Eaters." [References]. *Psychology of Addictive Behaviors, Vol.20,* 44–52.

33. Wade, T. D., Frayne, A., Edwards, S.-A., Robertson, T., and Gilchrist, P. 2009. "Motivational Change in an Inpatient Anorexia Nervosa Population and Implications for Treatment." *Australian and New Zealand Journal of Psychiatry, 43,* 235–243.

34. Vitousek, K., Watson, S., and Wilson, G. 1998. "Enhancing Motivation for Change in Treatment-Resistant Eating Disorders." *Clinical Psychology Review, 18,* 391–420.

35. Prochaska, J. and DiClemente, C. 1984. *The Transtheoretical Approach: Crossing the Traditional Boundaries of Therapy.* Homewood, IL: Dow Jones Irwen.

36. Blake, W., Turnbull, S., and Treasure, J. 1997. "Stages and Processes of Change in Eating Disorders: Implications for Therapy." *Clinical Psychology and Psychotherapy,* 4:186–191.

37. Ward, A., Troop, N., Todd, G., and Treasure, J. 1996. "To Change or Not to Change—'How' Is the Question?" *British Journal of Medical Psychology, 69,* 139–146.

38. Schmidt, U. and Treasure, J. 2006. "Anorexia Nervosa: Valued and Visible. A Cognitive-Interpersonal Maintenance Model and Its Implications for Research and Practice." *British Journal of Clinical Psychology, 45,* 343–366.

39. George, L., Thornton, C., Touyz, S., Waller, G., and Beumont, P. 2004. "Motivational Enhancement and Schema-Focused Cognitive Behaviour Therapy in the Treatment of Chronic Eating Disorders." *Clinical Psychologist, 8,* 81–85.

40. Katzman, M. A., Bara-Carril, N., Rabe-Hesketh, S., Schmidt, U., Troop, N., and Treasure, J. 2010. "A Randomized Controlled Two-Stage Trial in the Treatment of Bulimia Nervosa, Comparing CBT versus Motivational Enhancement in Phase 1 Followed by Group versus Individual CBT in Phase 2." *Psychosomatic Medicine, 72,* 656–663.

41. Willinge, A. C., Touyz, S. W., and Thornton, C. 2010. "An Evaluation of the Effectiveness and Short-Term Stability of an Innovative Australian Day Patient Programme for Eating Disorders." *European Eating Disorders Review, 18,* 220–233.

42. Rollnick, S., Miller, W. R., and Butler, C. C. 2008. *Motivational Interviewing in Health Care.* New York: The Guildford Press.

43. Treasure, J., Sepulveda, A. R., Macdonald, P., Whitaker, W., Lopez, C., Zabala, M. et al. 2008a. "The Assessment of the Family of People with Eating Disorders." *European Eating Disorders Review, 16,* 247–255.

44. Eisler, I., Szmukler, G., and Dare, C. 1985. "Systematic Observation and Clinical Insight—Are They Compatible? An Experiment in Recognizing Family Interactions." *Psychological Medicine, 15,* 173–188.

45. Eisler, I., Dare, C., Russell, G. F., Szmukler, G., Le Grange, D., and Dodge, E. 1997. "Family and Individual Therapy in Anorexia Nervosa: A 5-Year Follow-Up." *Archives of General Psychiatry, 54,* 1025–1030.

46. Szmukler, G., Eisler, I., Russell, G. F., and Dare, C. 1985. "Anorexia Nervosa, Parental 'Expressed Emotion' and Dropping out of Treatment." *British Journal of Psychiatry, 147,* 265–271.

47. Uehara, T., Kawashima, Y., Goto, M., Tasaki, S. i., and Someya, T. 2001. "Psychoeducation for the Families of Patients with Eating Disorders and Changes in Expressed Emotion: A Preliminary Study." [References]. *Comprehensive Psychiatry., 42,* 132–138.

48. van Furth, E., van Strien, D. C., Martina, L. M., van Son, M. J., Hendrickx, J. J., and van Engeland, H. 1996. "Expressed Emotion and the Prediction of Outcome in Adolescent Eating Disorders." *International Journal of Eating Disorders, 20,* 19–31.

49. Goddard, E., Macdonald, P., Naumann, U., Landau, S., Sepulveda, A. R., Schmidt, U., et al. 2011. "A Randomised Controlled Trial Examining the Effects of a Skills Training Programme for Carers of People with Eating Disorders." *British Journal of Psychiatry, 199,* 225–231.

50. Sepulveda, A. R., Todd, G., Whitaker, W., Grover, M., Stahl, D., and Treasure, J. 2009. "Expressed Emotion in Relatives of Patients with Eating Disorders Following Skills Training Program." *International Journal of Eating Disorders, 43,* 603–610.

51. Zucker, N. L., Ferriter, C., Best, S., and Brantley, A. 2005. "Group Parent Training: A Novel Approach for the Treatment of Eating Disorders." *Eating Disorders, 13,* 391–405.

SPOTLIGHT

In the next chapter by Kathy Kater, the author describes a model she has developed for teaching children about body acceptance and health as opposed to the usual weight-centered approach. She describes this approach as it relates to teaching HAES concepts to children. The emphasis in this model is on *health* rather than *weight*. It challenges the idea that appearance is the most important factor in our identity.

Chapter Nine

Promoting Health Instead of Size in Children: Teaching Kids to Care for Their Bodies

Kathy Kater

In the early 1960s, advertising campaigns promoting the "thin ideal" for females generated pervasive anxiety about weight among women that persists today. Body scrutiny, "fat talk," and the drive to be thin made restrictive eating "normal" for the vast majority of females, and became a rite of passage for adolescent girls. In the 1980s, increased marketing of the "lean/buff ideal" for males triggered concern about fatness, body dissatisfaction, and dieting in a growing number of men and teen boys as well. As the unhealthy, counterproductive, and even dangerous effects of this unrealistic trend were documented, individuals and organizations worked to raise awareness about the physical, mental/emotional, and financial costs—hoping it, and the diet industry it spawned, would fade.

But recently, even as research has continued to document that body dissatisfaction and the drive to be thin predictably lead to poor and disordered eating, diminished health, and weight *gain*, a new force for weight-worry has appeared. Everyone from public health practitioners to policymakers and members of Congress to celebrities and the media have unleashed ominous warnings about rising rates of fatness and massive campaigns to "prevent obesity" that are now driving weight stigma, fear of fatness, weight loss intentions, and "dieting" to a whole new level. As a result of these well-intentioned but ultimately misguided campaigns, almost no one escapes worry about weight today. Tragically, this includes a rapidly growing number of ever-younger children who wonder, "Am I fat?"

The consequences are severe, and will have the opposite effect than intended on both health and the economy. At a time when they should feel secure in their bodies' growth, most boys and girls today learn to worry about gaining weight, to harshly critique their "imperfect" sizes and shapes, and to feel it is their responsibility to guard against fatness by eating according to prescribed "food rules." Most of these children are not fat, but nonetheless are taught by well-intentioned adults to believe they should assume this vigilant stance prophylactically as part of the benevolent effort to eliminate obesity. Those with bodies that are chubby or fat learn to be very, very ashamed. If fear of weight gain and shame about fatness could somehow transform the eating and fitness habits of our population, conceivably this outcome could be defensible. But nothing could be further from the truth.

A growing child's inability to feel comfortable in his or her own skin is detrimental to the formation of his or her identity. Far from benign, children who are anxious or ashamed about weight begin to view their bodies from the outside, in—objectifying, comparing, and judging themselves against external standards—all too often disowning their very embodiment. In the process, they disconnect from internal cues that are perfectly attuned to what and how much their bodies need to eat, as well as the ways their bodies want and need to move naturally and joyfully in daily life. Missing this innate guide for lifelong health, they become even more vulnerable to the "noise" and pressures around them—much of it unhelpful. These children are *less* able to care for their bodies and *less* able to make normal, sound eating and activity choices—particularly in today's challenging food and entertainment environment.

The culturally mediated wish to be slim or lean plants the seeds for a host of body image, eating, fitness, and weight concerns that are extremely difficult to reverse once established. Kids who learn to worry about being or becoming fat are self-conscious, anxious, preoccupied by hunger and food, and inevitably unsure about what they need. Precisely at a time when their primary developmental task is to discover *who they are*, far too many learn to worry about *how they look* and the score on their BMI "report card."

Too few adults consider the ramifications to a child of getting a "failing" BMI score, or any other basis for body shame. Far from helping a child tune in to and feel motivated to respond to what is most needed to care for their bodies, a growing body of data shows the opposite: body dissatisfaction and shame reliably lead to despair and hopelessness on the one hand, and restrictive dieting for weight loss on the other. Neither motivates children to care for their bodies through positive eating and fitness choices.

What will drive healthy choices if not fear of fatness? Warnings about the dangers of childhood obesity lead many to believe that *more* worry about weight is needed, and that a *size-neutral* stance in regard to outcomes will lead to complacency about eating and fitness choices. This view is based on the widely held but false belief that critical body scrutiny and weight-worry can help. Individuals and organizations that are pushing current health agendas need to take a longer look at this faulty perspective. Since the thin-ideal became pervasive in the early 1960s, Americans have assumed more personal responsibility for their weight, claimed more weight-loss intentions, and engaged in more weight-loss efforts than previously imaginable. A multi-billion-dollar in-our-face weight-loss industry pressures us daily to join in or be left out. Could it be that if our children were just a little more fearful of or felt just a little worse about their fatness, they would improve their eating and fitness habits and childhood obesity would be eradicated? Do we need to test this hypothesis further?

The fact is, in the fifty years since weight was first framed as a "problem" with "weight control" cast as the solution, not only have eating disorders emerged to threaten those who are vulnerable, but rates of obesity and associated health risks have risen exponentially. While other environmental changes have certainly played a part, we cannot escape that the thinner we have tried to be, the fatter we have become. Clearly campaigns promoting "size prevention" (and therefore more weight stigma and fear of fatness) are not only ineffective in motivating healthier long-term eating and fitness choices, but they are also contributing to the problem. We must stop promoting this weight-focused approach to our children, and teach a more successful and humane way.

Promoting health instead of size. *The Model for Healthy Body Image and Weight* (MHBIW) [Figure 1] offers a comprehensive example of a weight-stigma reduction program for promoting health instead of size to children. It helps adults as well—educators, parents, health care providers, child-care workers, all who are our children's teachers—to resist cultural pressures that encourage body dissatisfaction and the counterproductive lifestyle habits they spawn. The evidence-based concepts in this model have been published in a popular and effective curriculum entitled *Healthy Bodies; Teaching Kids What They Need to Know*. Each of the eleven lessons teaches one of the MHBIW's child-friendly *Healthy Bodies Building Blocks* [Figure 2]. The program has demonstrated positive results in outcome studies with students in grades four through six, and it is endorsed by the U.S. Department of Health and Human Services' Office of Women's Health in their *Bodywise* information packet for educators. A companion book for parents, entitled *Real Kids Come in All Sizes: Ten Essential Lessons to Build Your Child's Body Esteem*, is also available to help parents reinforce the same principles at home. With this holistic model, problems inherent to a "right size/wrong size" paradigm can be avoided, as a more effective approach that also follows the maxim "do no harm" is embraced.

Development of a Comprehensive Model: The MHBIW is a proactive, universal, health-promotion model, based on the principle that positive body esteem and internal hunger and weight regulation are fully functional in healthy infants at birth. Ideally, all that is needed is a supportive environment for these to be maintained. Therefore, if problems occur among large numbers of people in a population, it is assumed that these are culturally mediated, not due to individual weakness or circumstance.

Concepts in the MHBIW are factual responses to a set of pervasive, distorted, or false culturally transmitted beliefs that together promote unhealthy body image, eating, fitness, and weight concerns in modern Western environments. This set of *toxic myths* serves as the seedbed out of which most problems take root and grow. The model provides eleven irrefutable prevention principles or "antidotes" that directly challenge the premises of these myths and empower resistance to their negative influence. In turn, healthier attitudes and behaviors

The Model for Healthy Body Image and Weight			
Conceptual Building Blocks	Foundation	Desired Outcome	Goal
Developmental change is inevitable. Normal changes of puberty include weight gain and temporary out-of-proportion growth; fat does not by itself define "overweight." Genetics and other internal weight regulators strictly limit the degree to which shape, weight, and body mass index (BMI) can be manipulated through healthy means. Restricted or restrained hunger (dieting) results in predictable consequences that are *counterproductive* to weight loss and interfere with normal hunger regulation.	Recognize and respect basic biology; understand what is *not* in our control regarding size, shape, weight, and hunger.	**Accept the innate body: " This is the body I was born to have."**	**Healthy Body Image** **Prevention of Unbalanced and Disordered Eating**
Balance attention to *many* aspects of identity. Looks are only one part. Consistently satisfy hunger with enough varied, whole some food in a stable, predictable manner. Limit sedentary choices to promote a physically active lifestyle at all ages. Choose role models that reflect a realistic standard.	Emphasize what *can* be influenced or chosen.	**Enjoy eating for health, energy, and hunger satisfaction. Create a physically active lifestyle for fitness, endurance, fun, relaxation, and stress relief.**	**Well-Fed, Fit, and Strong Bodies at Every Size**
Promote historical perspective on today's attitudes that promote body dissatisfaction. Teach critical thinking about media messages about appearance and food. Support each other in resisting unhealthy norms about weight, dieting, low-nutrient food choices, and a too-sedentary lifestyle.	Develop social and cultural resiliency.	**Develop autonomy, self-esteem, confidence, and the ability for critical thinking.**	

Figure 1

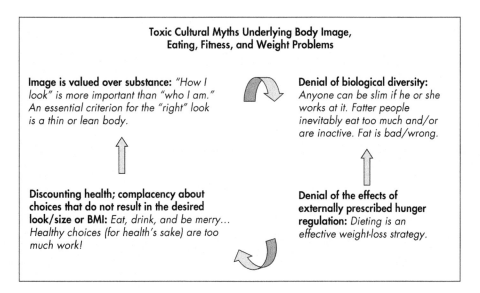

Toxic Cultural Myths Underlying Body Image, Eating, Fitness, and Weight Problems

Image is valued over substance: *"How I look" is more important than "who I am." An essential criterion for the "right" look is a thin or lean body.*

Denial of biological diversity: *Anyone can be slim if he or she works at it. Fatter people inevitably eat too much and/or are inactive. Fat is bad/wrong.*

Discounting health; complacency about choices that do not result in the desired look/size or BMI: *Eat, drink, and be merry... Healthy choices (for health's sake) are too much work!*

Denial of the effects of externally prescribed hunger regulation: *Dieting is an effective weight-loss strategy.*

Figure 2

can be maintained or reinstated. The antidotes teach a) the biological limits to manipulation of body size and shape through healthy means, b) behaviors that enhance health, body image, and self esteem, and c) actions for resiliency in the face of conflicting messages. (See Figure 1 for a representation of this organization.)

The MHBIW vigorously avoids short-term-only solutions. It rejects methods that appear to solve one problem, but at the expense of another. The goals and the means to reach them—healthy body image attitudes, healthy lifestyle choices, and healthy weights—are equally attainable for *all*, regardless of size, shape, weight, age, gender, socio-economic status, or cultural milieu. As such, the model is non-discriminatory, simple enough to be taught to children as well as adults, and equally useful for prevention or reversal of problems. Rather than promoting fear by warning children what to avoid, or delivering "rules" about what to do, concepts teach students to think about how cultural pressures conflict with the facts or truth regarding what can and cannot be controlled about size, shape, weight, health, body integrity, happiness, and overall wellbeing.

Interdependent Toxic Myths Are Challenged by the MHBIW Antidotes: As with any holistic prevention or treatment model, it is essential to keep all contributors to body image and eating and weight problems in mind in order to avoid solutions that conflict (Figure 3). The four toxic myths are summarized here, followed by the prevention principles or antidotes that challenge their unreliability.

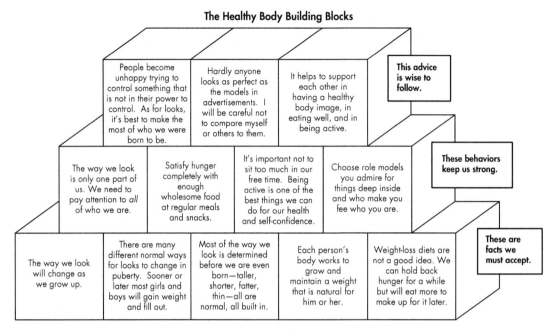

The Healthy Body Building Blocks

People become unhappy trying to control something that is not in their power to control. As for looks, it's best to make the most of who we were born to be.	Hardly anyone looks as perfect as the models in advertisements. I will be careful not to compare myself or others to them.	It helps to support each other in having a healthy body image, in eating well, and in being active.	**This advice is wise to follow.**

The way we look is only one part of us. We need to pay attention to *all* of who we are.	Satisfy hunger completely with enough wholesome food at regular meals and snacks.	It's important not to sit too much in our free time. Being active is one of the best things we can do for our health and self-confidence.	Choose role models you admire for things deep inside and who make you fee who you are.	**These behaviors keep us strong.**

The way we look will change as we grow up.	There are many different normal ways for looks to change in puberty. Sooner or later most girls and boys will gain weight and fill out.	Most of the way we look is determined before we are even born—taller, shorter, fatter, thin—all are normal, all built in.	Each person's body works to grow and maintain a weight that is natural for him or her.	Weight-loss diets are not a good idea. We can hold back hunger for a while but will eat more to make up for it later.	**These are facts we must accept.**

Figure 3

Myth 1—Based on the notion that image is more valuable than substance: "How I look" is more important than "who I am." An essential criterion for the "right look" is a thin or lean body.

Children learn that *beauty is only skin deep*, and *you can't judge a book by its cover*. But today's young students must be prepared to defend themselves in light of another adage: *One picture is worth a thousand words.* Since the explosion of visual media in the late 1950s, people no longer assume that other ordinary-looking people should be the basis for comparing their looks. Instead, millions of images of extraordinarily photogenic models, all chosen for their particularly appealing, slim look, have revolutionized the value placed on appearances in general and have created a mandate for a *lean* appearance in particular.

As children enter puberty, it is developmentally normal for them to begin to identify less with parents regarding certain issues and more with friends. Given the human need for inclusion, that which is perceived as culturally *normal* carries tremendous value. Playing on this human need for inclusion, intensive marketing of a generally unattainable, slim/lean appearance-ideals *as if* these are standard has been very effective in creating tremendous anxiety about appearance in general, and fear of fatness in particular in students who naturally want to be normal and fit in.

Many adults do not know that the *manufacturing of anxiety* about social acceptability is a purposeful marketing strategy. When awareness of this fact is systematically taught to elementary-age kids, they easily comprehend and are indignant to learn that insecurity about looks is a desired outcome for advertisers who then make money from products that promise to correct perceived deficiencies. Common responses include, "That just isn't right!" and "I know I'm not perfect, and will never expect to look like those models!"

The MHBIW provides three antidotes to help students to listen to their hearts, resist objectification, and develop resiliency in the face of pressures to compare themselves to unrealistic images.

Teach students to understand and resist body objectification:

> Acquire historical perspective on today's body image attitudes. It wasn't always this way, and doesn't have to always be this way. Understand that an emphasis on an "ideal look" is a formula for unhappiness.

> Develop a strong sense of identity based on a balance of *inner* qualities rather than on appearance. Who you are is more important than how you look.

> Become media literate and recognize advertising strategies. Think critically about media messages that encourage unrealistic, unhealthy body image attitudes and present low nutrient foods as the "cool way" to fulfill hunger needs.

> *Myth 2—Based on denial of biological diversity: Anyone can be slim if he or she works at it. Fatter people inevitably eat too much and/or are inactive. Fat is bad/wrong.*

For the thin-ideal to be widely embraced, facts pertaining to biological diversity of body size and shape must be dismissed, discounted, or denied. This denial has become pervasive. As a result children today learn that fatter people "must be doing something wrong" (must be overeating and/or sedentary). With this belief, weight bias freely develops. As a result, weight stigma has become normative, and anxiety about weight and the need to control it is rampant.

Weight will be influenced by lifestyle choices, but the idea that weight can be "controlled" through healthy means over the long term is false. This truth needs to be universally taught to children, who often grasp more easily than adults that only behaviors can be controlled, and weight is *not* a behavior. With elementary lessons on genetic influence, kids are able to learn that weight is an outcome of many complex variables, many of which are not in our power to choose. In light of this, the normal weight for individuals who eat well and are active will be very diverse, ranging from thin to fat. Again, as defenders of the truth, when presented with the facts, young students inevitably exclaim "it's just not right" to judge someone because of their size or in comparison to any external standard. The MHBIW offers three antidotes firmly grounded in biology regarding this:

Teach students the biological principles of growth and innate size diversity:

> Understand the normal, expected addition of body fat that is common during puberty and other developmental stages of life.

> Respect and appreciate the genetic diversity of body shapes and sizes.

> Understand how the internal weight regulatory system *limits* the extent of long-term control over weight that is possible.

Myth 3—Based on denial of the universal effects of externally prescribed hunger regulation: Dieting is an effective weight-loss strategy.

Whether for appearance or health, when a prescribed size (or "size prevention") is mandated, a means to attain it is needed. Because restricted eating results in weight loss in the short run, this is routinely used as evidence to support the belief that anyone could be slim(*mer*) if he or she worked at it through diet and exercise. Denial of the long-term results of dieting for weight loss is essential to keep the thin-ideal alive or to believe a normal BMI range is a viable goal for all.

Most people, including many medical providers, continue to blame a dieter's lack of will-power rather than accept that "dieting" is intrinsically flawed. But even very young children understand that when hunger is unsatisfied, it is like a starving caged lion. Universal, reliable, and predictable results (scientifically documented since the 1950s) can be expected: obsession and preoccupation with food, ravenous and uncontrollable hunger when food is made available, disconnection from internal hunger cues, moodiness, compulsive rebound eating, and regained weight (usually with added pounds).

Hunger demands to be fed and will subside naturally when it is satisfied. But this requires that children remain connected to their bodies in an accepting, positive, mindful way—tuned in and responsive to hunger and fullness cues. Suggesting to a child that they should eat less than hunger dictates teaches that they cannot trust and should not listen to internal regulatory cues, and that they must rely on external rules in order to be both healthy and acceptable in the eyes of others. Such a plan sets up an adversarial relationship with the body, and is a set-up for failure. The MHBIW includes one potent antidote to reinforce what students already know instinctually about denying hunger: If you are worried about getting enough, "… anyone would want to eat *so much more!*"

Teach children the well-documented facts about dieting for weight loss:

Recognize that there are predictable, counterproductive results when hunger is restricted according to an external plan. It's not hard to understand that 90% percent of weight lost through dieting is regained, usually with added pounds.

Myth 4—Based on discounting the value of health and complacency about lifestyle choices that do not result in the desired look: Eat, drink, and be merry. Healthy choices (for health's sake) are too much work.

In a context in which appearance, the drive to be thin, denial of the biological basis for size diversity, and the diet mentality dominate, the primary purpose of healthy habits for health's sake is easily lost. Too many children today grow up to believe the main reason to eat well and be active is to control weight. But the promise of a slim physique as the reward for a healthy lifestyle has backfired. When dieting and exercise are not sustainable or do not result in the promised slim/lean look, complacency about choices "just" for the sake of health are common. "Why should I eat healthy (or exercise) if it won't make me thin?"

Marketers capitalize upon this, promoting an ever-expanding array of cheap, readily available, highly flavored, seductively packaged, high-energy/low-nutrient treats as if these were the basis for a healthy diet, along with unending sedentary entertainment options. Awash in this environment, those who routinely override their internal hunger and weight regulatory systems, are poorly or erratically nourished, and lack basic fitness have increased exponentially. When the solution is another diet and more time at the gym, problems are perpetuated.

On the flip side, promoting weight loss or control as the goal of balanced nutrition and physical activity puts another group at risk: those who are naturally slim. "It doesn't matter what I eat. I've never been fat!" When the stated purpose for more nutritionally dense school lunches and more physical education is "to prevent obesity," the value of healthy choices *in their own right* is diminished.

Maintaining a self-nurturing lifestyle takes time and effort. If the primary purpose is to control weight, we can expect what we've gotten: a nation growing less healthy and in many cases fatter on feelings of failure or complacency. Instead, students can be taught that *health and well-being*—not size or shape—are more reliable and more important rewards for listening to their bodies' needs. With a size-neutral approach, body esteem, nutritional health, and physical fitness are achievable for every student at every size. Instead of food rules, students learn to pay attention to their own experience about what and how much to eat. If they are not free to "eat it all" (without judgment or fear of weight gain), how is it possible to learn how much is "enough"? The MHBIW suggests three antidotes to help children develop a personal stake in listening to and caring for their bodies:

Teach children of every size to embrace health and self-care as a value instead of size as a goal.

> Appreciate the value of balanced nutrition in its own right. Listen to internal cues and feel good about satisfying hunger completely with enough wholesome food. Enjoy all foods with mindful attention to outcomes.

> Appreciate the value of movement in its own right, and pay attention to the results. Listen to the body's need for enjoyable movement, and spend enough time and energy engaged in physical activity to maintain vitality at every stage of life. Enjoy of sedentary entertainment in ways that do not interfere with physical endurance, strength, vigor, and agility.

> Accept the size and shape that result from self-caring choices, purposefully maintaining a mindful, positive connection. Seek realistic role models that help you to feel good about who you are.

In practice, the MHBIW concepts are best conveyed through simple language using examples, stories, and experiential activities. Interested readers may find it helpful to obtain the *Healthy Bodies* curriculum for engaging methods of effectively teaching these concepts. *The Healthy Body Building Blocks* and *Ten Essential Lessons to Build Body Esteem in Children and*

Adults (Figure 4) demonstrate how the same MHBIW messages may be presented in diverse written formats. For more information, a sample lesson, and other associated handouts to copy for educational purposes, visit www.bodyimagehealth.org.

Conclusion: More remains to be learned about challenging the destructive messages that erode body esteem and cause eating and fitness habits to be devalued. However, in today's milieu of conflicting, counterproductive, and dangerous "solutions," the maxim, "first, do no harm," was never more relevant. A holistic, comprehensive, fundamentally sound, non-contradictory, non-discriminatory approach is essential to reverse the current trend. The MHBIW is a proven, common-sense model promoting health instead of size that satisfies these criteria.

To begin, accept what is *not in your control*:

1) Accept your body's genetic predisposition. All bodies are wired to be fatter, thinner, or in between. This includes fatter in some places and thinner in others. Regardless of efforts to change it, over time your body will fight to maintain or resume the shape it was born to be. You may force your body into sizes and shapes that you prefer, but you can't beat Mother Nature without a tremendous cost.

2) Understand that all bodies change developmentally in ways that are simply not in your control through healthy means. You may positively influence changes of puberty, pregnancy and lactation, menopause, and aging by making healthy lifestyle choices, but you will not "control" these changes, no matter how much you try.

3) Never "diet." Hunger is an internally regulated drive and demands to be satisfied. If you limit the food needed to satiate hunger completely, it will backfire, triggering preoccupation with food and ultimately an overeating or compulsive-eating response. You may lose weight in the short run, but 95% of weight that is lost through dieting is regained, plus added pounds. Dieters who go off their diets only to binge are not "weak willed." They are mammals whose built-in starvation response has kicked in—both physically and psychologically, going after what has been restricted. Scientific evidence has been available on this since the early 1950s, but most people are not aware of the biologically predictable, counterproductive results of "dieting."

Then focus your attention and energy *on what is within your power to achieve*:

4) Satisfy hunger completely with plenty of wholesome, nutrient-rich foods chosen from the core of the food pyramid—*eat well!* In today's world, surrounded by taste-stimulating, cheap, cleverly advertised, readily available, low-nutrient entertainment foods, learning to *feed* your body versus merely *eating* is an essential difference.

5) Limit sedentary entertainment. Move aerobically, if possible, on a regular basis. Everyone who is not medically inhibited, regardless of size, can and should develop a reasonable level of fitness and maintain it throughout the life cycle.

6) Understand that if you eat well and maintain an active lifestyle over time, your best, natural weight will be revealed. Set a goal to eat well and be active. Don't be swayed by whether or not this makes you thin. Healthy, well-fed, active bodies are diverse in size and shape, from fat to thin and everything in between. Don't let anyone tell you otherwise, not even your doctor, who may be caught in unhealthy cultural myths about weight.

7) Choose role models who reflect a realistic standard against which you can feel good about yourself. If the "Ugly Duckling" had continued to compare herself to the ducks, she'd *still* be miserable, no matter how beautifully she developed.

8) Maintain your integrity as a human being. In spite of advertisements seducing you to believe that "image is everything," *never* forget that how you look is only one part of who you are. Develop a sense of identity based on all the many things you can do, the values you believe in, and the person whom you are deep inside.

9) Become media savvy. Educate yourself about the hidden power of advertisements. Advertisers spend tons of money on strategies specifically designed to make you feel there is something wrong with you. Why? If they *first* advertise an unrealistic standard of beauty that leaves you feeling deficient by comparison, a product that promises to improve your condition is an easy sale. Don't be "sold" this bill of goods.

10) Encourage your friends and co-workers to join you in developing a healthy, realistic body image. Use the collective energy your group would have spent on hating your bodies to make the world a better place. Help the next generation to develop healthy body image attitudes and learn positive lifestyle habits too.

Figure 4. Ten Essential Lessons to Build Body Esteem in Children and Adults

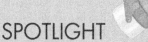

SPOTLIGHT

In the next chapter, Paula Quatromoni and Mary Ellen Bingham discuss a non-diet approach to health promotion for athletes, and offer a number of specific reasons that diets do not work with athletes. Using vignettes from clinical practice, this chapter emphasizes a client-centered counseling model that effectively uses motivational interviewing techniques and non-diet strategies that tailor nutrition education, goal setting, and intervention strategies to the athlete's individual needs and readiness to change. The authors discuss eating disorders in athletes, and appropriate treatment approaches, which include Motivational Interviewing techniques.

Chapter Ten

A Non-Diet Approach for Use with Athletes

Paula Quatromoni and Mary Ellen Bingham

WHY DIETS DON'T WORK FOR ATHLETES

Athletes are particularly vulnerable and willing to try diets. Whether hoping to gain a competitive edge, shave minutes off their time, or feel lighter as they train, athletes use their sport and their performance goals to justify dieting. Athletes are used to pushing themselves beyond their limits. They do whatever it takes to maximize their training and optimize performance. They push through pain and learn to ignore the body signals that tell them to stop and rest their bodies. Athletes know deprivation and they know sacrifice, making them prime candidates for dieting. They take advice from coaches, digesting every word as if it were gospel. They are bombarded with sport-specific products and supplements marketed directly at them, promising results even in the absence of an evidence base to support the claims.

It's not just that athletes are looking for quick fixes to get performance results. They are more than willing to put in the hard work and make dedicated changes to their diets in order to reach a goal. The problem is, athletes can easily become highly restrained and before long, their eating patterns are highly restrictive and regimented, include a very narrow range of a repetitive set of foods consumed every day, and are firmly linked to rigid rules that coincide with rigorous training protocols. Athletes also learn to block out internal stimuli like pain or fatigue to push their training to the limit. As such, they can effortlessly learn to ignore hunger and to dismiss satiety cues, replacing internal stimuli to eat with external stimuli to deprive. This reality makes many athletes "very good" at dieting.

Sports can be very black and white. Your team either wins, or it loses. You place first in a race, or you don't. Your time qualifies you for the finals, or it doesn't. You had a good training workout today, or you didn't. It is natural, then, for athletes to translate that black-and-white thinking that is so engrained in their training and performance onto their assessments of self. "I'm a winner, or a loser." "I'm a success, or a failure." "I'm fast, or I'm slow." "I'm thin (and fast), or I'm fat (and slow)." The black-and-white thinking doesn't stop there. It gets transferred onto food. There are "good" foods for athletes and there are "bad" foods. Good foods are things like sports drinks and power bars. Bad foods are defined differently by different people. Most often, they are foods with attributes that make them less healthy, like too much fat, sugar, or carbohydrate. Sometimes they are nutrient-rich foods, like meats and dairy. Sometimes they're bad because they make you fat. Sometimes it's because they're hard to digest or they make you feel poorly when you're training hard. Sometimes they earn the bad reputation simply because someone else said so. The same way that "good" foods are encouraged to athletes, "bad" foods are discouraged and freely discussed; sometimes with such palpable open criticism that being seen consuming such a food warrants commentary or public humiliation.

Bad foods are foods that other people can eat and enjoy, "but not me, because I'm an athlete!" Bad foods are just about everywhere and they can be impossible to avoid. Bad foods get pushed out of an athlete's diet, little by little, with the best of intentions. Regardless of the nutrients they provide, these foods are perceived as necessary to restrict or to avoid in order to reach a defined goal. Athletes mistakenly believe they can simply replace the micronutrients, like calcium and vitamin D when dairy is omitted, by taking supplements or by adding a sports shake. They move on and they rarely look back at the foods they've left behind, all in the name of sport. One example of this pattern is the adoption of a vegetarian or vegan eating pattern by many athletes. Vegetarians and vegans have unique nutritional needs. Add to that the specialized nutritional needs for an athlete, and the risk for nutritional inadequacy escalates. Without proper nutrition education, guidance, and meal-planning advice from a nutrition professional, athletes can easily become "uninformed vegetarians." These athletes run the risk of compromising their performance in sport and their overall physical health by shortchanging themselves of essential nutrients when faced with the physical demands of training and competition on top of routine needs for growth, repair, maintenance, and immunity.

It is no wonder then that athletes are tempted to diet. Athletes track numbers. They track seconds on a stopwatch; they track miles, laps, reps, and sets; they track wins and losses. It's a natural transition to track other numbers, like numbers on a scale, calories consumed, or calories burned off in a workout.. The same strategy that makes them successful in their sport has the potential to undermine them in the end, because athletes love diets. All too easily, they can become as obsessed with diets as they are with sport, and the two can become inextricably linked.

For some athletes and for some goals, the dieting approach might offer a desirable out-come, at least in the short run. But as a longer-term strategy, dieting is not the answer, no matter how tempting the idea is. Just as training for a triathlon is a long-term process, so too is healthful eating to fuel that athlete for that journey. There is no shortcut to getting in shape for a triathlon. Similarly, there is no shortcut to proper nutrition and crash dieting is not the solution. Here are three specific reasons diets don't work for athletes:

First, dieting is synonymous with weight loss. The myth that an athlete needs to be thin for optimal performance and athletic success is often a firmly held and widely touted belief. In reality, thin is not necessarily associated with peak athletic performance nor is larger neces-sarily associated with poor athletic performance.

Not all athletes need to lose weight, nor should they necessarily lose weight if performance in sport is their number-one goal. A commonly held belief is that thinner and smaller are equated with faster and better in many sports. This is inarguably a common belief expressed by athletes in sports such as gymnastics, track and cross country, swimming, and figure skat-ing. Yet is has also been articulated by soccer players, crew rowers, tennis players, and athletes in many other sports. Athletes will say it. Strength trainers will say it. Coaches will say it. Females will say it. Males will say it. This belief system can drive an athlete to extreme dieting with the solitary goal of achieving optimal performance in sport at any cost. The costs of dieting can be quite high for an athlete. They range from psychosocial stress to physical injury, from chronic hunger and fatigue to dehydration and disordered eating. Poor performance, which is inevitable under these circumstances, is blamed on the athlete's inability to reach goal weight, lack of adherence to the diet, or inadequate training and preparation in sport. Even injuries like repeated stress fractures are not necessarily linked back to chronic dieting or poor nutrition. They are often treated with rest, alternative training regimens, and medical interventions without ever addressing the underlying nutritional risk imposed by dieting that is compromising the athlete's bone health.

Second, dieting provides a scapegoat for criticism that pushes athletes further into the all-or-nothing black-and-white mode of thinking. It is perceived that athletes who don't look like they are at goal weight are "overweight" because they have no willpower, eat too much, and don't train hard enough. This belief makes the overweight athlete a target for differential treatment such as extra workouts or restricted access to food. These special treatments are often publicized and can be demeaning for the athlete, such as labeling the extra workout sessions, "the Chub Club." Just like everyone else, athletes naturally have different body shapes and sizes and different training and competitive regimens that influence body size and shape differently. For those reasons, moving toward acceptance of their bodies, what they can and cannot change, and how their bodies change under different training conditions can help athletes set more realistic goals and have better self-esteem. The non-diet approach can help athletes to embrace their bodies, to work with the strengths and the limitations of their bodies alike, and to value their bodies as contributors to their athletic prowess rather than viewing them as obstacles.

Finally, the belief that everyone can be thin, happy, and healthy by dieting is an understated myth when it comes to athletics. Dieting can be counterproductive for athletes and may compromise athletic performance if too restrictive, preventing proper fueling, adequate hydration, and recovery nutrition. Restrictive diets increase appetite[1], increase the frequency of obsessive thoughts about food[2], increase the risk of depression[3], and increase overeating in response to negative emotions and stress.[4,5] Not surprisingly, dieting often ultimately leads to weight regain, decreased self-esteem, and increased risk for disordered eating among athletes and non-athletes alike. In reality, health and happiness involve a dynamic interaction among mental, social, spiritual, and physical considerations, which are often overlooked among athletes, particularly those whose self-worth and happiness are strongly linked to athletic performance or body image.

Understanding the reasons diets don't work for athletes prompts consideration of an alternative paradigm: the non-diet approach. Also called Health At Every Size (HAES), mindful eating, attuned eating, and intuitive eating, this approach offers a paradigm that is notably different from the one built on the underlying faulty assumptions that diets work and that a diet is what's needed to achieve goals. The non-diet approach emphasizes eating in response to physiologic cues, like hunger and satiety, as regulators of food intake as opposed to dietary restraint, and enhancing body acceptance regardless of whether or not an individual is successful at weight loss.[6] The key features of HAES are that it is weight neutral; it teaches people to rely on internal signals and to eat intuitively rather than relying on external cues to eat; and it encourages positive body esteem in people of all shapes and sizes.[7]

THE NON-DIET APPROACH

The HAES non-diet approach to healthy eating and weight management has been widely described in the literature (and in this book). Studies on the effects of HAES interventions in overweight adult women show significant improvements in psychological outcomes including depression, reduction of disinhibition, susceptibility to hunger and/or binge-eating behaviors, and decreased tendencies to overeat compared to women on conventional diets.[6,8–13] While the HAES literature is relatively limited in scope and duration, the results of six randomized clinical trials and several studies that did not include a control group all show positive results and impressive retention rates specifically in HAES study groups.[6,8,9,11,12,14] Compared to weight-loss plans, the HAES approach is associated with statistically significant and clinically relevant improvements in physiological measures (blood pressure and blood lipids), health behaviors (eating behaviors, activity habits, and dietary quality), and psychosocial outcomes (self-esteem and body image).[15] The observation that psychological parameters are positively impacted even in the absence of significant weight loss in HAES intervention studies is particularly noteworthy. In fact, HAES is emerging as the standard of practice in the eating disorder field. The Academy of Eating Disorders, the National Eating Disorder Association, and other expert groups explicitly support the HAES non-diet approach to healthy eating.[16]

There is considerable evidence that intuitive eating can be learned and is associated with reduced eating disorder symptomatology.[14,17,18]

NON-DIET APPROACH FOR ATHLETES

A guiding principle of HAES is the promotion of eating in a manner that balances individual nutritional needs, hunger, satiety, appetite, and pleasure.[11] This principle makes HAES the ideal alternative to dieting for use with athletes. Developing skills to differentiate real feelings of hunger from external stimuli may be a key aspect of HAES that is particularly relevant for athletes. HAES teaches an athlete to rely on internal regulation through the process of intuitive eating which encourages increased awareness of the body's response to food. In this way, the athlete learns to make food choices that reflect his or her own "body knowledge."[15] Specifically, HAES encourages athletes to connect what they eat to how they feel in the short and medium term. HAES encourages the individual to pay attention to food and the body's physiologic response to it, mood, concentration, energy levels, fullness, appetite, satiety, and comfort eating. In this model, food is valued for its nutritional, psychological, sensual, cultural, social, and in the case of athletes, performance-related attributes.

The HAES focus on body acceptance is another relevant theme for athletes. Critics of HAES fear that encouraging body acceptance will cause an individual to eat with abandon and disregard dietary considerations altogether, leading to weight gain.[15] This, however, has been disproven by the evidence among the populations studied to date. Not a single randomized trial testing the HAES plan has resulted in weight gain.[11,12,14,19] Several studies show that intuitive eating is associated with lower body mass index (BMI).[17,20,21] Further, in studies that reported dietary quality or eating behavior outcomes, improvements or at least maintenance was observed, not worsening.[6,8,11,12,14,22–26] This finding is in direct contrast to what is seen when people are put on conventional diets; over time, even in the most carefully executed clinical studies with plenty of resources to support education, counseling, and behavior change, participants gain back the weight that was lost.[27–33]

To our knowledge, HAES has not yet been described in published observations or interventions involving athlete populations, in spite of its obvious applicability and utility within the niche of sports nutrition. This is an important area for future research and professional development. The HAES paradigm readily extends to athletes and their unique circumstances. In the remainder of this chapter, clinical applications of the non-diet approach to working with athletes will be described in detail, as this model is extended to the athlete population and informed by clinical practice. Table 1 summarizes the underlying assumptions in the traditional weight loss paradigm, the HAES principles, and how these principles are adapted for athletes.

Experts propose that traditional dieting that encourages dietary restraint may be particularly contraindicated for women with a history of chronic dieting.[6] That same caution could be extended to athletes as a group at high risk for adverse dieting outcomes. Using the same three arguments laid out previously that link dieting to feelings of failure[6], consider the following realities from the context of the athletes' unique vulnerability. First, restrictive eating has a history of failing to achieve long-term weight loss[27,35–37] and this failure has been damaging to self-esteem.[38] From the sports-psychology literature, it is known that low self-esteem, sub-par self-confidence, and mental unpreparedness can do as much to undermine an athlete's performance as poor nutrition, improper hydration, and inadequate physical conditioning. Second, weight-loss failure may be damaging to a person's overall self-image, particularly for those who place an inordinate amount of importance on their weight and body shape when evaluating themselves as a person.[39] This is particularly true of athletes who define their self-worth not only in terms of their weight and body shape, but also in terms of their athletic performance, which, in their mind or in the mind of their

Table 1. Comparing Underlying Assumptions

Traditional Weight Loss Paradigm	Health At Every Size	Health At Every Size for Athletes
Everyone needs to be thin for good health and happiness.	Thin is not intrinsically healthy and beautiful, nor is fat intrinsically unhealthy and unappealing.	Thin is not necessarily associated with peak athletic performance nor is larger necessarily associated with poor athletic performance.
People who are not thin are "overweight" because they have no willpower, eat too much, and don't move enough.	People naturally have different body shapes and sizes and different preferences for physical activity.	Athletes naturally have different body shapes and sizes, and different training and competitive regimens influence body size and shape differently. Similarly, athletes in different sports with different training regimens have unique nutritional needs that set them apart from athletes in other sports and from non-athletes.
Everyone can be thin, happy, and healthy by dieting.	Dieting often ultimately leads to further weight gain, decreased self-esteem, and increased risk for disordered eating. Health and happiness involve a dynamic interaction among mental, social, spiritual and physical considerations.	Dieting can be counterproductive for athletes and may compromise athletic performance if too restrictive in a way that prevents proper fueling, adequate hydration, and recovery nutrition. Dieting often ultimately leads to weight re-gain, decreased self-esteem, and increased risk for disordered eating among athletes. Health and happiness involve a dynamic interaction among mental, social, spiritual and physical considerations which are often overlooked among athletes, particularly those whose self worth and happiness are strongly linked to athletic performance.

Adapted with permission from Robison J. Health at Every Size: Toward a New Paradigm of Weight and Health. MedGenMed. 2005; 7(3):13.

coach, may be firmly tied to their weight or body shape/size. And finally, restrictive eating has the potential to intensify the dieting and overeating/binge-eating cycle.[4,40] This cycle is the hallmark of the beginning stages of disordered eating. Since athletes are particularly vulnerable to disordered eating and experience eating disorders at a higher rate than the general public[41], this aspect of dieting is quite problematic in the setting of athletics. It is therefore likely that athletes have a low potential for success using traditional dieting approaches. Athletes will likely be better served by a non-diet approach that focuses on positive messages of inclusion that will reduce restrictive eating behaviors and improve overall health and athletic performance.

Recently, the American College of Sports Medicine (ACSM) and the Academy of Nutrition and Dietetics (AND)[42] updated their statement on weight management strategies for athletes based on a prior summary of evidence[43] and these expert professional groups do not recommend dieting. Rather, their strategies are in line with a non-diet approach to health promotion for athletes. Their guidelines emphasize setting personal and realistic weight and body composition goals; encouraging less focus on the scale and more on healthful habits such as making quality food choices and managing stress; monitoring progress by measuring changes in exercise performance and energy level, the prevention of injuries, normal menstrual function, and overall well-being; and helping athletes develop lifestyle habits that achieve and maintain a healthful weight that is self-defined rather than defined by their sport, coach, teammate, or for any other reason. Athletes are advised not to go on diets, even in the short term. It is recommended that athletes not skip meals, especially breakfast; avoid becoming overly hungry; be prepared by having nutritious snacks available throughout the day, as in "book-ending" workouts with nutrient-dense snacks pre- and post-exercise; not deprive themselves of favorite foods or set unrealistic or rigid dietary rules, but rather to keep eating patterns flexible and goals achievable; avoid categorizing foods as "good" and "bad"; undertake some self-assessment in order to identify their own personal dietary challenges and to plan strategies for dealing with them; and work toward making lifelong dietary changes to sustain a healthful weight and optimal nutritional status.

Letting go of firmly held beliefs about dieting and nutrition for sports performance can be frightening for athletes. As it feels precarious for anyone to relinquish old habits and shift attitudes toward a new way of thinking, it can be particularly difficult for athletes to challenge conventional wisdom or depart from a coach's advice. Replacing entrenched habits and dieting belief systems with a new, non-diet strategy requires trust, commitment, and assistance. The role of the professional sports nutritionist is to provide those tools to assist athletes in making the journey toward embracing the HAES way of life.

Spotlight: A male collegiate track star became obsessed with a new strategy that he believed would help him lose weight and consequently post faster race times. His goal was to get the daily dose of nutrients he needed but consumed in the smallest gram weight amount of food possible. His strategy was aimed specifically at minimizing the weight of food in his GI tract, believing that he would run faster if he were lighter, including inside his visceral organs. In spite of the fact that his body fat was measured at 3.1% (where 3%–5% is considered "essential fat" for a male[44]) and his BMI was 21 (indicating that he had substantial muscle mass on his 6' frame), he considered himself "fat and slow" and in need of weight loss. Daily, he took several vitamin/mineral supplements including calcium, vitamin D, iron, and B-vitamins. For food, he ate only sports bars and a couple of daily servings of fruit to provide the minimal amount of calories, protein, carbohydrates, and fats that would sustain him. Sports bars had a "halo effect" for this athlete, perceived as nutritionally superior to other food choices simply because they are marketed to athletes. When used, they are meant to be used as snacks and as convenient grab-and-go foods to enhance fueling or recovery nutrition, not as meal replacements.

In this example, sports bars were misused to an extreme based on a faulty belief system that "lighter means faster" and that these "super foods" made specifically for athletes will "do no harm" and will somehow provide all the nutrition an athlete needs if the right number of them are eaten over the course of the day. This athlete created the illusion for himself that he was in fact eating meals, by varying his choice of sports bars flavors, brands, and varieties throughout the day and carefully planning which bars to consume at which meal. Needless to say, the success of this strategy was limited not only by the faulty nutrition principles upon which it was based, but also by the athlete's inability to restrict himself from real food to this extreme extent for very long. This scenario describes only one of several cycles of disordered eating that this athlete succumbed to during a six-year career as a collegiate athlete. Over the course of six years, this athlete worked with a sports nutritionist to address his chronic need to diet and to lose weight in order to be the best athlete he could be. He cycled through periods of recovery, readiness to change, and improved nutrition that were highlighted by incredible achievements on the track. He also experienced several periods of relapse where he reverted to restrictive eating so severe that he became weak, injured, underperforming, and depressed. The importance of ongoing education, counseling, support, and monitoring by nutrition professionals is underscored by this example. The other lesson here speaks to the success of the non-diet approach. With the help of the nutritionist, when he was able to break free from the dieting mentality and work on sports nutrition goals that normalized and embraced healthy eating patterns that included whole foods, disentangled fact from fiction, and addressed faulty belief systems, he achieved his goals both on and off the track. He later acknowledged that his work with a sports nutritionist in college saved his track career, and he described it as both life-changing and life-saving.

ASSESSMENT AND COUNSELING
STRATEGIES FOR ATHLETES

There are several tools that a dietitian uses to assess nutritional risk in clients. The broad domains of nutritional assessment include Anthropometry, Biochemical, Clinical, and Dietary assessments. With athletes, all of the conventional tools apply. However, it is important that the sports nutritionist know her clientele well, choose carefully from among her assessment and monitoring tools, introduce and sequence them appropriately according to the unique needs of the individual client, and remain flexible with the understanding that some tools work well whereas others can completely sabotage an ongoing working relationship with an athlete. Interactions that are successful are those in which the nutrition professional is knowledgeable and competent in dealing with sport-specific nutritional needs and challenges; is a patient and reflective listener; uses motivational interviewing techniques effectively (refer to Chapter 3); and acts as a facilitator of change rather than as an authoritative expert who tells the client what he or she needs to do. Putting athletes on the scale and computing BMI in the first visit is not appropriate as a standard of practice to apply to every athlete who walks through the door. Focusing on the scale, rather than on performance goals or even body fat as a more appropriate anthropometry tool, is a mistake made by some clinicians. Similarly, assuming that restoration of body weight in an athlete suffering from anorexia is the hallmark of recovery is a faulty assumption. Psychopathology, unhealthy relationships with food, and chaotic eating patterns linger long after weight is restored and require ongoing counseling and support for most individuals to effectively move into and remain in recovery. Finally, making assessments and recommendations that are not based on relevant facts in the athlete's daily life is another surefire way to sabotage the working relationship when the dietitian instructs rather than assesses; talks rather than listens and observes.

In general, while interdisciplinary collaboration with other sports medicine professionals is often required, it is important that the nutrition professional not medicalize the situation right off the bat, particularly when assessing disordered eating in athletes. Athletes perceive themselves as healthy, fit, strong, and sometimes, super-human. Even those with eating disorders that meet clinical diagnostic criteria do not typically consider themselves to be sick, weak, or suffering. The benign perception of disordered eating is unusually high among athletes who often consider their eating behaviors and dieting strategies necessary components of their training regimen and badges of honor that demonstrate their commitment as an elite athlete. When suggesting a referral to sports psychology for a college-aged athlete struggling with the psychopathology of disordered eating, a common response is, "I'm not that bad! I don't need to see a therapist."

Spotlight: A female collegiate athlete is referred by her coach for nutrition assessment because he considers her notably underweight. The athlete reports to the dietitian,

"In high school, they made me see a nutritionist. She told me I had an eating disorder. So my parents said that I didn't have to go back." That single interaction effectively ended this athlete's involvement with nutrition assessment, education, counseling, or rehabilitation before it even got started. After a few years of working with a less-confrontational professional who took an approach that was more sensitive to where the athlete was coming from, this athlete finally acknowledged that she was suffering from anorexia athletica, which is a disorder characterized by excessive, obsessive exercise and restriction of food intake. When she finally admitted to herself that she did, in fact, have an eating disorder, she defined it in a category reserved for athletes, as if her eating disorder were more noble than regular anorexia nervosa. Regardless of how she defined the disorder for herself and for others, the fact that she acknowledged the disorder and was now committed to recovering from it was heavily influenced by the approach that a different clinician took with this client.

ASSESSING DIETARY INTAKE

When obtaining dietary recalls from athletes, it is important to utilize the motivational interviewing strategy of avoiding close-ended questions and asking open-ended ones. One strategy is to say to the client, "Walk me through what you consider to be a typical day for you, and tell me about the foods and beverages you ate." This kind of open invitation to talk allows the client to speak from the perspective that is personally most salient when it comes to their eating habits. Where they choose to start and what they choose to share actually tells the nutritionist a lot. Allow the client to recall and report as much as they want before going back and asking for clarification or details such as the contents or the timing of specific meals and snacks. Listen for the broad strokes, then go back and carefully probe for details. Avoid questions or comments that imply that you are judging the client.

Food records can be extremely valuable tools but the choice to use them will depend on the type of client. For some clients, recording everything they are eating can be a trigger for disordered eating or may not yield honest reports. It is very important to assess whether or not this will be a valuable tool for your client. The value of a food record is often less about counting calories or monitoring portion sizes and more about acquiring information regarding the client's behavioral patterns, nutritional quality and variety of foods consumed, meal/snack times, emotional cues, and responses to eating. Food record forms that contain columns for clients to note their feelings associated with eating episodes are particularly useful and can stimulate interesting discussion by uncovering important clues that the client might otherwise not readily report in a counseling session. In addition, information about self-perceived hunger and satiety levels before and after eating can be extremely valuable for athletes to report on a food record. You can provide the client with a hunger and satiety scale where a value of 1 represents "starving" and 10 represents "completely stuffed" (refer to Chapter 13). This exercise is particularly important for athletes who no longer recognize or respond to hunger and satiety cues because they have blunted these perceptions as a part of either restrictive eating or binge-eating disorders.

> **Spotlight**: A female runner recorded that at 10 p.m., she ate 10 cherry tomatoes. In the "feelings" column, she wrote a single word: GUILTY. When the nutritionist said, "tell me about this," the athlete responded that she felt guilty for having broken her rule, which was not to eat any food after 8 p.m. This information was critical for quickly identifying a red flag related to rigid rules governing this athlete's food intake pattern. While cherry tomatoes were a nutritious, fat-free food eaten in a very appropriate portion, the athlete was wracked with guilt over eating even a healthy food outside the parameters she had defined for herself, ruled by the clock.

COUNSELING ACCORDING TO READINESS TO CHANGE

Athletes are highly motivated to make changes that they believe will enhance their performance or support their training goals. With this in mind, they are sometimes more willing to jump into action than other clients who present for nutrition services. It is important, however, to carefully assess a client's readiness to change[45] before setting goals and deciding on strategies for behavior change. For example, a client may willingly seek nutrition counseling because she is eager to change her diet, more specifically, to learn how to further control and restrict her food intake or how to tailor a low-calorie diet that will help her drop body fat to be a faster sprinter in the pool. When upon assessment the nutrition professional uncovers disordered eating and makes a referral to sports psychology, the athlete may be completely resistant to the mental health intervention. So while this athlete was very ready to change her eating behaviors (to the extent and in the direction she personally had in mind), she was not ready to address the psychopathology that underscored her eating disorder. Careful assessment, done with the aid of motivational interviewing and other techniques, can lead to accurate assessment of a client's readiness to change and appropriate tailoring of intervention strategies accordingly. The following vignettes provide illustrations of strategies according to stages of change.

> A softball player who is sent to the dietitian by her coach comes to the appointment out of obligation and makes it clear that she doesn't want to be there. "What I'm doing is working just fine. I've been bulimic since I was 13, that day when my father made a comment to me at the breakfast table about my breasts developing. This is just what I do. I almost passed out on the erg machine last week. But it was

no big deal. I figured it would happen sooner or later." This athlete is in the **Pre-Contemplation** stage of readiness. In short, she is not ready to change anything. She does not consider her eating disorder to be a problem, nor has she explored the root causes of her disorder. A female soccer player is distressed by increase in the size of her thighs as a result of the strength and conditioning program she's subjected to in college. Suddenly, her jeans no longer fit, at least not during the in-season period of the year when training is at its peak. Perceiving this enlargement of her body, she thinks she needs to diet. She is overwhelmed because she knows she needs carbs in her diet to fuel her workouts and can't imagine doing what it takes to starve herself all day long and only allow herself salad at dinner. This athlete is in the **Contemplation** stage of readiness. She is thinking about making changes but is somewhat paralyzed from doing so, in part because she has defined "fit and healthy" in terms of "all or nothing." This is a common mindset for athletes and it can have a detrimental effect on performance and on behaviors. If she is fit and strong (i.e., has big thighs from strength and conditioning), then she's "too big" to be attractive or to look good in her jeans. If she diets to fit into those jeans again, she'll have to dramatically cut a lot of food from her diet and that could affect her social life, her focus in school, and maybe even her performance on the field. Unable to do anything because of the high stakes associated with several unappealing options, the athlete just lives in a state of stress. A nutrition professional can help this athlete using tools of assessment, education, and counseling to address this black-and-white thinking and being to work on small, manageable changes with client-driven goal setting. A female runner seeks nutrition advice to improve her diet, but she doesn't really know how to go about it and isn't quite sure what she needs to change. She is actively searching for information to better understand how nutrition can enhance her performance. She observes her teammates and listens to their advice; however, she is concerned because some of what she observes borders on unhealthy eating, in her opinion. Yet, she is unsure if this is what it takes to be an elite athlete. She spends lots of time reading about professional athletes and wonders "what do they eat?" This athlete is in the **Preparation** stage of readiness; she is open to ideas and suggestions but has not yet been able to implement any changes. She is also quite impressionable and is so eager to get it right that she could fall prey to fad diets, gimmicks, or disordered eating. She's not at all sure where to start, but through careful assessment, the dietitian identifies protein adequacy as an obvious goal since the athlete eats a low-fat, high-carbohydrate diet that is pretty rich in fiber but quite lacking in protein. By skipping lunch, she is missing a midday opportunity of specifically getting protein into her diet. The client might be willing to set a very specific goal, "To add a midday eating episode that includes protein." The nutritionist can help the client take ownership for this goal by using the Importance/Confidence Scaling technique, (refer to Chapter 3). This evaluation can lead to an in-depth discussion of strategies to enhance the client's confidence through knowledge of food sources of protein, skills to plan, purchase, or prepare protein foods for a midday meal, and self-monitoring to ensure follow through on goal setting.

Athletes who walk through the door and are already embracing healthy eating have fully bought into the concepts of performance nutrition and are actively making conscious choices to eat well are in the **Action** stage of change. Nonetheless, these athletes need guidance to fine tune their strategies or may need specific advice, like for recovery nutrition, tips for dealing with GI distress on game day, or guidelines for hydration. Goal-setting tools and traditional education and counseling strategies to provide knowledge, build skills, and enhance confidence in making behavioral changes are appropriate for use with these athletes. Nutritionists help athletes in action to identify useful resources to improve the quality of their diets, like tips for purchasing food and planning meals on a limited budget, recipes for quick meals that get more vegetables into their daily diets, or recommendations for healthy choices in restaurants when eating on the road when their team travels for away games. Each of these goals will enhance athletic performance and can be achieved via small, realistic changes. A focus on intuitive eating is an appropriate skill for athletes who are in action. This refers to eating in response to hunger and satiety cues, and to feed yourself when you are hungry and to stop eating when you are satisfied and full (see chapters 2 and 15 for more on intuitive eating). Athletes who are practicing new dietary behaviors and are working to sustain them are in the **Maintenance** stage of change. These athletes still benefit from working with nutrition professionals so that they can discuss and acknowledge what is going well for them and identify new goals that become apparent over time. The role of the nutritionist is to support ongoing behavioral changes and to praise and reinforce achievements. Focusing on skills that support intuitive eating is highly relevant for athletes in the maintenance stage of change. An ongoing working relationship with a nutrition professional allows the client to explore contributors to successful maintenance of healthy eating as well as potential challenges and obstacles, like social situations, interpersonal dynamics, or food environments. Finally, athletes who go back to old (unhealthy) dietary behaviors that are counterproductive to their personal goals and may sabotage performance are in **Relapse**. This stage of change is normal and is expected, particularly early in the continuum of change. Athletes need help understanding that relapse is both normal and expected. Their all-or-nothing mindset may convince them otherwise and can lead to feelings of failure and hopelessness. These negative reactions can worsen a relapse and may cause the athlete to fall far back to the pre-contemplation stage. Some athletes can move through relapse and back into action, but many cannot. The importance of a consistent therapeutic process to guide the athlete through relapse cannot be overstated in this situation. For athletes with disordered eating, several periods of relapse may occur throughout a typical recovery journey that may span five years or more. Nutrition professionals can help the athlete to explore contributors to relapse and problem-solve how to manage triggers.

CONCLUSION

Athletes have unique nutritional needs related to intake, assessment, counseling, and intervention strategies. At the core of a successful strategy for meeting the special needs of athletes is a trusting and honest working relationship with a nutrition professional. A non-diet approach to healthy eating is advocated, with client-driven goal setting and tools of motivational interviewing guiding the pursuit of individualized goals. Strategies that promote positive and empowering messages that encourage athletes to focus on foods to include to maximize nutrition rather than to focus on foods to restrict or avoid are recommended. Nutritionists are expected to provide action-oriented guidance and skills that build behavioral competency to help athletes get the hydration and the nutrients they need from whole foods consumed in the context of a balanced meal plan. Special expertise in identifying and treating disordered eating is important for nutrition professionals working with athletes. Where possible, involvement of other health professionals is recommended to establish a multidisciplinary collaborative team that can most effectively serve the best interests of the athlete.

References

1. Doucet E, Imbeault P, St. Pierre S, et al. 2000. "Appetite After Weight Loss by Energy Restriction and a Low-Fat Diet-Exercise Follow-Up." *Int J Obes Relat Metab Disord.*, 24:906–14.

2. Hart KE and Chiovari P. 1998. "Inhibition of Eating Behavior: Negative Cognitive Effects of Dieting." *J Clin Psychol.*, 54:427–30.

3. Chaput JP, Drapeau V, Hetherington M, Lemieux S, Provencher V, and Tremblay A. 2007. "Psychobiological Effects Observed in Obese Men Experiencing Body Weight Loss Plateau." *Depress Anxiety*, 24:518–521.

4. Polivy J and Herman CP. 1985. "Dieting and Binging. A Causal Analysis." *Am Psychol.*, 40:193–201.

5. Polivy J. 1996. "Psychological Consequences of Food Restriction." *J Am Diet Assoc.*, 96:589–592.

6. Bacon L, Keim NL, Van Loan MD, et al. 2002. "Evaluating a 'Non-Diet' Wellness Intervention for Improvement of Metabolic Fitness, Psychological Well-Being and Eating and Activity Behaviors." *Int J Obes Relat Metab Disord.*, 26:854–65.

7. Aphramor L. 2010. "Validity of Claims Made in Weight Management Research: A Narrative Review of Dietetic Articles." *Nutrition Journal*, 9:30–8.

8. Provencher V, Begin C, Tremblay A, Mongeau L, Boivin S, and Lemieux S. 2007. "Short-Term Effects of a 'Health-At-Every-Size' Approach on Eating Behaviors and Appetite Ratings." *Obesity*, 15:957–966.

9. Ciliska D. 1998. "Evaluation of Two Nondieting Interventions for Obese Women." *West J Nurs Res.*, 20:119–35.

10. Nauta H, Hospers H, and Jansen A. 2001. "One-Year Follow-Up Effects of Two Obesity Treatments on Psychological Well-Being and Weight." *Br J Health Psychol.*, 6:271–84.

11. Bacon L, Stern JS, Van Loan MD, and Keim NL. 2005. "Size Acceptance and Intuitive Eating Improve Health for Obese, Female Chronic Dieters." *J Am Diet Assoc.*, 105:929–36.

12. Rapoport L, Clark M, and Wardle J. 2000. "Evaluation of a Modified Cognitive Behavioural Programme for Weight Management." *Int J Obes Relat Metab Disord.*, 24:1726–1737.

13. Higgins LC and Gray W. 1998. "Changing the Body Image Concern and Eating Behaviour of Chronic Dieters: The Effects of a Psychoeducational Intervention." *Psychol Health*, 13:1045–60.

14. Provencher V, Begin C, Tremblay A, et al. 2009. "Health-At-Every-Size and Eating Behaviors: 1-Year Follow-Up Results of a Size Acceptance Intervention." *J Am Diet Assoc.*, 109:1854–61.

15. Bacon L and Aphramor L. 2011. "Weight Science: Evaluating the Evidence for a Paradigm Shift." *Nutrition Journal*, 10:9–21.

16. Medical News Today. 2009. "Eating Disorder Organizations Join Forces to Urge Focus on Health and Lifestyle Rather Than Weight."

17. Tylka T. 2006. "Development and Psychometric Evaluation of a Measure of Intuitive Eating." *J Couns Psychol.*, 53:226–40.

18. Kristeller J and Hallett C. 1999. "An Exploratory Study of a Meditation-Based Intervention for Binge Eating Disorder." *J Health Psychol.*, 4:357–63.

19. Goodrick GK, Poston WSC II, Kimball KT, Reeves RS, and Foreyt JP. 1998. "Nondieting versus Dieting Treatment for Overweight Binge-Eating Women." *J Consult Clin Psychol.*, 66:363–8.

20. Smith T and Hawks S. 2006. "Intuitive Eating, Diet Composition and the Meaning of Food in Healthy Weight Promotion." *Am J Health Educ.*, 37:130–6.

21. Hawks S, Madanat H, Hawks J, and Harris A. 2005. "The Relationship Between Intuitive Eating and Health Indicators Among College Women." *Am J Health Educ.*, 36:331–6.

22. Tanco S, Linden W, and Earle T. 1998. "Well-Being and Morbid Obesity in Women: A Controlled Therapy Evaluation." *Int J Eat Disord.*, 23:325–39.

23. Miller WC, Wallace JP, Eggert KE, and Lindeman AK. 1993. "Cardiovascular Risk Reduction in a Self-Taught, Self-Administered Weight Loss Program Called the Nondiet Diet." *Med Exerc Nutr Health*, 2:218–23.

24. Steinhardt M, Bezner J, and Adams T. 1999. "Outcomes of a Traditional Weight Control Program and a Nondiet Alternative: A One-Year Comparison." *J Psychol.*, 133:495–513.

25. Carrier KM, Steinhardt MA, and Bowman S. 1993. "Rethinking Traditional Weight Management Programs: A 3-Year Follow-Up Evaluation of a New Approach." *J Psychol.*, 128:517–35.

26. Omichinski L and Harrison KR. 1995. Reduction of dieting attitudes and practices after participation in a non-diet lifestyle program. *J Can Diet Assoc.*, 56:81–5.

27. French SA, Jeffrey RW, Forster JL, McGovern PG, Kelder SH, and Baxter J. 1994. Predictors of weight change over two years among a population of working adults: The Healthy Worker Project. *Int J Obes.*, 18:145–54.

28. Stice E, Cameron RP, Killen JD, Hayward C, and Taylor CB. 1999. Naturalistic weight reduction efforts prospectively predict growth in relative weight and onset of obesity among female adolescents. *J Consult Clin Psychol.*, 67:967–74.

29. Coakley EH, Rimm EB, Colditz G, Kawachi I, and Willett W. 1998. "Predictors of Weight Change in Men: Results from the Health Professionals Follow-Up Study." *Int J Obes Relat Metab Disord.*, 22:89–96.

30. Bild DE, Sholinksy P, Smith DE, Lewis CE, Hardin JM, and Burke GL. 1996. "Correlates and Predictors of Weight Loss in Young Adults: The CARDIA Study." *Int J Obes Relat Metab Disord.*, 20:47–55.

31. Korkeila M, Rissanen A, Kapriio J, Sorensen TIA, and Koskenvuo M. 1999. "Weight-Loss Attempts and Risk of Major Weight Gain." *Am J Clin Nutr.*, 70:965–73.

32. Neumark-Sztainer D, Wall M, Guo J, Story M, Haines J, and Eisenberg M. 2006. "Obesity, Disordered Eating, and Eating Disorders in a Longitudinal Study of Adolescents: How Do Dieters Fare 5 Years Later?" *J Am Diet Assoc.*, 106:559–68.

33. Field AE, Austin SB, Taylor CB, et al. 2003. "Relation Between Dieting and Weight Change Among Preadolescents and Adolescents." *Pediatrics*, 112:900–6.

34. Robison J. 2005. "Health At Every Size: Toward a New Paradigm of Weight and Health." *Med Gen Med.*, 7(3):13–15.

35. Heatherton TE, Herman CP, and Polivy J. 1991. "Restraint, Weight Loss, and Variability of Body Weight." *J Abnorm Psychol.*, 100:78–83.

36. Klesges RC, Klem ML, Epkins C, and Klesges LM. 1991. "A Longitudinal Evaluation of Dietary Restraint and Its Relationship to Changes in Body Weight." *Addict Behav.*, 16:363–8.

37. Tiggemann M. 1994. "Dietary Restraint as a Predictor of Reported Weight Loss and Affect." *Psychol Rep.*, 75:1679–82.

38. Polivy J and Herman CP. 1999. "The Effects of Resolving to Diet on Restrained and Unrestrained Eaters: The 'False Hope Syndrome.'" *Int J Eating Disord.*, 26:434–47.

39. McFarlane T, Polivy J, and McCabe RE. 1999. "Help, Not Harm: Psychological Foundation for a Nondieting Approach Toward Health." *J Social Iss.*, 55:261–76.

40. Lowe MR. 1993. "The Effects of Dieting on Eating Behavior: A Three Factor Model." *Psychol Bull.*, 114:100–21.

41. Sundgot-Borgen J and Torstveit MK. 2010. "Aspects of Disordered Eating Continuum in Elite High-Intensity Sports." *Scand J Med Sci Sports*, 20(Suppl. 2):112–21.

42. American Dietetic Association, Dietitians of Canada, American College of Sports Medicine, Rodriguez NR, Di Marco NM, and Langley S. 2009. "American College of Sports Medicine Position Stand. Nutrition and Athletic Performance." *Med Sci Sports Exerc.*, 41(3):709–31.

43. Manore MM. 1996. "Chronic Dieting in Active Women: What Are the Health Consequences?" *Womens Health Issues*, 6:332–41.

44. Clark N. 2003. *Nancy Clark's Sports Nutrition Guidebook.* (3rd ed.) Champaign, IL: Human Kinetics. page 182.

45. Norcross JC, Krebs PM, and Prochaska JO. 2011. "Stages of Change." *J Clin Psychol.*, 67(2):143–54.

SPOTLIGHT

In the next chapter, Michelle Neyman Morris discusses the idea of moving away from a weight-centered approach to health and toward a HAES paradigm, specifically in the education and training of dietetics professionals. Her argument that being overweight is the last acceptable prejudice in western culture is important. Dietitians have long been trained to focus on "weight management," which really means losing weight and keeping it off. As noted in previous chapters of this book, trying to influence people to lose weight does not work for many reasons. Morris makes the case that dietetics professionals in particular should shift the paradigm away from a weight-centered idea, and discusses the possible consequences of such changes in attitude and approach.

Chapter Eleven

The Social Justice Imperative for a HAES Paradigm Shift in Dietetics Education and Practice

Michelle Neyman Morris

"Myths about weight are so deeply entrenched that it may be difficult to imagine an alternative and have the courage and means to move toward it." - Linda Bacon, *Health at Every Size: The Surprising Truth About Your Weight*

"It is hard for people to accept the HAES paradigm. People like to believe that being fat is only temporary and that they can escape weight oppression if they just try hard enough, and that they will find happiness when they are thin. It's easier to focus on weight control rather than challenging cultural prejudice." - Reflections of an undergraduate after learning about the HAES paradigm

PRIVILEGE AND OPPRESSION

As noted in previous chapters, increasing evidence points to the need for a paradigm shift away from the conventional weight-based health model and toward a Health at Every Size® approach. The lack of efficacy among weight-loss diets in the long term, and subsequent physical and psychological health risks associated with diets and weight cycling, e.g., increased cortisol levels and perceived stress, depression, reduced self-esteem, body dissatisfaction and increased risk of disordered eating,[1-4] provide ample evidence to call a truce in the "war on obesity." In addition, a *social justice* case for a paradigm shift toward a HAES approach can also be made.

Pharr suggests that those engaging in the work of social justice do so because of a fundamental belief in the value and dignity of every human being, each deserving respect, equality, and justice.[5] Such a view encompasses a broad definition of human rights, which ensures access for all to the basic necessities including food, clothing, and shelter, as well as education, healthcare, safety, and a living wage. These values ideally lead to communities and institutions that support people in maximizing their human growth and potential regardless of race, class, gender, sexuality, or religion. HAES allies believe it is time to add size to this list.

When people are reduced to any single dimension of identity, this typically serves to exclude and silence them, positing them as "other" and as inferior to the norm to which they are compared.[6] Sociologists refer to the "social construction" of reality in which these dimensions are significant only within the systems of privilege and oppression where they were created. Such privilege "exists when one group has something of value denied to another group simply because of the groups they belong to, rather than because of anything they've done or failed to do."[6] Furthermore, all oppressions are interrelated and systemic, based in institutions and general society, where members of the dominant group exert power and control over the subordinate group.[5] Our current health model places thin individuals in the dominant position and overweight and obese individuals as subordinate. Hence, those with "thin privilege" move in the world without the stigma reserved for those classified as overweight or obese.

A history of oppression in this country has led to movements advocating for civil rights for people of color, for women, those with disabilities, and lesbians and gay men. Because of the intersection of all oppressions, we risk lacking integrity if we demand civil rights for one group of people but then perpetuate oppression against others. This sentiment was perhaps best articulated by the Rev. Martin Luther King Jr. during the civil rights movement in his 1963 Letter from Birmingham Jail, "Injustice anywhere is a threat to justice everywhere."[7] In addition, oppressive beliefs become internalized in both victims and perpetrators, thus imposing limitations on us all, regardless of group status. This internalized oppression is evident today in our fat-phobic society and in no small measure fuels an increasingly hostile and violent war on obesity. Recognizing this, size-acceptance advocates have rejected the terms "overweight" and "obesity" and have reclaimed the word "fat" in order to strip it of its pejorative connotation, just as other terms were reclaimed by previously marginalized groups. "Fat" will thus be the term used throughout this chapter.

WEIGHT STIGMA AND DISCRIMINATION

Body-weight discrimination is as prevalent as racial discrimination in our country.[8] While over 60 percent of Americans are considered fat, there is currently no federal legislation to ensure equitable treatment and protection against weight-based discrimination. Instead, fat

Americans are routinely denied access to educational opportunities as well as full access in the workplace and health care settings.[9] Some make the argument that weight loss, especially among children and adolescents who may be especially prone to bullying,[10] is the best defense against discrimination. Yet it would be preposterous to ask any other member of a subordinate group to leave that group for the dominant group in order to escape discrimination. Instead, legislation exists to ensure that those in privileged positions do not deny any individuals their fundamental rights. Why should this be any different for fat Americans? And, what role might each of us play, consciously or unconsciously, in perpetuating their oppression?

Welsh examined the intersections of gender, class, and size oppressions and asserts that a "good health imperative" fuel the war on obesity, especially among women.[11] While feminists agree that it is wrong to equate a woman's value with her looks (including weight), it is acceptable to encourage that same woman to lose weight for "health" reasons. Welsh argues that this good-health imperative glosses over structural socioeconomic reasons for poor health and weight disparities, also known as social determinants of health. In doing so, the individual and her poor choices are identified as the focus. In particular, poor women, who tend to be the primary caretakers of children and suffer disproportionally from nutrition-sensitive diseases, are targeted—thus the war on obesity is not gender or class neutral, since women are disproportionately targeted. Weight stigma and discrimination also contribute to stress, which is related to poor health outcomes, in fact the very chronic diseases associated with "overweight".[12]

A focus on weight and providing simplistic messages such as "eat less, exercise more" are certainly easier than addressing the root causes of income and health inequality in our society. This becomes particularly salient as Kirkpatrick describes the rise of food insecurity and increased need for food assistance resulting from the economic recession.[13-15] Poverty, food insecurity and hunger, and access to quality health care are problems rooted in systemic privilege and oppression and are not addressed so long as we're distracted by prejudicial beliefs that overweight individuals are necessarily unhealthy, and that individuals alone have the power to change their weight. This "personal responsibility" approach negates the substantial role that genes, the built environment, and neurophysiology play in determining our weight,[16] as well as the barriers to eating well that current food policy imposes, especially among low-income Americans. This sets the stage for obesity to be judged as an individual character flaw with morality implications and as long as this is the case, discrimination against fat people will continue.

Weight stigma and discrimination also contribute to rising health care costs. While it is more common to hear that fat Americans are driving up health care costs, it should be noted that using Body Mass Index (BMI) as a proxy for health is not without cost. In one analysis, 42% of healthy people (55 of 132 million) in the "overweight" or "obese" categories were deemed unhealthy and treated with unnecessary tests and procedures, while 18% of those with abnormal cardiometabolic profiles (16 of 92 million) in the "normal weight" category were overlooked, potentially resulting in higher medical costs later.[1] Thus, those with "thin privilege" also suffer the consequences of oppression, by erroneously assuming that they don't need to worry about eating well or being physically active, and this is reinforced by health care providers who are making treatment decisions based on weight.

PUBLIC HEALTH AND NUTRITION POLICY IN THE U.S.

Those in positions of power to set the agenda for nutrition and public health policy in this country are not without bias. For example, the International Obesity Task Force (IOTF) was the driving force behind setting a BMI of 25 as the cutoff for "overweight"[16] *even though most epidemiologic studies indicate that overweight individuals live longer than "normal" weight individuals.*[17,1] It should be noted that the IOTF receives funding from Hoffman-La Roche and Abbott Laboratories (makers of the weight-loss drugs Xenical and Meridia, respectively, and funders of obesity research). Thus, corporate interests having much to lose with a HAES paradigm shift, unduly influence both the research agenda and public-health nutrition policy. Challenging size discrimination requires vigilance in exposing funding sources for the research that leads to messages about weight.

At the federal level, the United States Department of Agriculture is responsible for not only developing and promoting dietary guidance (e.g., Dietary Guidelines for Americans and MyPlate),[18] but also for ensuring the livelihood of farmers and ranchers. This not-so-subtle conflict of interest is also evident in the U.S. Farm Bill, illustrating the power of the food and agriculture industries to influence nutrition and nutrition-education policy.

These industries perpetuate what is in the best interests of their dominant position, including providing the consumer with an abundance of cheap and highly processed food products.[19,20] Satter provides a critique of U.S. nutrition policy and dietary guidance systems, suggesting that they contribute to distorted eating attitudes and behaviors, and recommends the alternative HAES approach.[21]

DIETETIC EDUCATION AND PRACTICE

Among health care professionals, Registered Dietitians (RDs) are positioned as the "nutrition experts" and as such may be complicit in the oppression of larger people. A standard educational path is required for becoming a RD. First, a student must complete an accredited undergraduate Didactic Program in Dietetics. Then they must complete an accredited Dietetic Internship consisting of 1,200 hours of supervised practice in clinical, administrative, and community nutrition settings. Finally, they must pass the national registration exam. Throughout this training, the government-developed dietary guidance and traditional weight-management techniques for "overweight" individuals are taught and used (e.g., portion control, calorie restriction, energy expenditure). Weight management is included in the profession's Nutrition Care Process standardized language[22] and post-credentialing certificates in Weight Management are available.

Dietetic education and training in weight management are problematic for several reasons. First, conventional weight management has a high long-term failure rate,[23,1] and as evidence-based practitioners it seems unreasonable to continue prescribing what we know does not work. Yet, this seems to be the case and confirmation bias may cloud the judgment of researchers and practitioners. Aphramor's literature review of *The Journal of Human Nutrition and Dietetics* from 2004–2008 found that while an energy-deficit approach to weight management has a high long-term failure rate, this approach is still prevalent among research in the field.[24] Furthermore, the research often lacks critical examination of the controversies in the evidence base and optimistic claims frequently misrepresent available data. Aphramor concludes that dietetic literature on weight management fails to meet evidence-based standards.

Second, standard weight-management prescriptions for fat people (e.g., calorie control, restriction of certain foods, exercise for the purpose of burning calories) are some of the very behaviors used to diagnose eating disorders in thin people, for which chronic dieting is a risk factor.[25,26] This is concerning not only for the clients RDs serve, but also for dietetic students. Dietetics is a predominantly white, middle class, female-dominated profession, and the intersections of privilege and oppression operate in this system as well. Dietetic education and training reinforces the internalization of the "thin ideal" and resulting body dissatisfaction that most women are subjected to beginning early in life,[27,28] and supports "helping people lose weight." It should then come as no surprise that dietetic students suffer from disordered eating at higher rates than the general population.[29] While the American Dietetic Association's Position Paper on the Treatment of Eating Disorders (ED) acknowledges the value of the HAES paradigm in treating ED clients, this does not extend to the general population or dietetic students.[30]

Finally, dietetic education and training along with internalized oppression contributes to the weight bias seen among dietetic students. Puhl, Wharton, and Heuer investigated the attitudes of U.S. dietetic students toward "obese" persons and tested whether or not a patient's weight influenced their health evaluations.[31] Participants (92% female, ethnicity not provided) completed the online Fat Phobia Scale to assess weight bias. They also read mock health profiles, differing by weight status and gender, and were asked to make a judgment about the patient's health status. The authors reported that participants displayed a moderate amount of fat phobia and that "obese" patients were judged to be less likely to comply with treatment recommendations and to have poorer diet quality and health status, *despite equivalent nutritional and health information provided across weight categories.* The authors conclude that increasing emphasis on weight bias in dietetics curricula is warranted. Others have noted similar bias among other health professions.[32,33]

The Code of Ethics for the Profession of Dietetics outlines responsibilities to the public, clients, and profession.[34] It stipulates that practitioners use evidence-based principles and current information in their practice and includes a statement prohibiting discrimination, although weight is not included in the list of protected categories. Nor is it included in statements related to valuing diversity.

Pharr notes that it is often easier to talk about diversity than shared power.[5] Dietetic educators, practitioners, and students concerned with social justice must examine the systems of privilege and potential conflicts of interest that influence the nutrition and public health agenda in our country. In addition, corporate influence must be acknowledged. Ultimately, pharmaceutical companies, the diet, beauty, and growing weight-loss surgery industries all stand to benefit from the stigmatization and discrimination of fat people. These industries can make money and maintain their positions of privilege only if consumers internalize the message that FAT=BAD and are willing to spend money in an attempt to become THIN and GOOD. In the past, women were predominantly targeted to change their physical appearance in order to gain status (privilege). More recently men, representing a major source of yet-untapped revenue, are targeted as potential consumers of products and procedures to address their own "weight-management" concerns.

It should also be noted that the leadership of the Academy of Nutrition and Dietetics (AND), formerly the American Dietetic Association (ADA), and professional organization of registered dietitians, routinely establishes partnerships and accepts money from the industrial food complex in order to subsidize their professional meetings and advance their endeavors. Thus, RDs attending conferences to learn about the latest evidence-based research and practice are also bombarded with messages and free products from corporations such as Coca-Cola, McDonald's, General Mills, NutriSystem, Monsanto, and Cargill, Inc.[35] While the "all foods can fit" mantra supports the idea that these companies' products can be part of a healthy diet, the corporations are surely more concerned with their bottom line and shareholders' profit rather than supporting dietary variety. Some RDs voice concern that the "nutrition experts'" messages are being co-opted by food industry. They also view these relationships as a conflict of interest, which is addressed in the Code of Ethics for the profession, yet those in privileged leadership positions are allowed to decide what constitutes a conflict, and to date, none have been noted.

HAES EVIDENCE BASE AND DIETETICS EDUCATION AND PRACTICE

There is limited but growing evidence of the efficacy of HAES interventions in improving health behaviors and physiological and psychosocial outcomes without the deleterious side effects related to dieting and weight cycling.[36–40,1]

If after examining the HAES evidence base we conclude that a paradigm shift is warranted, we must not presume this will be an easy process. Discomfort is likely to ensue when we examine our own positions of privilege, biases, and internalized oppression. In addition, discomfort may arise when we consider new perspectives that lead to cognitive dissonance and requires giving up old ways of knowing and thinking. Honoring and acknowledging that discomfort with our students, colleagues, and clients is a crucial step if we wish to be truly effective social-justice change agents.

Critically examining our own weight (and other) biases and asking students to do the same is also critical to the process. Use of the on-line Implicit Association Test can lead to powerful discussions and shed light on the internalized oppression around weight we have been socialized to accept and perpetuate.[41] Many trained in the dietetics profession may be called to do additional work on healing their relationships with food and their bodies.

It stands to reason that dietetic practitioners may question how a HAES paradigm shift will impact their careers, and their very identity as a RD, especially if much of their career was spent managing weight. The employer/employee power dynamic must also be acknowledged. RDs who have greater autonomy or are in positions of career privilege may more easily navigate a paradigm shift with their boss or organization's culture without risk to their livelihood. If a RD has focused on weight management using traditional methods, they may also wonder what else can be done and what role will they now play as a member of the health care team. But there is much to do: facilitating behavior change using a HAES approach and the tools of motivational interviewing can lead to health improvements.[42] The focus is put on behaviors that the patient or client has control over, instead of weight. And, referrals can be made for facilitating health-enhancing behavior change outside the RD scope of practice.

Among dietetic students, in addition to identifying their own internalized weight bias, they may be required to process conflicting information from instructors who vary in their support of the HAES tenets. We should not shy away from this reality, but use it as an opportunity for rich discussion and critical examination of the systems that define the standard curriculum. In addition, once we start talking about embodiment, or how we live in our bodies, we challenge the way power is embedded in academic institutions generally, and in the nutrition and dietetic fields specifically. Typically, a mind–body split is required of academics, students, and evidence-based practitioners, with intellectual pursuits being prized to the almost complete exclusion of body knowledge. Yet from a HAES perspective, it is imperative that we honor our bodies and the wisdom they hold. Classroom discussion questions might include: what counts as "knowing" and hence "evidence" in dietetics practice? Where does dietetic culture render silence and who decides that? What role might experiential knowledge play in a socially just paradigm? What do those in power and deciding our profession's agenda stand to lose if power is more equitably shared? And what might we all gain?

These types of questions are already being asked by the Critical Dietetics movement, which arose out of a 2009 research workshop held at Ryerson University. Critical Dietetics endorses the HAES paradigm and is informed by transdisciplinary scholarship from the natural and social sciences and humanities and recognizes that the knowledge that enables an understanding of health is socially, culturally, historically, and environmentally constructed.[43] Critical

Dietetics aims to examine our assumptions, explore power relations, and acknowledge that there are no value-free positions, thus creating space for a socially just scholarship and pluralistic development of the profession.

The HAES tenets are making their way into dietetics curriculum and practice as well as in other fields as described by Watkins and Concepcion,[44] (refer to Chapter 12) Education intervention research is beginning to emerge, and more is needed. Brown reported that combining a PowerPoint presentation with reading a peer-reviewed HAES intervention publication led to improved knowledge and attitudes regarding HAES as an evidence-based approach among fitness and health students in a disease prevention course.[45] Using the same validated survey tool as Brown, Neyman Morris, Roitman, and Schneider evaluated the impact of reading and discussing *Health at Every Size: The surprising truth about your weight*[16] on the knowledge and attitudes of senior level dietetics majors enrolled in a community nutrition course.[46] Intervention subjects significantly increased their understanding of ($p < 0.001$), and perceived ability to counsel individuals ($p < 0.05$) and design programs ($p = 0.001$) using a HAES approach to health promotion from pre to posttest. In addition, intervention subjects were significantly less likely to agree that it will be their responsibility as a health professional to help end the obesity epidemic by promoting caloric restriction for overweight and obese people ($p < 0.05$).

Individual HAES tenets such as intuitive or mindful eating can also be incorporated in dietetics curriculum. Clifford, Welden, and Neyman Morris reported that the use of Tribole and Resch's *Intuitive Eating*[47] in a nutrition counseling and education course and Koenig's *The Food and Feelings Workbook*[48] in a lifecycle nutrition course led to significant improvements in Intuitive Eating Scale (IES) scores ($p < 0.001$).[49] IES scores were also significantly and positively correlated with higher levels of self-reported body satisfaction. Moving beyond dietetics and health majors, Neyman Morris, Rios, Bacon, Clifford, and Gray reported that community college students using a HAES-based introductory nutrition textbook[50] significantly improved their mean IES scores and reported positive changes in their shopping and cooking habits and motivators for food choices following the intervention compared to controls.[51] In addition, Alber's *eat, drink, and be mindful* workbook[52] was successfully incorporated in the graduate-level nutrition education curriculum at California State University, Chico in spring 2012, and exposed students to the HAES principles of size acceptance and mindful eating. A HAES general education course, requiring Matz and Frankel's *The Diet Survivor's Handbook*,[53] was offered for the first time in fall 2012 at the same institution. In these courses, students are exposed to the HAES paradigm and are required to critically examine its evidence base.

HAES RESOURCES

Additional research to strengthen the evidence base not only for HAES interventions but also related to student learning outcomes is needed. In addition, HAES continuing professional education opportunities for practitioners offered through AND are warranted. Educators, students, and practitioners wishing to learn more about the socially just HAES paradigm can engage with organizations, including the Association for Size Diversity and Health (www.sizediversityandhealth.org), the National Association to Advance Fat Acceptance (www.naafa.org), Critical Dietetics (www.criticaldietetics.org), and HAES Community (www.haescommunity.org). These professional organizations endorse the HAES tenets, provide on-line resources, conferences, and opportunities for advocacy, networking, and community building—which is essential for those called to challenge the current weight-based health paradigm and discrimination. HAES RDs and other nutrition professionals may also join a listserv specially tailored to their needs by sending an email to: HAESRD-subscribe@yahoogroups.com

HAES ADVOCACY

Dietetic professionals and students are uniquely positioned to be HAES allies advocating for equality at every size. The dietetics profession is bound by a Code of Ethics[34] that requires evidence-based practice, critical thinking, avoidance of any conflict of interest, and respecting diversity. The HAES paradigm is consistent with these values and offers a socially just alternative to the traditional weight-based health paradigm. Many students begin their dietetic education with a profound desire to "help people." Our common humanity requires that we acknowledge and challenge all systems of oppression, and seek comprehensive solutions to multifaceted problems that create barriers to good health for all. When we focus on weight, we miss the opportunity to ask critical questions about the power and privilege that fails to recognize every individual as equally deserving of dignity and respect, and to support them in maximizing their health and human potential. How might we use our privilege as educated professionals to advocate for a HAES paradigm shift in order to best meet the needs of students, practitioners, and the public?

> *"The classroom, with all its limitations, remains a location of possibility. In that field of possibility we have the opportunity to labor for freedom, to demand of ourselves and our comrades, an openness of mind and heart that allows us to face reality even as we collectively imagine ways to move beyond boundaries, to transgress. This is education as the practice of freedom."* – bell hooks, *Teaching to Transgress: Education as the Practice of Freedom.*[54]

"When you have believed for 22 years that your body is inadequate, trying to look at it kindly and treating it with love almost feels like breaking the rules. HAES emphasizes the importance of loving and respecting ourselves and our bodies for all the amazing things they do for us each day. What we love and respect we treat well. I think that might be the main point—love and respect yourself, treat yourself well." - Reflections of an undergraduate after learning about the HAES paradigm

References

1. Bacon, L. and Aphramor, L. 2011. "Weight Science: Evaluating the Evidence for a Paradigm Shift." *Nutrition Journal*, 10, 9.

2. Herman, P. and Polivy, J. 1980. "Restrained Eating." In Stunkard, A. (Ed.) *Obesity*. (pp. 208–225). Philadelphia, PA: Saunders.

3. Matz, J. "In Consultation: Beyond the Diet Mentality." http://www.psychotherapynetworker.org/recentissues/923-in-consultation. Accessed August 17, 2012.

4. Tomiyama, A., Mann, T., Vinas, D., Hunger, J., DeJager, J., and Taylor, S. 2010. "Low Calorie Dieting Increases Cortisol." *Psychosomatic Medicine*, 72(4), 357–364.

5. Pharr, S. 2010. "Reflections on Liberation." In Adams, M., Blumenfeld, C., Castaneda, C., Hackman, H., Peters, M., and Zuniga, X. (Eds.) *Readings for Diversity and Social Justice, 2nd Ed.* (pp. 591–598). New York: Routledge.

6. Johnson, A.G. 2010. "The Social Construction of Difference." In Adams, M., Blumenfeld, C., Castaneda, C., Hackman, H., Peters, M., and Zuniga, X. (Eds.) *Readings for Diversity and Social Justice, 2nd Ed.* (pp. 15–20). New York: Routledge.

7. King, M.L. 1963. "Letter from a Birmingham Jail." http://coursesa.matrix.msu.edu/~hst306/documents/letter.html. Accessed August 20, 2012.

8. Puhl, R., Andreyeva, T., and Brownell, K. 2008. "Perceptions of Weight Discrimination: Prevalence and Comparison to Race and Gender Discrimination in America." *International Journal of Obesity*, 1–9.

9. Puhl, R. and Brownell, K. 2001. "Bias, Discrimination, and Obesity." *Obesity Research*, 9, 788–805.

10. Washington, R. 2011. "Childhood Obesity: Issues of Weight Bias." *Preventing Chronic Disease*, 8(5), A94.

11. Welsh, T. 2011. "Healthism and the Bodies of Women: Pleasure and Discipline in the War Against Obesity." *Journal of Feminist Scholarship*, 1, 33–48.

12. Moore, C. and Cunningham, S. 2012. "Social Position, Psychological Stress, and Obesity: A Systematic Review." *Journal of the Academy of Nutrition and Dietetics*, 112, 518–526.

13. Kirkpatrick, S. 2012. "Understanding and Addressing Barriers to Healthy Eating Among Low-Income Americans." *Journal of the Academy of Nutrition and Dietetics*, 112, 617–620.

14. Coleman-Jensen, A., Nord, M., Andrews, M., and Carlson, S. 2011. "Household Food Security in the United States in 2010." Washington, DC: US Department of Agriculture. Economic Research Report No. 125.

15. Feeding America. 2010. "Hunger in America 2010." http://feedingamerica.org/hunger-in-america/hunger-studies/hunger-study-2010.aspx/. Accessed August 17, 2012.

16. Bacon, L. 2010a. *Health At Every Size: The Surprising Truth About Your Weight.* Dallas, TX: BenBella Books Inc.

17. Flegal, K., Graubard, B., Williamson, D., and Gail, M. 2005. "Excess Deaths Associated with Underweight, Overweight, and Obesity." *Journal of the American Medical Association,* 293(15), 1861–67.

18. United States Department of Agriculture. "Dietary Guidelines" and "MyPlate." http://fnic.nal.usda.gov/dietary-guidance. Accessed August 20, 2012.

19. Nestle, Marion. 2007. *Food Politics: How the Food Industry Influences Nutrition and Health.* Berkeley, CA: University of California Press.

20. Simon, Michele. 2006. *Appetite for Profit: How the Food Industry Undermines Our Health and How to Fight Back.* New York: Nation Books.

21. Satter, E. 2012. "Dietary Guidelines and Food Guide Pyramid Incapacitate Consumers and Contribute to Distorted Eating Attitudes and Behaviors." http://www.ellynsatter.com/resources/diet.pdf. Accessed August 17, 2012.

22. Academy of Nutrition and Dietetics. Nutrition Care Process. http://www.eatright.org/healthProfessionals/content.aspx?id=7077#.UC6izo4ih0d. Accessed August 17, 2012.

23. Mann, T., Tomiyama, J., Westling, E., Lew, A., Samuels, B., and Chatman, J. 2007. "Medicare's Search for Effective Obesity Treatments: Diets Are Not the Answer." *American Psychologist,* 62, 220–233.

24. Aphramor, L. 2010. "Validity of Claims Made in Weight Management Research: A Narrative Review of Dietetic Articles." *Nutrition Journal,* 9, 30.

25. National Eating Disorders Association (NEDA). http://www.nationaleatingdisorders.org/. Accessed August 17, 2012.

26. EAT-26 Self-Test. http://www.eat-26.com/. Accessed August 17, 2012.

27. Ahern, A., Bennett, K., Kelly, M., and Hetherington, M. 2011. "A Qualitative Exploration of Young Women's Attitudes Towards the Thin Ideal." *Journal of Health Psychology,* 16, 70–79.

28. Dohnt, H. and Tiggemann, M. 2006. "Body Image Concerns in Young Girls: The Role of Peers and Media Prior to Adolescence." *Journal of Youth and Adolescence,* 35(2), 141–151.

29. Worobey, J. and Schoenfeld, D. 1999. "Eating Disordered Behavior in Dietetics Students and Students in Other Majors." *Journal of the American Dietetic Association,* 99, 1100–1102.

30. American Dietetic Association. 2011. "Position of the American Dietetic Association: Nutrition Intervention in the Treatment of Eating Disorders." *Journal of the American Dietetic Association,* 111, 1236–1241.

31. Puhl, R., Wharton, C., and Heuer, C. 2009. "Weight Bias Among Dietetics Students: Implications for Treatment Practices." *Journal of the American Dietetic Association,* 109, 438–444.

32. O'Brien, K., Puhl, R., Latner, J., Mir, A., and Hunter, J. 2010. "Reducing Anti-Fat Prejudice in Pre-Service Health Students: A Randomized Trial." *Obesity,* 18(11), 2138–44.

33. Schwartz, B. 2003. "Weight Bias Among Health Professionals." *Obesity Research,* 11, 1033–39.

34. American Dietetic Association. 2009. "American Dietetic Association/Commission on Dietetic Registration Code of Ethics for the Profession of Dietetics and Process for Consideration of Ethics Issues." *Journal of the American Dietetic Association,* 109(8), 1461–67.

35. Academy of Nutrition and Dietetics. (2012). Food and Nutrition Conference & Expo. Member Product Marketplace http://s19.a2zinc.net/clients/Academy/fnce2012/public/Content.aspx?ID=1302&sortMenu =103000. Accessed August 17, 2012.

36. Bacon, L., Keim, N., Van Loan, M., Derricote, M., Gale, B., Kazaks, A., and Stern, J. 2002. "Evaluating a 'Non-Diet' Wellness Intervention for Improvement of Metabolic Fitness, Psychological Well-Being and Eating and Activity Behaviors." *International Journal of Obesity,* 26, 854–865.

37. Bacon, L., Stern, J, Van Loan, M., and Keim, N. 2005. "Size Acceptance and Intuitive Eating Improve Health for Obese, Female Chronic Dieters." Journal of American Dietetic Association, 105, 929–936.

38. Provencher, V., Begin, C., Tremblay, A., Mongeau, L., Corneau, L., Dodin, S., Boivin, S., and Lemieux, S. 2009. "Health-At-Every-Size and Eating Behaviors: 1-Year Follow-Up Results of a Size Acceptance Intervention." *Journal of the American Dietetic Association,* 109, 1854–1861.

39. Ciliska D. 1998. "Evaluation of Two Nondieting Interventions for Obese Women." *Western Journal of Nursing Research,* 20, 119–135.

40. Rapoport, L., Clark, M., and Wardle, J. 2000. "Evaluation of a Modified Cognitive-Behavioural Programme for Weight Management." *International Journal of Obesity,* 24, 1726–1737.

41. Project Implicit. https://implicit.harvard.edu/implicit/. Accessed August 9, 2012.

42. Aphramor, L. 2011. "Dietetics, Weight Science and Ethics: Time to Look Again?" *NHD Magazine,* 70, 10–13.

43. Critical Dietetics: A Declaration. 2009. http://www.criticaldietetics.org/PDF/Critical%20Dietetics%20 Declaration.pdf. Accessed August 9, 2012.

44. Watkins, P. and Concepcion, R. 2023. "Teaching HAES to Health Care Professionals and Students." In Wellness, Not Weight: Health At Every Size and Motivational Interviewing".

45. Brown, L. 2009. "Teaching the 'Health At Every Size' Paradigm Benefits Future Fitness and Health Professionals." *Journal of Nutrition Education and Behavior,* 41(2), 144–145.

46. Neyman Morris, M., Roitman, A., and Schneider, J. 2010. "Reading 'Health at Every Size': The Surprising Truth About Your Weight Improves Non-Diet Approach Knowledge and Attitudes Among Dietetics Students." *Journal of the American Dietetic Association*, 110(9), Supplement, A57.

47. Tribole, E. and Resch, E. 2003. *Intuitive Eating: A Revolutionary Program That Works* (2nd ed.). New York: St. Martin's Press.

48. Koenig, K. 2007. *The Food and Feelings Workbook: A Full Course Meal on Emotional Health.* Carlsbad, CA: Gurze Books.

49. Clifford, D., Welden, V., and Neyman Morris, M. 2009. "A Pilot Study to Evaluate the Impact of Non-Diet Approach Books on Intuitive Eating Scores Among Dietetics Students." *Journal of the American Dietetic Association,* 109(9), Supplement, A55.

50. Bacon, Linda and Aphramor, Lucy. Eat Well: For your Self, For the World. BenBella Books, Dallas. Forthcoming 2014.

51. Neyman Morris, M., Rios, L., Bacon, L., Clifford, D., and Gray, K. 2012. "Impact of 'Eat Well: For Your Self, For the World' Text and Curriculum on College Students' Attitudes and Eating Habits." *FASEB Journal*, 26, 634.2.

52. Albers, S. 2008. *Eat, Drink and Be Mindful: How to End Your Struggle with Mindless Eating and Start Savoring Food with Intention and Joy.* Oakland, CA: New Harbinger Publications, Inc.

53. Matz, J. and Frankel, E. 2003. *The Diet Survivor's Handbook: 60 Lessons in Eating, Acceptance and Self-Care.* Naperville, IL: Sourcebooks, Inc.

54. hooks, b. 1994. *Teaching to Transgress: Education as the Practice of Freedom.* New York: Routledge.

55. Hawks, S., Madanat, H., Smith, T., and De La Cruz, N. 2008. "Classroom Approach for Managing Dietary Restraint, Negative Eating Styles, and Body Image Concerns Among College Women." *Journal of American College Health*, 56(4), 359–366.

SPOTLIGHT

The focus of the next chapter, by Patti Lou Watkins and Rebecca Concepcion, is on teaching HAES principles to students and health care providers. The authors review the relevant existing literature describing ways of teaching HAES, both to students and to practicing health care providers. They then provide a thorough review of existing programs on this topic, and discuss future needs for education of health care providers and students.

Chapter Twelve

Teaching HAES to Health Care Students and Professionals

Patti Lou Watkins and Rebecca Concepcion

T he preceding chapters have elucidated the tenets of Health At Every Size (HAES) and provided an evidence-based rationale for this approach. The ability of HAES interventions to improve health without the concomitant stigma and side effects associated with weight-centered programs provides the impetus for training practitioners in this model. This chapter examines curricula for teaching HAES principles so that educators might design their own courses for those who will, or currently do, work within health care professions.

A RATIONALE FOR HAES EDUCATION

Although weight bias occurs across societal institutions, it is perhaps most harmful when enacted within health settings by professionals entrusted with promoting the physical and psychological well-being of the populace they serve. Nevertheless, Puhl and Heuer[1] report that physicians hold negative attitudes toward "obese" patients, blaming them for their circumstance and prescribing weight-loss interventions that, according to Mann et al, are bound to fail.[2] Medical school appears to be a training ground for anti-fat sentiment as obese patients are the most common targets of students' derogatory humor.[3] Practicing and student nurses also hold negative attitudes toward obese patients and, like physicians, advocate dieting as a course of treatment.[4] Carryer contends that despite their devotion to holistic care, nurses have adopted the reductionist view that "obesity" is synonymous with "disease," thus weight loss must be accomplished at all costs, with this stance engendering weight bias.[5] Dietitians to whom medical personnel refer patients also harbor weight bias. Both dietetics students and practicing dietitians report anti-fat attitudes.[6,7] Stone and Werner found that, consistent with other health professionals, dietitians blamed patients for their weight status, with such beliefs manifesting in shorter sessions, less effort, and more negative behavior toward obese patients.

Weight-biased attitudes also exist among college students enrolled in sport, exercise, kinesiology, health promotion, recreation, and physical education majors who may ultimately work in a variety of health-related settings.[8,9,10] These students tend to believe that their future charges must attain a "normal" weight, likely the result of educational curricula that link excess weight to poor physical and mental health.[9] D'Abundo observed this weight-centered approach among aerobics instructors.[11] Despite a wellness philosophy, instructors repeatedly accentuated appearance goals to be accomplished via weight loss. This focus on weight is apparent in child populations as well. Greenleaf and Weiller found physical educators to maintain moderate anti-fat attitudes, with the vast majority of their sample endorsing the belief that being "normal" weight is vital to children's health.[12] These researchers described their sample as participating in an "ideology of blame" that "places sole responsibility on fat individuals for their lot in life" (p. 418). Such pejorative attitudes have not been lost on their recipients. Participants in Sykes and McPhail's qualitative analysis characterized their experiences as fat children in physical education classes as predominantly negative, often "traumatizing."[13]

Psychologists and students training to enter this discipline are not immune to weight bias. McHugh and Kasardo explain that theories of weight are based on the unquestioned assumption that being fat is pathological, perhaps even worthy of diagnostic status as a mental illness.[14] They warn that anti-fat attitudes among therapists may result in less effort or lower expectations of clients along with weight-loss recommendations lacking the scientific support that the field touts as its hallmark. Despite evidence challenging the notion that obesity is synonymous with disease, McHugh and Kasardo contend that psychology education at both undergraduate and graduate levels is still quite tied to the medical model that views fat, rather than fat oppression, as the problem.[14]

Given the extent of weight bias among health care students and professionals as well as the misguided treatment prescriptions stemming from traditional weight-based models of health, researchers have suggested novel types of training for persons entering these careers. First and foremost, they recommend educational approaches aimed at reducing weight bias and, as Peters and Jones (2010) suggest, explicitly framing body weight as a diversity issue. Carryer offers that nurses should be re-educated in methods by which they learn to "focus more directly on constructive nutrition for people regardless of body size and to promote active rejection of the diet industry" (p. 96).[5] In order for nurses to assume this position, she contends they must acknowledge and overcome their own internalized weight bias. D'Abundo echoed this sentiment with respect to female aerobics instructors, advising that their training incorporate feminist pedagogy such as the promotion of well-being over appearance, personal comfort and options within the class, and social engagement with group members to disarm weight-based attitudes and behaviors.[11] Sykes and McPhail support teacher education that leads to re-conceptualizations of the relationship between weight and health.[13] They stress that teachers become sensitized to the dire consequences of weight bias on children's well-being, especially when coming from trusted adults such as themselves. Puhl and Heuer suggest that health care professionals take a more compassionate approach to obese patients rather than persist in disdainful attitudes toward this population.[1] Chambliss et al. advocate education and certification courses teaching client-centered approaches that facilitate practitioners' empathy toward obese individuals.[8] Stone and Werner agree that practitioners need to learn empathy, explicitly suggesting that dietitians in this case be provided with educational tools such as Motivational Interviewing (MI) to accomplish this goal.[7] Emmons and Rollnick make a case for training generalist health practitioners in MI, as this technique has potential to do away with heavy-handed advice-giving regarding health behavior change, possibly diffusing the belittling tone of communications with clients regarding their weight.[15] Poirier et al. also advocate the use of MI, sharing an example of training medical students in this method so that they may provide information about weight and health in a less judgmental fashion.[16] These recommendations are consistent with the HAES paradigm that McHugh and Kasardo invoke when discussing alternative instructional approaches for health care students and practitioners.[14] O'Reilly and Sixsmith also endorse HAES education coupled with anti-weight-bias training as a means of ameliorating the damaging consequences of weight-centered approaches to health.[17] The following sections review existing efforts to disseminate HAES-based pedagogical practices.

TEACHING HAES TO COLLEGE STUDENTS

HAES concepts have made their way into the curricula of college classes in recent years. Watkins, Farrell, and Doyle[18] reviewed Fat Studies courses that incorporate lessons on HAES, utilizing chapters from *The Fat Studies Reader* (e.g., Burgard 2009)[19, 20] among other readings such as journal articles from *Health At Every Size* (http://www.bulimia.com/client/client_pages/haespdfs.cfm). HAES is a key component of the emergent field of Fat Studies that addresses weight bias on a broader scale, viewing body size as a form of human diversity subject to oppression akin to—and intersecting with—gender, race, social class, sexual orientation, age, and ability. Watkins et al. review other courses in the humanities as well as the health sciences that are heavily reliant on HAES principles.[18]

Psychology courses have also begun to incorporate HAES concepts. For instance, Escalera describes ways in which she integrated HAES material into her health psychology class.[21] Importantly, she evaluated students' reactions to this approach, finding that self-reported weight bias decreased by term's end. Similarly, Watkins, Doyle-Hugmeyer, and Belle evaluated quantitative and qualitative outcomes of "Women, Weight, and Body Image," a class taught by the first author that incorporates HAES ideas.[22] Like Escalera, Watkins et al. found that students exhibited statistically significant improvement on weight-bias questionnaires throughout the term. Furthermore, excerpts from assignments indicated that they understood HAES principles and could apply these to their own lives. One student who described herself as 5'3" and weighing 150 pounds said "I am considered obese if I go to the doctor." However, during the class, she had "come to realize it's not about the number on the scale, it's about the shape I am in, how I feel. If you are healthy, then you are healthy." In addition to grasping the notion that weight and health are not synonymous, students seemed to appreciate weight bias as a social justice issue. One student remarked, "We are not all meant to look, think or even weigh the same. People can be healthy even if they do not look 'thin.' Most importantly, everyone is deserving of a basic level of respect and dignity." Watkins also examined student responses to HAES concepts related to their professional aspirations as behavioral health scientists.[23] Despite education to the contrary, students seemed receptive to these new ideas and willing to draw upon them in their future work lives.

Co-author Rebecca Concepcion teaches a general nutrition class that incorporates HAES into traditional "weight-management" content by introducing the topic of weight diversity via the Frontline documentary, *Fat*.[24] In this film, various experts discuss genetic influences on weight as well as provide evidence for the concept of "fit and fat." As illustration, the film features the case of a "clinically obese" man who has completed nearly 300 triathlons. His physician testifies to his excellent health, acknowledging that obesity does not inevitably equate with disease and early mortality. Similarly, researcher Steven Blair discusses his own overweight status and inherently stout build, along with his running routine of 35 miles per week and his high level of metabolic health. *Fat* helps students begin to separate the constructs of weight and health, providing scientific support for concepts consistent with HAES and stimulating lively discussion among students who share their own experiences and observations on these topics. An equally persuasive resource requiring less class time is *Body of Works*.[25] This photo essay depicts internationally ranked athletes in training gear accompanied by weight, waist circumference, body fat, performance measures, and calorie intake. Initially, students are impressed with the size and ability of these athletes, but are then pushed to imagine how the larger power athletes would appear obese in their street clothes. The instructor asks students to consider how the athletes might be perceived should their physical capabilities not be known and how well the commonly held stereotypes for overweight people fit these athletes. Helping students challenge their assumptions about body size and shape as well as to understand that they are not indicative of health or physical function is ultimately the goal of this activity.

In addition to courses that encompass HAES concepts, Watkins et al. identified two classes centered on HAES,[18] Michael Loewy and Nathaniel Pyle's clinical psychology course, "Professional Skills Workshop: Body Image and Health at Every Size" and Dawn Clifford's nutrition and food science course, "Health at Every Size: A Non-Diet Approach to Wellness." The former course aims to sensitize graduate students to diversity issues surrounding body shape and size and to facilitate their ethical treatment of clients, adhering to a HAES rather than a weight-centered approach to psychotherapy. Consistent with previous recommendations for reducing bias, this course positions weight as a form of human variation subject to oppression, possibly intersecting with oppression related to other areas of difference. According to the syllabus, it employs feminist and social constructionist perspectives to break down dominant discourse surrounding weight and to entertain alternative points of view. Apart from promoting ethical practice principles, the class seeks to enlighten students about biases and ethical transgressions in "obesity" research. For instance, the course illuminates the fact that studies are often funded by weight-loss corporations and, not surprisingly, conclude that obesity is a risk factor for an assortment of disorders, with weight-loss approaches warranted as a remedy—sometimes in stark contrast to the data they actually produce. Fall 2012 marked the debut of the latter course, which is designed to provide an overview of the HAES paradigm. Topics include size discrimination, cultural influence on body dissatisfaction, and adoption of enjoyable physical activity and mindful eating. This course, which satisfies the university's U.S. Diversity and Writing Proficiency requirements, frames weight-based oppression as a social justice issue, with students expected to "Describe how body weight is an area of human difference subject to privilege and discrimination that intersects with other systems of oppression in the U.S. based on gender, race, class, age, sexual orientation, and ability." Students will be responsible for explaining the HAES model and generating potential applications of its use in their field. The course also entails a service learning assignment in which students will use social media to communicate HAES tenets. Because it fulfills general education requirements, this course is expected to attract students from a variety of majors. A research study will compare outcomes from this course to those from a basic nutrition course, tracking changes in students' eating attitudes, body esteem, and weight bias as a function of the curricula.

More recently, Diedrichs and Barlow evaluated the impact of a brief intervention on pre-service health students.[26] Their two-hour class presentation did not aim to specifically communicate HAES principles, but aimed to reduce weight bias by presenting information on its consequences in health care and the multiple determinants of body weight, such as genetics, which lie beyond individual control. The lecture also contained material on size acceptance, "addressing issues related to nutrition and physical activity with all clients regardless of size" (p. 852). A control group received a lecture reflecting mainstream notions about obesity that emphasized lifestyle factors as etiological elements and targets of change via traditional weight-loss treatments. As predicted, only the intervention group altered their anti-fat attitudes, with improvements still evident at three-week follow-up. Rukavina, Li, and Rowell assessed the efficacy of a six-week intervention that entailed both lecture and service learning components to improve undergraduate kinesiology students' anti-fat attitudes.[27] This intervention, embedded within a fitness testing class, aimed to raise awareness about weight bias in health care, to evoke empathy for obese people, and to eliminate blame for poor health status or lack of health behaviors. It also attempted to reshape participants' professional practice ideals from "athletic" and "diet and exercise to lose weight" to "health-related fitness" and "healthy lifestyle at every size" (p. 99). Quantitative results showed reduced weight bias following the intervention. From a HAES perspective, qualitative results seemed mixed. Although some quotes drawn from term papers suggested that students understood that people can be healthy regardless of weight status, other comments belied this conclusion. Many students still adhered to the belief that healthy lifestyles, and health itself, boil down to individual choice.

Indeed, the perception that socially responsible citizens must modify their behavior in the name of health—and that such behavior change is within the purview of the individual—is difficult to relinquish. Welsh refers to this moral imperative as "healthism," a disciplining of the body in pursuit of physical well-being that she deems as damaging as disciplinary practices undertaken for aesthetic purposes.[28] While Welsh concedes that the HAES movement constitutes an improvement over the "war on obesity," perhaps in reducing the risk of eating disorders as a function of dieting for weight loss, it is still "replete with a set of prescriptions about proper and improper attitudes and behaviors" (p. 43). Given these concerns, how are we to view individuals who face environmental barriers to health behavior change or those who simply choose not to make health a personal priority, let alone those who engage in healthy behaviors yet have poor metabolic health? Lee, a literary scholar and fat activist, questions whether or not discussions about weight bias should be kept separate from discussions about health to avoid stigmatizing fat people who do experience health problems.[29] That is, how do we refrain from designating and differentiating "good fatties" from "bad fatties" based on their health habits or status? Avoiding talk of health while teaching about weight bias is an all-but-impossible task for those of us working within health-related fields. However, we, the authors, agree that presenting students with the concept of healthism and urging them to bear this in mind as they proceed along their professional path is an integral part of teaching about HAES in college courses.

TEACHING HAES TO HEALTH CARE PROFESSIONALS

The examples of HAES-based education and its potential to affect health care students' attitudes about weight and intentions toward practice are quite encouraging. But while an increasing number of college courses incorporate these lessons, many heath care professionals presently working in their respective fields were not exposed to this perspective during their training. Fortunately, programs and materials geared toward professional audiences are now becoming available. These range from films and websites, to provider training sessions, to empirically validated multi-lesson courses.

Much of the impetus for developing HAES training for professionals seems to stem from concern that traditional weight-based practice may produce body image distress and disordered eating. Burgard describes how practitioners typically consider calorie-counting, food restriction, excessive exercise, and frequent weighing to be problematic when enacted by "normal" or "underweight" individuals, yet laud these same behaviors when exhibited by "overweight" and "obese" persons.[30,31] In fact, practitioners often prescribe these behaviors considered pathological in one population to another population as a means of health promotion. Cliff and Wright exemplify this issue by examining the impact of a health and physical education curriculum on tenth-grade girls.[32] They observed that discourses around obesity and eating disorders were conflated. While the instructor decried eating disordered behavior such as maintaining a preoccupation with food, she concurrently issued messages about the importance of monitoring fat intake and avoiding weight gain. These researchers describe "a kind of practical paralysis" as teacher and students tried to make sense of the curriculum's mixed messages surrounding food, weight, and health, concluding that "Well-meaning professionals who are invested in the welfare and long-term health of their students seem to have at least some sense that the body pedagogies that they mobilise in the name of obesity have potentially dangerous repercussions for many young people." As such, they call for resources to help teachers negotiate these issues, lamenting the scarcity of available tools to do so.

The recently developed web-based program, *The Student Body: Promoting Health at Every Size*, may fill this niche. McVey, Gusella, Tweed, and Ferrari created this training module that they disseminated to elementary school teachers and public health practitioners working in schools.[33] The program was designed to inform participants about the many influences on children's body image including over-emphasis on weight as a marker for health, weight-monitoring, pressure to diet, and weight bias, all of which might be communicated via the media, peers, school-sanctioned activities, and by the participants themselves as powerful adult role models. The salience of adult influences is captured in this bit of program content, "Some adults (parents or teachers) might be overly concerned about their own physical appearance, which can inadvertently rub off on children" (p. 7). Furthermore, the program cautioned participants about discussing dieting or making jokes about fattening foods given the detrimental effect this could have on students. Following the 60-day intervention, McVey et al. found that teachers who received the program displayed significantly improved knowledge about restrictive dieting and peer influences on dieting behavior and body image. Public health practitioners who received the program demonstrated significant improvements in self-efficacy to confront weight bias. McVey et al. suggest one of the most important results of the intervention was participants' increased appreciation of how their own behavior might adversely impact students. Undeniably, instructors' verbalizations and behavior regarding their own body dissatisfaction can undermine curricula that otherwise emphasize health over weight-loss and appearance goals (e.g., Cliff and Wright 2010; D'Abundo 2009).[32,11] Hague and White also developed a web-based intervention aimed at reducing weight bias among education majors and certified teachers, most specializing in health/fitness or elementary education.[34] This non-diet, health-centered educational module addressed controversies surrounding the etiology of "obesity, risks associated with weight-loss efforts, sociocultural pressures to be thin, and negative effects of weight bias. Additionally, it offered "strategies to help children deal with the social stigma of obesity" along with "intervention techniques to promote bias-free behavior in the school setting" (p. 60). Intervention participants evidenced significant improvements in anti-fat attitudes at treatment's end and at six-week follow-up.

The film, "Dieting: At War with Our Bodies", represents another means of introducing health care professionals to HAES.[35] This documentary depicts a collection of women participating in a HAES support group and includes commentary from researchers presenting scientific support for this model. Omichinski describes how the film has been received during its various screenings, often featured at *International No Diet Day* events.[36] For instance, in Iceland, the film was part of a program that included lectures on the cult of thinness that organizers advertised especially to area health and fitness practitioners. Reportedly, the film generated much enthusiasm and discussion, including continued conversation via the web. Another media-based source of HAES information is the website, *Teaching Tolerance* (www. tolerance.org). Founded in 1991 by the Southern Poverty Law Center, this organization is devoted to reducing prejudice across categories of difference and providing an equitable school experience for children of all ages. The website provides teachers with information and resources to accomplish this end, including material targeting size bias, with some units specifically invoking HAES. The site supplies teachers with grade-relevant classroom activities to convey lessons. For example, an activity entitled "Many Shapes and Sizes" for early grades involves the teacher reading the book, *Shapesville*, and having students trace their own shapes on sheet of butcher paper that they decorate and discuss in terms of what is special and unique about the diversity of their bodies.[37] The Association for Size Diversity and Health's website (https://www.sizediversityandhealth.org/Index.asp) is a virtual repository for information about HAES. This site includes numerous audio/visual and print resources, many directed toward professionals seeking to integrate HAES principles into their practice. For instance, one document spells out guidelines for therapists who work with fat clients. Others advance ideas for addressing and preventing weight-based bullying among children and teens. The resources on both of these websites are available to the general public and largely free of charge.

CONCLUSION

Weight bias is a widespread phenomenon in health care that translates to a range of problems for recipients, such as developing eating disorders, eschewing physical activity, and avoiding medical visits. However, pedagogical approaches designed to train students and professionals to operate from a HAES perspective are now emerging, with these having the potential to reduce weight bias while facilitating health behavior change. Some scholars and educators endorse training in MI methods to aid in this endeavor. Instructional methods span the gamut from full-term college courses centered on HAES, to one-time lectures, to media resources. We hope that the information conveyed in this chapter stimulates further efforts to introduce health care students and professionals to HAES. Finally, we support increased empirical evaluation regarding the outcome of such training in terms of knowledge acquisition, acceptance, and, perhaps most importantly, implementation of HAES principles in day-to-day practice.

References

1. Puhl, R. M. and Heuer, C. A. 2009. "The Stigma of Obesity: A Review and Update." *Obesity, 17*, 941–964.

2. Mann, T. A., Tomiyama, J., Westling, E., Lew, A., Samuels, B., and Chatman, J. 2007. "Medicare's Search for Effective Obesity Treatments: Diets Are Not the Answer." *American Psychologist, 62*, 220–233.

3. Wear, D., Aultman, J. M., Varley, J. D., and Zarconi, J. 2006. "Making Fun of Patients: Medical Students' Cynical Humor in Clinical Settings." *Academic Medicine, 81*, 454–462.

4. Poon, M. Y. and Tarrant, M. 2009. "Obesity: Attitudes of Undergraduate Student Nurses and Registered Nurses." *Journal of Clinical Nursing, 18*, 2355–2365.

5. Carryer, J. 2001. "Embodied Largeness: A Significant Women's Health Issue." *Nursing Inquiry, 8*, 90–97.

6. Puhl, R. M., Wharton, C., and Heuer, C. A. 2009. "Weight Bias Among Dietetics Students: Implications for Treatment Practices." *Journal of the American Dietetic Association, 109*, 438–444.

7. Stone, O. and Werner, P. 2012. "Israeli Dietitians' Professional Stigma Attached to Obese Patients." Qualitative Health Research, 22, 768–776.

8. Chambliss, H. O., Finley, C. E., and Blair, S. N. 2004. "Attitudes Toward Obese Individuals Among Exercise Science Students." *Medicine and Science in Sport and Exercise, 36*, 468–474.

9. Greenleaf, C., Martin, S. B., and Rhea, D. 2008. "Fighting Fat: How Do Fat Stereotypes Influence Beliefs About Physical Education?" [Supplement 2] *Obesity, 16*, S53–S59.

10. Peters, D. M. and Jones, R. J. A. 2010. "Future Sport, Exercise and Physical Education Professionals' Perceptions of the Physical Self of Obese Children." *Kinesiology, 42*, 36–43.

11. D'Abundo, M. L. 2009. "Issues of Health, Appearance and Physical Activity in Aerobic Classes for Women." *Sport, Education, and Society*, 14, 301–319.

12. Greenleaf, C. and Weiller, K. 2005. "Perceptions of Youth Obesity Among Physical Educators." *Social Psychology of Education, 8*, 407–423.

13. Sykes, H. and McPhail, D. 2008. "Unbearable Lessons: Contesting Fat Phobia in Physical Education." *Sociology of Sport Journal, 25*, 66–96.

14. McHugh, M. C. and Kasardo, A. E. 2012. "Anti-Fat Prejudice: The Role of Psychology in Explication, Education, and Eradication." *Sex Roles, 66*, 617–627.

15. Emmons, K. M. and Rollnick, S. 2001. "Motivational Interviewing in Health Care Settings: Opportunities and Limitations." *American Journal of Preventive Medicine, 20*, 68–74.

16. Poirier, M. K., Clark, M. M., Cerhan, J. H., Pruthi, S., Geda, Y. E., and Dale, L. C. 2004. "Teaching Motivational Interviewing to First-Year Medical Students to Improve Counseling Skills in Health Behavior Change." *Mayo Clinic Proceedings, 79*, 327–331.

17. O'Reilly, C. and Sixsmith, J. 2012. "From Theory to Policy: Reducing Harms Associated with the Weight-Centered Health Paradigm." *Fat Studies: An Interdisciplinary Journal of Body Weight and Society, 1*, 97–113.

18. Watkins, P. L., Farrell, A. E., and Doyle-Hugmeyer, A. 2012. "Teaching Fat Studies: From Conception to Reception." *Fat Studies: An Interdisciplinary Journal of Body Weight and Society, 1*, 180–194.

19. Burgard, D. 2009. "What Is 'Health at Every Size'?" In E. Rothblum and S. Solovay (Eds.), *The Fat Studies Reader* (pp. 41–53). New York: New York University Press.

20. Isono, M., Watkins, P. L., and Lee, E. L. 2009. "Bon Bon Fatty Girl: A Qualitative Exploration of Weight Bias in Singapore." In E. Rothblum, and S. Solovay (Eds.), *The Fat Studies Reader* (127–138). Berkeley, CA: University of California Press.

21. Escalera, E. A. 2009. "Stigma Threat and the Fat Professor: Reducing Student Prejudice in the Classroom." In E. Rothblum and S. Solovay (Eds.), *The Fat Studies Reader* (pp. 205–212). Berkeley, CA: University of California Press.

22. Watkins, P. L., Doyle-Hugmeyer, A. D., and Belle, M. 2010, November. "A Fat Studies Approach to Teaching About Body Image." Paper presented at the National Women Studies Association annual meeting, Denver, CO.

23. Watkins, P. L. 2012, July. "Teaching Fat Studies: Intersections with Behavioral and Health Sciences." Paper presented at Fat Studies: Reflective Intersections, Wellington, NZ.

24. Thompson, A. (Producer). 1998, November 3. "Fat." *National Public Broadcasting; Frontline.* Transcripts retrieved from http://www.pbs.org/wgbh/pages/frontline/shows/fat/etc/script.html.

25. New York Times. 2008, July 30. Bodies of Work. *The New York Times Magazine.* Retrieved from http://www.nytimes.com/slideshow/2008/07/30/magazine/803BODIES_index.html.

26. Diedrichs, P. C. and Barlow, F. K. 2011. "How to Lose Weight Bias Fast! Evaluating a Brief Anti-Weight Bias Intervention." *British Journal of Health Psychology, 16*, 846–861.

27. Rukavina, P. B., Weidong Li, W., and Rowell, M. B. 2008. "A Service Learning Based Intervention to Change Attitudes Toward Obese Individuals in Kinesiology Pre-Professionals." Social Psychology of Education, 11, 95–112.

28. Welsh, T. L. 2011. "Healthism and the Bodies of Women: Pleasure and Discipline in the War Against Obesity." *Journal of Feminist Scholarship, 1*, 33–48.

29. Lee, J. 2012, July. "Embodying Stereotypes: Memoir, Fat and Health." Paper presented at Fat Studies: Reflective Intersections, Wellington, NZ.

30. Burgard, D. 2005. "Blinded by BMI." *Health At Every Size, 19*, 45–53.

31. Burgard, D. 2006. "We Should Know Better." *Health At Every Size, 20*, 83–88.

32. Cliff, K. and Wright, J. 2010. "Confusing and Contradictory: Considering Obesity Discourse and Eating Disorders as They Shape Body Pedagogies in HPE." *Sport, Education and Society, 15*, 221–233.

33. McVey, G., Gusella, J., Tweed, S., and Ferrari, M. 2009. "A Controlled Evaluation of Web-Based Training for Teachers and Public Health Practitioners on the Prevention of Eating Disorders." *Eating Disorders, 17,* 1–26.

34. Hague, A. L. and White, A. A. 2005. "Web-Based Interventions for Changing Attitudes of Obesity Among Current and Future Teachers." *Journal of Nutrition Education and Behavior, 37,* 58–66.

35. McNabb, C. and Finley, A. (Producers). 2006. "Dieting: At War with Our Bodies" [DVD]. Available from www.nedic.ca/resources/videos.shtml.

36. Omichinski, L. 2006. "HUGS: The Journey to Building Momentum and Unity for Health At Every Size." *Health At Every Size 20,* 119–131.

37. Mills, A. and Osborn, B. 2003. *Shapesville.* Carlsbad, CA: Gurze Books.

38. Bacon, L., Stern, J. S., Van Loan, M. D., and Keim, N. L. 2005. "Size Acceptance and Intuitive Eating Improve Health for Obese, Female Chronic Dieters." *Journal of the American Dietetic Association, 105,* 929–936.

39. Brown, L. B. 2009. "Teaching the 'Health At Every Size' Paradigm Benefits Future Fitness and Health Professionals." *Journal of Nutrition Education and Behavior, 41,* 144–145.

40. Friedman, S. 2012, February. "Celebrating All Shapes and Sizes: Helping Children and Teens Feel Good About Their Bodies and Themselves." Paper presented at the Columbia River Eating Disorder Network annual conference, Portland, OR.

41. Polensek, N. 2012, February. "Rethinking Obesity: How to Talk So Your Patients Will Listen and How to Listen So Your Patients Will Talk." Paper presented at the Columbia River Eating Disorder Network annual conference, Portland, OR.

42. Sturtevant, D. and Kinavey, H. 2012, February. "Health At Every Size: Practical Applications in the Clinical Setting." Paper presented at the Columbia River Eating Disorder Network annual conference, Portland, OR.

INTRODUCTION TO PART THREE, COMMUNICATING A NON-DIET APPROACH TO PATIENTS/CLIENTS

There are many ways to describe and explain the HAES model, Motivational Interviewing, and non-diet concepts. The choice depends upon your setting, the population with whom you work, and your own understanding of these ideas and approaches. We present a variety of approaches to members of the lay public and to health care providers working with them.

PART THREE

COMMUNICATING A NON-DIET APPROACH TO PATIENTS/CLIENTS

SPOTLIGHT

In the first chapter of Part 3, Judith Matz and Ellen Frankel write from the perspective of the therapist working with clients who have difficulty in their relationship with food. This may be a diagnosable eating disorder or simply "disordered eating." The latter expression refers to people who struggle with food in their lives, but these problems do not meet the diagnostic criteria for an eating disorder. The authors discuss the concepts of hunger, fullness, and satiety, and offer practical solutions to common problems that clients present as they attempt to transition from a dieting mentality to a "non-diet" approach. They offer examples of client interactions which help to illuminate the ideas and concepts in the chapter.

Chapter Thirteen

Principles of Attuned Eating

Judith Matz and Ellen Frankel

Consider the following questions:

- Do you know when you are hungry?
- Do you eat when you are hungry?
- Do you ask yourself what you are hungry for?
- Do you do your best to get what you are hungry for?
- Do you stop when you are full/satisfied?

To the extent you answered "yes" to these questions, you are in tune with your body's natural hunger signals. To the extent that you replied "no" to these statements, you may be out of touch with your true hunger needs. When a client comes to you to work on binge or compulsive eating problems, her response will be "no" to these questions as they apply to the majority of her eating.

[The non-diet approach to treating overeating helps clients normalalize their relationship with food.] The concepts of attuned eating address the questions of when, what, and how much to eat. Researchers, dietitians, and therapists developed these ideas based on the understanding that human beings have natural, internal instincts that can reliably direct them in regulating their food choices. Clients who display symptoms of binge or compulsive eating have lost their innate ability to regulate their hunger and satiation. Regardless of whether this lack of attunement comes from years of dieting, the use of food to manage feelings, or both, the first step in the process of ending overeating is for clients to relearn how to accurately listen to and trust their bodies' signals.

The ideas presented in this chapter are meant to be guidelines that help people work their way out of overeating problems. Unlike diets where rules must be strictly followed to achieve results, and the dieter is judged as good or bad based on adherence, we offer a process whose principles form a solid basis toward normalizing eating and resolving psychological issues. Clients have a tendency to want to turn these guidelines into a new set of rules, preferring the structure of an external source to the idea of relying on themselves to direct their eating. There is frequently a wish to make the non-diet into a new diet! Instead, the attuned eating approach offers a road map, and the path for each client will be unique to her own set of circumstances.

HUNGER

The first step in helping your client become an attuned eater is to help her identify physiological hunger. If you ask a binge or compulsive eater how she decides when to eat, you will find that her reach for food has very little to do with internal cues. She may tell you that she tries to eat at certain times of the day; many foods in her world are too hard to resist; various feelings trigger emotional eating; she eats every time she turns on the TV; or that she just loves to eat. Your task at this point is to assist your client in discovering the signs of physiological hunger so that she can begin to reconnect her hunger needs with the act of feeding herself. It is also helpful to remind your client that food actually tastes better when she is physically hungry.

Identifying Physical Hunger

If you ask people how they know when they are hungry, typical responses include: growling stomach, weakness, emptiness in stomach, lightheadedness, headache, irritability, and poor concentration. All of these answers indicate physical sensations, and the ability to recognize these sensations is essential in your client's ability to move in the direction of attuned eating. Symptoms such as weakness, lightheadedness, headaches, irritability, and poor concentration indicate that a person has waited too long to eat and is now physically uncomfortable. While a growling stomach can indicate physical hunger, stomachs can growl at other times, such as during digestion. Therefore, presenting the concept of emptiness in the stomach provides a more accurate cue for clients returning to normal eating.

The Hunger Scale helps people learn to identify different levels of hunger and fullness:

HUNGER SCALE

Starving
Very Hungry
Hungry
Somewhat Hungry
Not Hungry/Not Full
Somewhat Full
Full
Very Full
Stuffed

This scale intentionally uses words to help clients label different levels of hunger and fullness so that they can build their ability to notice internal states. Your client may also find it useful to assign numbers to the Hunger Scale, so that 1 means "starving," 5 means "not hungry/not full," and 10 means "stuffed." Using this method, a client would ideally keep herself in the range of about 3 to 7 so that she does not become too hungry or overfull. At the same time, these numbers should not be turned into new diet rules where a client reports that she is "good" because she ate at a 3, or "bad" because she ate to a 9. Rather, both forms of the hunger scale offer guidelines to discuss her journey toward becoming an attuned eater.

Probably everyone has had the experience of waiting too long to eat and reaching the range of "starving" on the Hunger Scale. When a person reaches the starving level, she feels desperate to put food in her body and can no longer determine what foods her body craves. At this point, anything will do; your client is likely to eat whatever is available, and she will eat more than her body needs. This is a normal, physiological response.

Between "starving" and "not hungry/not full" there is a wide range of possible physiological signals. Although at first your client may say that she cannot tell the difference in her degree of hunger, over time she will begin to recognize the nuances in her hunger signals. People vary in where they prefer to respond to themselves, and this variation can occur for the same person on different days or at different times of the day. The optimal times for making a decision to eat fall into the ranges of "somewhat hungry," "hungry," or moving into "very hungry." Under these conditions, your client can begin to recognize her body's message that she needs to eat, without the unnecessary discomfort that comes from waiting too long. She will now be in a position to determine what type of food her body craves.

Responding to Non-Physical Hunger

Although the goal for your client is to eat when she is physically hungry, the nature of binge and compulsive eating means that there will be times when she is unable to wait. As you teach your client about the difference between physiological and psychological hunger, it is important to offer her another way to respond to her overeating. "I'm out of control," or "I'm fat and disgusting" can be replaced with compassionate words such as, "This is the result of the deprivation of diets," or, "I'm reaching for food and I'm not physically hungry. Something must be making me uncomfortable right now and this is the best way I know to calm myself." Although she may quickly return to the familiar, critical voice, over time she will come to believe that she is not inherently bad for her need to turn to food. In part, the messages that you convey to her will help her internalize a new voice that is full of compassion and free of judgment.

Responding to Physical Hunger

The primary goal for your client early in treatment is to check in with her stomach and try to wait for physical hunger. Clients sometimes assume that their hunger will become obvious to them, but this is not always the case. Suggest to your client that she can check in with her stomach every so often, perhaps in 15-minute intervals. If she notices physiological hunger, instruct her that she must respond by eating. Developing the hunger/food connection is essential to breaking into overeating patterns.

Most people can eventually rediscover physical hunger, but the process will vary from person to person. In order to help your client find that attunement, she will need to give up preconceived notions about when she is supposed to eat. If she is not hungry first thing in the morning, let her know that it is okay to wait for a cue from her body. If she notices her hunger at 9:00 am, she will need to respond by eating. Her eating will proceed in this manner throughout the day. If her lunch break occurs at 12:00 and she is hungry, she will eat; if not, she will wait until later. Attuned eating means letting go of the concept of mealtimes and replacing external structure with internal cues. One caveat is for the client who is so disconnected from her internal cues of physical hunger that she does not experience any hunger in the morning and therefore goes through much of her day without eating. Unfortunately, as her body becomes ravenous, she is at high risk of bingeing later in the day, resulting in becoming too full in the evening; when she wakes up the next morning chances are she will not experience hunger yet again, thereby perpetuating the cycle. Suggest to your client that she experiment with eating in the morning, even if she does not truly feel her physical hunger, in order to "recalibrate" her appetite and move toward tuning into her internal cues.

The Case of Cary

Cary learned from her diet programs that she should never eat past 7:00 pm. She recalled that when ordering a pizza for dinner one night, she at three quarters of it, leaving her feeling stuffed and uncomfortable. She reasoned, however, that she would not be able to eat again until tomorrow morning. She feared becoming hungry later in the evening, and therefore ate more than she needed.

As Cary learned about attuned eating, she told herself that she could eat whenever she was physically hungry. This meant that if her stomach signaled hunger at 10:00 pm, she could and would respond. Cary found that she needed only a couple of slices of pizza to satisfy her when she ate early one evening. She trusted that she would attend to her needs for food if they arose. That night, Cary became hungry again around 9:00 pm. There was plenty of leftover pizza, which appealed to her. Cary ate half a slice of the pizza, and she put the rest away.

As you discuss the concept of using physiological hunger as the best indicator of when to eat, clients may express concerns about the feasibility of eating when they are hungry because their lifestyle specifies certain times of day that they are supposed to eat. First and foremost, your client must understand that in order to have a good chance of eating when she is physically hungry, she must have food available to her. If she allows herself to wait for hunger, but cannot get something to eat, she will become very uncomfortable. As a result, she may engage in prophylactic eating in which she turns to food in order to prevent hunger at some future time. She must think about herself the way she might think about a young child. When parents know they will be away from home for a period of time, they bring a bottle or food for the child. No one expects the child to suffer through her hunger; in fact, both parents and child end up miserable when unprepared. The client must also view her own hunger as so important that she will go to the trouble of bringing food with her when she is away from her home.

Perhaps your client tells you that she only has a certain time to eat at work or wants to have dinner with her family. These concerns are very important and need to be addressed. As with all aspects of the guidelines presented for normalizing eating, it is useful to start with a problem-solving approach to difficulties. If these ideas fail in helping your client implement the behaviors useful in ending overeating, then it may become necessary to explore deeper meanings.

In general, people can be very creative in finding ways to allow themselves to eat when they are hungry, if they truly believe that they are entitled to do so. For example, Sheila used the refrigerator provided to the staff at her office to keep yogurt, bread, and lunch meat. In addition, she kept a couple of cans of soup and some frozen entrees at work. Now that she no longer needed to go out to a restaurant to order food, she was able to eat when she noticed she was hungry, rather than becoming constricted to her one-hour lunch break. As a teacher, Gwen decided to eat in front of her second grade class if she became hungry. With a sense of fairness, her students were also allowed to keep a snack at their desk. Greg called his wife prior to leaving work to let her know whether or not he thought he would be hungry when he arrived home. Although the family mealtime was usually around 6:00, the couple agreed that if Greg was not hungry, he would join the family for conversation, and put together his own meal later in the evening when he was ready to eat.

MAKING THE MATCH

The next task in becoming an attuned eater requires your client to identify what she is hungry for when her physiological hunger occurs. Previously, your client made food choices primarily in response to what she "should" or "shouldn't" eat. Foods such as apples, salads, and vegetables were deemed "good" while she considered pizza, cake, and ice cream to be "bad." Eating rarely had to do with what her body actually craved, and the idea that she can trust her body to tell her what to eat is likely to feel frightening to her. Ultimately, when it comes to making a match, your client needs to answer the following questions: How will this food feel in my body? Is this the way I want to feel?

Presenting the Concept

Initially, your client is likely to have a difficult time making matches. Reassure her that this challenge is to be expected, and that you understand that it will take her time and practice to relearn how to listen to her body's natural cues. Eventually, the ability to recognize her hunger and decipher the food(s) she needs will become second nature for her. At the same time, even normal eaters must stop for a moment and give some thought to what they are hungry for. While as a dieter she has been quick to negate her true physical hunger, she must now feel entitled to spend time thinking about her needs. It is important for you to convey to her that you trust that over time she will develop her natural ability to recognize what her body craves.

You can begin the process of helping your client understand the concept of matching by asking her if she can remember a time where she was hungry and got exactly what she wanted. Most people can recall an experience, either recent or in the past, when they clearly knew what they were hungry for. Explore that memory with your client so that she can begin to connect her own desires with eating and satisfaction. For example, Lisa reported that when she was on vacation with her partner, she just had to have a steak and potatoes. After checking with the hotel concierge, they found a restaurant known for its steaks. Because she was on vacation, Lisa relaxed her diet rules and allowed herself to get exactly what she wanted. The steak tasted great to her and felt very good in her stomach. She remembers this as a very satisfying eating experience, although she also remembers telling her partner, "I probably shouldn't have eaten a steak because it's so fattening. When we get home, I'm really going to have to get back on my diet."

The therapist can explain to the client that this is exactly the type of experience she will want to try to collect. Congratulate her for listening to her body so well, and emphasize that this is an excellent example of how listening to her body provides great satisfaction both physically and psychologically.

Learning the Strategies

There are several strategies you can share with your client as she begins this challenging task. At the moment she experiences physical hunger, she can ask herself "If I had a magic wand and could summon whatever I wanted to eat, what would I choose?" This question eliminates obstacles, either real or the outcome of resistances, such as not having the food available or not having the time to prepare a particular dish. Instead, your client has made a first step toward identifying a food preference at a particular moment. Ideally she will be able to get the exact food she craves; regardless, she has begun to realize that her body can speak to her, if only she can listen.

Often, clients will find that even after asking what they truly want to eat, they are still unable to discriminate among food options. Teach your client that she can ask herself a series of questions that will help her in the process of learning about herself as an attuned eater. Specifically, does she want something hot or cold? Crunchy, mushy, or smooth? Salty, spicy, or bland?

Your client's choice will have something to do with how she imagines the food will taste in her mouth; after all, there is no reason to eat food that does not taste good to her. However, she must also think beyond taste and imagine how the food will feel in her body. Is it too light or too heavy? Can she tell if her body craves protein, fat, or carbohydrates? The idea of truly paying attention to her body is a novel idea for someone caught in the diet/binge cycle. At first she may say that she just does not know what she really wants to eat; she loves all food. However, over time and with gentle coaxing to listen to herself, your client will discover that she can collect attuned eating experiences.

The Case of Michelle

Michelle, a new group member, told the other participants that she never knows what she wants to eat. In fact, she was noticing some hunger as she sat in the group, but "didn't have a clue." The therapist took this opportunity to work with Michelle on the process of identifying the match.

Therapist: Michelle, can you tell if you want something hot or cold?

Michelle: I don't know.

Therapist: Think about how the food will feel in your body. Temperature is usually the easiest to figure out.

Michelle: Something warm would feel better.

Therapist: O.K. Can you tell if you want something substantial or solid, like meat, or something mushy?

Michelle: (responding immediately) Soft.

Therapist: Soft like soup, or soft like pasta?

Michelle: I actually want something more like a burrito. That's soft and warm, but the spicy sounds good too.

Therapist: Fine. Now take a moment to imagine the burrito in your stomach. Does it seem just right?

Michelle: It feels pretty good.

The therapist asked Michelle if she would be able to provide herself with a burrito following the group, and Michelle assured the group that she knew a restaurant that had just the kind that she liked. Hopefully, Michelle identified the correct food to satisfy her craving. If so, she will have collected an attuned eating experience that will serve as a building block toward her new way of feeding herself. Unlike diets in which one "binge" means failure and then "starting over," encourage your client to view her hunger and matching as a process of gathering experiences, which she carries with her forever. Whether she collects one, five, or ten experiences between sessions with you, she has begun to move in the direction of attuned eating.

Let's consider the possibility that the burrito did not satisfy Michelle's craving. Instead, she reports at the next meeting that her stomach felt upset. Michelle needs help processing the experience to understand what happened. She explains that the burrito felt too greasy after all; the cheese did not sit well in her stomach. By asking her if she can remember what would have made the food feel better in her stomach, Michelle reveals that she thinks a fajita would have been a better match because she liked the warmth and spiciness of the burrito, but didn't need the cheese. In this manner, Michelle learns to listen to herself and see that her body provides important feedback for her. Rather than berating herself for not making the perfect match, Michelle can adopt a compassionate view of herself. She is engaged in relearning how to eat, which will take some time after the many years of ignoring herself and looking toward external sources. Furthermore, Michelle will need to repeatedly hear from the therapist that each eating experience provides an opportunity to learn something about herself as an eater. If she feels satisfied, she gains the knowledge that she can tune in to her physical hunger. If she misses the mark, she can ask herself where she misinterpreted her signals so that she is in a stronger position to make a match the next time she feels stomach hunger. After years of dieting, it is no longer a matter of being "good" or "bad," but rather a process of listening, experimenting, and learning.

Encourage your client to make use of this process of matching each and every time she is hungry. Although your client may typically search the refrigerator or cabinets to see what is available, or look at the restaurant menu first, she will actually increase her ability to make a match by tuning into her stomach *before* she limits her possibilities. If she realizes she is hungry for egg salad and it is available, then she will be able to make a great match. If she decides she is hungry for egg salad, but there is none available, she can use that as a starting point to making a "good enough" match; perhaps she really wants eggs, and having them scrambled or an omelet will come the closest. Or, if she really wants the feel of the salad, she might choose to have the tuna salad that is available. By starting with her stomach, your client has a much greater likelihood of determining what will truly satisfy her hunger.

Ending "Good/Bad" Thinking

As you encourage your client to listen to her body to tell her what to eat, she faces a major obstacle. She has already categorized foods as good and bad, fattening and nonfattening, or healthy and unhealthy. This division of food interferes with listening to her body's true needs because she judges the food before allowing herself to have it. Therefore, the next task in the process of helping your client return to normal eating is to work with her on the process of "legalizing" foods.

Normal eating means eating a wide variety of foods. Sometimes our body craves protein; at other times we want something sweet. Sometimes we need vegetables; at other times we require starchy foods. Imagine for a moment that what you ate would have no effect on your weight. What would stay the same about your food choices? What might change? This is a question that can be useful to your clients. Although the initial fear may be, "I would only want junk food," most people realize very quickly that their body naturally desires a wide variety of foods.

Presenting the Concept

In order to help your client stop the judgments about food that prevent her from considering her body's needs, instruct her that *for the purpose of ending overeating* she will need to give herself permission to eat all types of foods. Obviously, foods are not nutritionally equal; however, as she gives herself full permission to eat what she is hungry for, she will become in charge of her relationship with food. It is helpful to remind your client that the deprivation she currently experiences as the result of trying to stay away from forbidden foods actually causes her to eat more of them than she needs when she breaks through her food restraints. Conversely, the pressure she feels to eat certain foods, such as fruits and vegetables, may actually cause her to reject them, even when they are what she craves. Ultimately, as your client learns to listen to her body to tell her what to eat, she will find that all types of foods can make a good match.

The Case of Devin

Devin, the newest client in the group, is trying to learn to listen to her hunger. With the encouragement of her therapist, Devin tells herself that all foods are now legal. When she is hungry, her task is to ask exactly what she is hungry for, and do her best to obtain that food. When Devin arrives home from work, she realizes that her stomach feels empty. She asks herself what would feel just right at that moment. The chocolate cake that she often eats is available; however, when Devin really checks in with her stomach, she finds that some stir fry chicken would feel better in her body. She reassures herself that if she gets hungry again later in the evening, she will once again make a match. If chocolate cake is what her body craves at that time, she can have some. The stir fry chicken tastes very good to her and feels just right in her stomach. Devin has made a match and collected a stomach hunger experience, without feeling any deprivation. After all, if she was hungry for the cake, she would have had it. If she becomes hungry for the cake, she will have it.

One of the biggest misinterpretations of this method of normalizing eating is a false belief that the instruction to clients is to eat whatever they want whenever they want. The true goal of attuned eating is for people to *eat what they are hungry for when they are physically hungry*. The results of these statements are dramatically different. A person who eats whatever she wants whenever she feels like it will move no closer to ending her binge or compulsive eating. She will feel out of control because she skipped over the step of connecting her eating to internal, physiological cues.

On the other hand, a client who begins to reconnect her hunger with her food choices will feel an immediate sense of calmness in relation to these attuned eating experiences. She will discover that she does not always crave the foods that make her feel out of control. She will probably be surprised by some of the foods that make good matches for her. Because this process can be fraught with psychological meaning for the binge or compulsive eater, the guidance of a therapist may prove invaluable as she navigates her hunger signals and any complicated issues and obstacles associated with her eating.

Matching Revisited

In this chapter, we have focused on letting go of "good" and "bad" thinking so that your client can make matches with food based on what will feel most satisfying in her stomach, which is the essence of becoming an attuned eater. Making decisions about what to eat can also take into consideration other factors such as particular health concerns or philosophical beliefs. Matching is an empowering action that can take place on many levels as your client decides from the inside out what will truly nourish her.

FULLNESS

So far, we have addressed the when and what in the process of normalizing eating. The final aspect of physiological-based eating involves knowing when to stop. While packaged foods provide serving portions, these amounts do not necessarily correspond to your client's hunger needs. Restaurants, which offer varying serving sizes, cannot predict the exact amount of food its patrons require on a particular visit. It is by tuning in to her stomach that your client will discern when she is ready to stop eating.

Identifying Fullness

Earlier in the chapter, we provided the Hunger Scale that gives a range of experiences that your client will have as she tunes in to her stomach. When a client first comes to see you for help, chances are that the majority of her eating experiences leave her in the very full to stuffed range. Point out to her that for now, she needs to be aware of how this makes her body feel. Is she uncomfortable? Is that okay with her?

Most clients find that they have an easier time recognizing their signals for hunger than noticing their signals of fullness. For all attuned eaters, in order for there to be a signal to stop, there needs to have been a signal to start. If your client turns to food for reasons other than physical hunger, she will be unable to rely on an internal cue to stop her overeating. Likewise, matching plays an important role in the ability of stopping. If your client eats exactly what she is hungry for when she is hungry, she will find a moment when her stomach feels satisfied. If she can pay attention to this signal, she will accomplish the task of stopping when full.

Binge and compulsive eaters will often describe eating experiences where they actually know what their body craves. However, they judge the food as "bad" and try to eat their way around it. Ultimately, they do not feel satisfied by their other choices and either return to the forbidden food after all, or keep eating the undesired foods in an attempt to become satisfied. As a result, their stomach becomes overfull, but they do not feel satisfied.

Teaching the Strategies

As your client focuses on the task of learning to stop when full, you can offer her some suggestions to aid in this process. In the past, the biggest cause of her overeating was a belief, conscious or unconscious, that certain foods would be taken away from her; either literally by the next diet, or in her mind as the result of her judgment that she should not be eating them. Now, she can remind herself that the foods she desires will always be available to her. Nothing and no one will ever take it away from her again. This will help her feel safe enough to begin to consider putting down her fork or spoon when she feels satiated.

Furthermore, you can advise your client to remind herself that the sooner she stops eating, the sooner she will become hungry again, leading to the next eating experience. This is a very important concept to your client who, by definition of being a compulsive eater, needs to go to food often. This frequent contact with her internal cues promotes her attuned eating. Since these guidelines are meant to be flexible, your client should determine when she feels satisfied. If, however, she feels physically uncomfortable, she has clearly eaten more food than her body needs.

Remember to AIM

As clients work toward noticing and honoring their fullness, the steps of Attunement, Intention, and Mindfulness (AIM) can support their ability to stop eating at the moment of satisfaction.

Attunement occurs as your client notices her physical hunger and honors it by choosing food(s) that satisfy her. Before she begins to eat, it is helpful for her to set an *intention* about how full she wants to feel at the end of her eating experience. She can then visualize the food she is about to eat as she thinks about the level of comfort she wants to achieve when she finishes eating, as well as 15 or 20 minutes later. She may want to start with the amount of food on her plate that she imagines will satisfy her—with full permission to get more if needed. Or, if there is more food on her plate than she thinks she will need, such as at a restaurant, she can move some aside as a reminder to check in with her stomach before proceeding to eat the remainder. While at first your client may say that she really has no idea how much food it will take to feel full without overeating, remind her that this is a time of experimentation; the more she practices, the stronger the connection between her stomach and her mind will become.

Mindfulness is a term used to describe the process of bringing awareness to an experience without judgment, distraction, or expectation. Bringing that mindfulness to the process of attuned eating deepens the pleasure of the experience as your client savors the taste and sensation of food without judgments. She will also become better able to notice her satisfaction level so that she can decide to stop eating when she reaches the level of fullness that feels comfortable.

Clients usually report that once they eat in accordance with their bodies' signals for hunger and satiation, they are surprised by how little food it takes to feel satisfied. This presents clients with an interesting struggle; on the one hand, they feel much more in charge of their eating and achieve physical and psychological satisfaction, yet they must also grieve the loss of consuming more food. The ability to tolerate this situation varies among clients who often feel that are giving up a "best friend." Even as clients mourn the loss of the amount of food in their life, the incentive to continue to move in the direction of attuned eating stems from the quality of these new eating experiences in comparison to the distress of their compulsive eating or bingeing. It is useful to remind your clients that while they may need less food during any given eating experience, the next opportunity to eat is just around the corner. Unlike other addictions such as smoking or alcoholism where the goal is to completely give up the substance, people cannot live without food. With this approach to ending binge or compulsive eating, clients do not have to give up the very thing they love. Instead, they get to have exactly what they want day in and day out.

As you teach or support your client in the process of learning to eat when she is hungry, eat what she is hungry for, and stop when she is full, you enable her to build an internal structure by which she can organize her eating. She is no longer as susceptible to the latest diets and fads that eventually lead to the next binge. She can replace her chaotic eating style with a consistent and reliable method of evaluating her food choices as she experiences the joy of developing a healthy relationship with food.

SPOTLIGHT

Molly Kellogg writes eloquently in the next chapter, describing the use of Motivational Interviewing with the HAES and "non-diet" concepts. Here you will find specific ways of using MI with patients and clients to help move them toward a HAES approach to wellness. Molly offers a wide variety of realistic sample conversations with clients to illustrate the ideas presented.

Chapter Fourteen

Integrating Motivational Interviewing and the Non-Diet Approach

Molly Kellogg

Motivational interviewing and the Health At Every Size paradigm are well suited to each other. Both the spirit and the specific skills employed in a motivational interview further the broad goal of health for the client. MI provides us the specific strategies and a way of being with our clients that guide them toward a sustainable lifestyle that maximizes their health.

THE SPIRIT OF MI

The **spirit of MI** is captured in four terms:

- Partnership
- Acceptance
- Compassion
- Evocation

Partnership implies working together, working with and for the client. The old model of being the expert and telling clients what is best for them is one of the things we leave behind when we shift into work with HAES. We partner with our clients to find the ways that they will uniquely walk down the path toward true health. We may have information and advice that may be useful to our clients. But our expertise is secondary to what the clients know about themselves and to the process they will go through on their journey.

To understand **acceptance**, it can be further broken down:

Worth: A key tenet of MI is a rock-solid belief that clients have value and worth just for being alive. When paired with HAES, this is extended to include that the worth is not tied to weight.

Empathy: This means accurately "getting" our clients, truly see their world as they see it. This part may be a challenge if much of what we hear is rooted in the diet mentality. We can work to carefully hear how clients see the world while also evoking deeper yearnings that come from a broader concept of health.

Autonomy: This means accepting that all people have a right and ability to direct their own lives, make their own choices. Our clients can and will choose the path that seems right to them. If we attempt to force our view and beliefs on them, we will ultimately fail. This includes forcing a non-diet process.

Affirmation: This means intentionally choosing to focus on what is right and what is working. Adopting a strengths perspective is both respectful of our clients and most effective. The HAES model is by its nature strengths-based. It assumes that much of what clients are already doing is health-promoting and it encourages us to build on what is working already to guide the clients toward health and self-esteem.

Compassion is not sympathy. It is being and acting fully for the benefit of the other person. This focus on the best interests of our clients has led many of us to the HAES paradigm. We see it as an approach that takes into account the whole person and all the best interests of that person.

Evocating speaks to both the spirit with which we engage with clients as well as the process. An evocative spirit implies that the majority of the answers are in the client, not in us. By our words and actions we say to our clients that they have what is needed to move toward greater health and that together we will find it.

THE TECHNIQUES OF MI

Shifting to a HAES approach to self-care involves profound changes for our clients. These changes include attitudes, priorities, and values as well as behaviors. MI techniques are uniquely designed for working with people who are considering profound change. They include an assumption that change is not easy and that taking time and care with the process will be more satisfying.

We will look at the techniques and at examples of how they might sound with our clients. Then, to put it all back together, we will look at the four processes that form a motivational interview.

As was discussed in Chapter 3, the set of basic techniques in MI goes by the acronym OARS: Open questioning, Affirming, Reflective listening, and Summarizing. Here are examples of how the OARS techniques can be used with a HAES approach:

Open questions allow you to invite the client who is focused on weight to see a bigger picture. For example:

- "If we are successful here, how do see your life in the future?"
- "Tell me about your dreams for your life."
- "Tell me more about how that would look."

To bring out what the client already knows about the downside of dieting:

- "Tell me your experience with diets."
- "And then what happened?"
- "Tell me more about what it feels like when you are on a diet."

To focus on strengths:

- "Tell me about times you have made permanent changes in taking care of yourself."
- "How did you do it? What worked?"
- "What self-care behaviors are second nature for you?" Some clients may not understand this question and may need examples, such as brushing teeth, putting on lotion.

To guide clients to the next step to take:

- "How might you practice that this week?"
- "What might be your first step toward that goal?"
- "How do you see yourself using this appetite scale (or journal)?"

What you choose to **affirm** has a profound effect on your clients. To affirm, you notice strengths or efforts and reflect them back. Sometimes you reframe what you have heard to pick out a larger strength. Examples in a HAES model:

- "You've thought a lot about this since our last visit. You are someone who takes things to heart."
- "You notice what is going on in your life and how it affects your eating."
- "You know which foods tend to satisfy you and which ones usually don't."

- "You are someone who learns from your experience."
- "You are capable of distinguishing between eating for appetite and for emotions."
- "You already have the skill of scheduling self-care actions in your phone."
- "You have lots of habits in place that contribute to your health."
- "You are someone who cares about both your physical and mental health."
- "When you set your mind to something, you follow through."

As in any type of counseling, careful **reflecting** encourages the client to continue the thought process forward. You could notice change talk that moves in the direction of HAES behaviors and reflect it. Refer to Chapter 3 for how to recognize change talk. You could focus on HAES-consistent outcomes as they emerge. This might sound like: "You like this feeling of being more relaxed when you think about food." Or, "You find your mind functions better at work since you have given yourself permission to have a snack in the midmorning."

Complex reflections can highlight insights clients have and guide them toward more. For example:

- "You've noticed that the diet 'voice' in your head gets louder when you have been around that friend."
- "You dislike the feeling of guilt when you eat something 'forbidden' and see that giving yourself permission to eat anything will allow that to fade away."
- "You like this person you are becoming and continue to search for ways to like her more."

Summarizing allows you to reflect the clients' main points again. You also use summaries to segue into asking for focus or to wrap up and remind the clients what they plan to do this week.

One format for summaries:

- Introduction: Reflect something about the situation as you heard it from the client
- Include some things you heard are important to this person
- Reflect again some strength and efforts
- Repeat any ability statements you heard
- Wind up with the plan as stated by the client (if there is one)
- Ask for confirmation or a key question that will move you to the next process

Here is an example of a summary at the end of a first session:

So, Eric, you came in here today very concerned about this new diagnosis of high blood pressure and figuring that I would tell you to stop eating everything you love and to lose weight. You are someone who is proud of your health and want to do all you can to avoid using medication to bring down your blood pressure. Being around for a long time to provide for your family is a bedrock value for you. You are an organized person and know that you have made some health changes in the past that have become habits. You have been on rigid diets before and have learned from them that they backfire. You are ready to use this journal to take a good look at how your eating goes now. You've decided to fill out these three columns for now. Next time we will see what you can learn from these observations and will look more at what you can do for your blood pressure that does not involve rigid dieting. What have I missed?

THE FOUR PROCESSES OF MI

Whatever kind of counseling you are doing, it is useful to have in mind an overall format for a session. In a traditional diet approach, this may be assessment of the client's current diet, formation of a diet plan, and helping the client work out how to do the diet plan.

When you first adopt the HAES approach, sessions can seem less structured. The four processes of motivational interviewing provide a loose structure to follow that encourages lasting change while remaining profoundly client-centered. This format encourages you to maintain the spirit of partnership, acceptance, compassion, and evocation throughout. The four processes can be seen as phases. However, they do not necessarily flow in order. You shift back and forth among them as needed with a general movement toward the final process of planning.

Engagement is always first. You bring yourself into the world of the client, even if it's painful. It can be tempting to work to bring the client into your worldview. Especially when you so strongly believe in a non-diet approach and that it is best for this person. It *is* possible to truly hear how much a person wants to weigh less and how painful it is live in this body while also attending to what is OK in that person's life and looking for the signs of readiness for a HAES perspective.

Engagement includes searching for efforts toward health and strengths this person has and affirming them. It means attending to what is working now in the person's life. Both MI and HAES are strengths-focused paradigms.

Focusing is the process of guiding clients to clarify the picture of where they are headed and then to focus further on the specific steps they will take to get there. All of the OARS techniques further this process. The initial focusing may include discussion of long-term life goals and experiences with dieting. You may reflect some of these experiences and ask for elaboration. For example: "I hear you say that the times you have been on diets you find yourself enjoying life less. Tell me more about that."

We know that a commitment to not diet is only the beginning of the HAES process. When clients decide to turn their backs on dieting, it is time to guide them toward practicing the specific behaviors that will support their new, expansive view of health. These may include gaining skill at recognizing appetite and satiety, legalizing all foods, finding new ways to cope with stress, planning days so as to avoid extreme hunger, and speaking up for themselves with others. This process of focusing on just one or a few behaviors at a time is an ongoing process that you will go through again and again as you work with a person to make this significant life shift. The order in which a person works on the elements of self-care inherent in HAES will vary. You and the client will revisit focusing each time one behavior is becoming established and the client is ready to take on another.

Based on your experience, you may have suggestions on the most effective order to address behaviors. Your expertise here is valuable *and* clients know themselves in ways you cannot. In MI, the commitment to client autonomy leads you to help clients find the focus that is right for them at this time. This does not mean you withhold advice. When you believe your advice is warranted, you ask permission to provide it and then elicit a response, deferring to the client's choices. For example: "I have an idea of how to proceed now. Would you like to hear it?" When the client says yes, you say: "Most of my clients find that beginning with attending to this appetite scale provides a strong foundation for normal eating. What are your thoughts on this?"

You may choose to give a menu of options from your experience working in the HAES manner. For example: "Now that you are feeling more confident about attending to appetite, we could bring in a new focus. What are your thoughts, or would you like some ideas from me?" If the client wants ideas, you say: "You mentioned times you turn to food to calm down and you also wanted to get better at ending meals when you have had enough. How would it be to focus on one of them?"

When a session is wandering, part of your role is to notice this lack of focus and suggest reorienting. This is a conversation about change. Is it focused enough to be effective? If not, interject: "Let's step back for a moment and check in on how we are doing here. I'm wondering if we are talking about the most important thing today. Of all these things, which is most important to address right now?"

This focusing process strikes a balance between actively directing the client and simply following. Guiding is midway between the two and allows for both client autonomy and your expertise.

Evoking occurs throughout your work. What you choose to evoke at a given time will vary. In initial sessions, you will work to evoke values, big goals, what the person knows from past experience, what has worked before to reach bigger goals, what in life is good and working well. Most people find it useful to revisit these larger goals frequently. Some clients will bring them up on their own, voicing the big picture themselves to keep focused on HAES. Other clients will need you to bring their attention back over and over to what initially motivated them to adopt the HAES approach and how far they have come. For example: "I hear your discouragement today. Might we revisit some of the things you said to me in the first visit in December? We could also take a look at how your life is now compared with last fall."

Throughout the HAES counseling process, you will evoke a client's creativity to choose how to proceed or to come up with what might work in a stuck place. It's tempting to share your ideas as soon as you see the place for them. Working in an MI manner includes acknowledging that clients are the experts on their lives. This means evoking the client's ideas and offering yours only if needed and with permission. For example: "You've noticed that you are really hungry when you get home from work and then tend to overeat and end up quite full. What thoughts do you have for handling this in a new way?"

Often the client will generate workable ideas. You will then simply reflect the plan you hear, perhaps guiding the client to make the plan a bit more specific. When the client comes up with a plan without you making any suggestions, the client's self-efficacy is enhanced.

Planning is the final process. People are more apt to follow through with a proposed behavior if they have a clear plan and have expressed it to someone. Planning proceeds best when engagement is good, a focus has been agreed upon, and at least some reasons to change have been evoked. Moving to planning too soon will disrupt engagement. Failing to guide toward a plan misses an important opportunity to support clients in their change process.

How to tell when a client is ready to talk about specific behavioral changes? You will hear some change talk and perhaps some tentative ideas of how to proceed. The most effective way to shift the conversation toward planning is to summarize the conversation so far and follow that with a key question. Ideally your summary will include only a few of the reasons to not move forward toward HAES and include every one of the reasons to change. For example: "You called me last week because you are sick of the dieting roller coaster and want to address your eating in a sustainable way. The diet-and-regain process has been painful and embarrassing to you. You know that big weight swings are not good for your health and at your stage in life you want to focus on health. You are willing to shift focus to health instead of weight. You know that you are a person who can make big changes because of your successful career change and you have a supportive family. You have done some reading about intuitive eating and want to give it a try. Might we talk about some next steps now (or tell me what you see as your first step in that direction)?"

As with all clients, you have a role in guiding them to plans that are SMART (Specific, Measurable, Achievable, Relevant, and Time-bound). You might do this with questions such as: "How might that look this week?" "Which days will you go for those walks?" "How confident are you that you will bring your lunch?" "What can you tell me about how that fits into your larger goal?" "When do you see yourself doing that journaling?" You can also help a client see that each plan is just for now and that this is a step-by-step process.

USING MI IN DIFFICULT SITUATIONS

We all encounter clients who tell us that if they change their body (lose weight), it will change their life for the better and a focus on weight loss alone is all they wish from us. MI reminds us that arguing will get us nowhere. It will only bring up more of the same.

Here is an example of a session that gets off track as the counselor holds her belief in HAES above her commitment to client autonomy. She misses opportunities to engage with the client.

Client: I really want to lose weight. Every time I do I feel so much better about myself.

Counselor: It sounds like you have yo-yo dieted many times. How many times? (Closed question)

Client: Well, I wouldn't really say it's been that many.

Counselor: Well, you know that dieting just doesn't work. At least 95 percent of those who lose regain it, so let's focus instead on what you can do to stay healthy. (Advice without permission)

Client: I am healthy, now at least. That's not the point. I need to get this weight off. I hate the way I look. I mean, look, it's disgusting, and at this weight I can't shop in the regular stores.

Counselor: Focusing on appearance doesn't work in the long run. I can tell that you have gotten caught in the diet/binge cycle and there is only one way out. Focusing on eating what you really want and learning to follow your internal signals of hunger and satisfaction are how to get out of the yo-yo dieting syndrome. (Pushing one choice)

Client: What? If I ate what I wanted, I'd be a whale. That's what I'm doing when I'm not dieting and you can see what happens.

Here the counselor provides uninvited opinions and advice and uses closed questions. The conversation quickly becomes an argument. The counselor is then further from engagement than she was at the beginning and the client is less willing to adopt a new approach.

How can you approach this conversation in an MI-consistent manner? This would mean staying embedded in a belief in client autonomy and compassion for the client's situation. You begin as MI always does, with engagement. The more you attend to "getting" your clients, seeing the world as they do, the less apt you are to veer off into argument. We don't abandon our belief in the value of the non-diet approach. That faith is based on our experience and that of our past clients. Part of our role is to share our opinion. Within the framework of MI we don't share our experience until we sense engagement and have permission to add our input.

Notice the difference here, when the counselor primarily reflects and asks open-ended questions and gives opinions and advice only after receiving permission. An assumption of client autonomy is assumed throughout.

Client: I really want to lose weight. Every time I do I feel so much better about myself.

Counselor: You would really like to feel better about yourself. (Reflection)

Client: It's embarrassing for all my friends to see me regain the weight I lose. I want to lose it permanently this time, especially since my doctor says I may be headed for diabetes.

Counselor: Losing and regaining is painful, and you have a reason to focus on your health now. (Complex reflection)

Client: Yes, and I hate how I look.

Counselor: Your appearance is important to you. Tell me more about how the losing and regaining doesn't feel so good. (Reflection and asking for elaboration)

Client: Well, I begin to lose weight and feel great. I'm proud of myself and begin to get compliments. But I feel deprived and the food gets boring. I slip here and there, and before I know it, I've gained the weight back. Then I feel worse than I did before. I'm good at so many things in my life. Why can't I do this?

Counselor: You like the sense of achievement when you diet and you've also learned that depriving yourself backfires eventually. You want to find a way to be proud of yourself without feeling worse in the long run. You are someone who doesn't give up when you really want something and you haven't yet found a way to feel successful with your eating. (Summary from client's perspective with a reframe)

Client: Yes, that's what is so frustrating and embarrassing about this.

Counselor: Many of my clients have shifted their attention to health and enjoyment instead of weight, and it has improved their lives. Would you like to hear more about this? (Offering a fact and an open-ended question)

Client: Oh, so that's what you do? Tell me about it.

Counselor: There is another path that leads to feeling much more competent about eating. By leaving restrictive eating behind, practicing eating according to appetite, and focusing on finding foods that satisfy, people begin to be more comfortable eaters and also feel better about themselves. It's your choice. What are your thoughts about this path? (Offering advice after permission followed by an open-ended question)

In this conversation, the counselor encourages the client to voice her distress and makes sure the client knows she heard it while highlighting the insights and concerns that might allow a paradigm shift.

What about when a client who has initially embraced the HAES paradigm, then voices ambivalence? This may sound like:

- "That's not going to work."
- "I am happier at meals, but I'm still eating too much."
- "This isn't working. I'm not losing weight."
- "I've decided to go on this two-week diet that my friend told me about."

The MI approach of rolling with what you hear fits well here.

- "It's your choice what ideas you try out."
- "You know yourself and what will fit for you."
- "You're frustrated that your body remains the same size as you work to normalize your eating."

Offer to step back to take a look at the bigger picture.

- "Tell me again (or more) about the effect of focusing on losing weight."
- "Tell me how this fits into your long-term goals."
- "Remind me of what you have learned over the years about what works for you."

You might also provide a summary of what you have heard that points out the client's HAES process so far and how it seems to be getting off track. For example: "Let me summarize what I see here. You came hoping I would help you diet again. You realized that this dieting process doesn't work in the long run and decided to give the new approach a try. As you have focused on feeding yourself in this new respectful way, you have noticed how much more relaxed you feel around food and that most of the time you end up eating less than you did when you were trying to diet. You have noticed that there are still times you turn to food for comfort, and we have just begun to look at other ways to care for yourself. Your blood sugars have been more consistent and your doctor agreed to not increase your medication. This week you had good news about your son getting engaged and this reminded you how much you would like to weigh less. This led you to think about dieting again. So, where does this leave you right now?"

The spirit, techniques, and processes of MI support you as you gain skill in working with a HAES approach. Just as your clients work through many stages when shifting toward acceptance, you, too, can choose to see your process as a counselor as ongoing. Over and over you can revisit skills and concepts and practice them. As one skill or stance becomes second nature, you can look for another to practice.

SPOTLIGHT

The next chapter by Dawn Clifford provides a description and rationale for application of the "Eating Competence Model" developed by Ellyn Satter. This approach to "normal" eating is a non-diet one that emphasizes internal regulation of eating. The model includes four characteristics of competent eating, including eating attitudes, food acceptance, internal regulation, and contextual skills. It is a holistic approach to feeding oneself that includes food choice, acceptance of one's body, and learning to feed oneself regular and predictable meals and snacks. The chapter describes the Satter model from the point of view of the individual and how these ideas can practically fit into everyday life. Examples of meals, snacks and shopping lists are included, to help the reader in operationalizing the concepts included in this model.

Chapter Fifteen

Becoming a Competent Eater

Dawn Clifford

INTRODUCTION

L indsay and Jenna are best friends. These 14-year-olds enjoy many of the same things including softball, dance class, Facebook, music, and talking about boys. However, their relationships with food are very different.

Lindsay calls herself a picky eater, eating only grains, cheese, and a few select fruits. She has a solid, athletic build, but notices that her thighs aren't quite as petite as Jenna's. Lindsay's mom is on Weight Watchers, so Lindsay has started reading the materials she leaves around the house and paying attention to calories on food labels. Lindsay complains that when her mom is dieting, there's never any "good food" in the house.

Jenna's house, on the other hand, always has a wide variety of foods. In addition to preparing balanced meals most days of the week, Jenna's mom makes homemade cookies once a week. When Lindsay is over at Jenna's house and there are cookies in the oven, she can hardly contain herself, often eating five or six cookies with her glass of milk. Lindsay doesn't understand how Jenna can just eat one or two and be satisfied.

Jenna is very different from Lindsay when it comes to eating. Jenna loves all foods with the exception of liver and mushrooms. She cooks with her mom on occasion and enjoys developing new and tasty creations in the kitchen. As Jenna goes through puberty, she notices her body developing curves and her mother reassures her that this is a natural process of growing up, so Jenna doesn't give it much thought.

Jenna and Lindsay are similar in many ways, and yet very different in their relationships with food and their bodies. How did they end up this way? Is a person born with a certain relationship with food, or are there environmental factors at play?

The Satter Eating Competence Model (ecSatter) is an evidence-based model that can be used to describe one's relationship with food.[6] Ellyn Satter, a registered dietitian, licensed social worker, and expert in child feeding and adult eating, developed the model after decades of experience working with children and adults. The model has been empirically tested with many audiences, and outlines the components that make up an individual's relationship with food. (For more n the Satter Model, refer to Chapter 1, by Marsha Hudnall, "A Mindful, Non-Died Approach to Eating).

So what is a competent eater anyway? At first glance, one might think that a competent eater is someone who eats all the "right" foods with plenty of fruits, vegetables, whole grains, and lean protein sources. Perhaps you're thinking that a competent eater knows how many calories are needed and keeps track of nutrients like fat, sugar, and fiber. In actuality, research shows that individuals who are greatly concerned about the nutritional details are often not very eating-competent at all. As it turns out, nutritionally obsessed individuals often have a great deal of anxiety regarding food selection and a negative relationship with food.

Eating Competence Overview

According to Satter, competent eaters are relaxed about eating, enjoy eating a variety of food, provide themselves with regular and rewarding meals and snacks, and eat in response to hunger and fullness cues. The ecSatter is made up of the following four subcategories:

1. **Eating Attitudes**. Having a positive relaxed attitude about eating with minimal feelings of guilt or anxiety.
2. **Food Acceptance**. Enjoyment in eating a variety of food, including nutritious food, and willingness to try new foods.
3. **Internal Regulation**. Attending and responding to internal cues such as hunger, appetite, and satiety.
4. **Contextual Skills**. Planning and providing regular, reliable meals and snacks of preferred food at predictable times.

The ecSatter describes a holistic approach to eating. While nutrition is briefly mentioned in the model, it centers on giving oneself permission to eat enjoyable foods along with discipline to plan and prepare regular feedings. Therefore, it may be surprising to readers that competent eaters actually have lower blood cholesterol levels than individuals who are not considered competent.[5] In addition, competent eaters have lower BMIs and are more satisfied with their body weight.[13]

Are competent eaters born or created? Attitudes about food and body are largely shaped by family, friends, and society. Parents are especially influential. In their attempt to get their children to eat or not eat, there is often pressure at the table. A simple comment such as, "you have to eat your broccoli if you want to eat dessert" seems innocent, but can actually be quite damaging in the long run. Pressuring a child to eat can cause anxiety at the table, ultimately negatively influencing eating attitudes, food acceptance, and an individual's attention to hunger and fullness cues.

While you can't change the past, your brain can be re-wired so that you can enjoy a future as a competent eater. In the following section, each of the categories of the ecSatter model will be described, and specific strategies will be provided so that you can begin your journey toward becoming a competent eater.

THE ROAD TO EATING COMPETENCE

The road to becoming a competent eater isn't easy and will not happen overnight. In this section each of the four components of the ecSatter will be discussed. Tips will be provided to get you started on the journey. However, these tips are merely a starting place. As you read each section, you may realize that some tips are easier to implement than others. Be patient with yourself; behavior change isn't easy. **The goal of this section is to increase your awareness of the process and to break it down into smaller, more manageable pieces.**

GUILT-FREE EATING: EATING ATTITUDES

Dieters, also known as restrained eaters, often experience feelings of guilt surrounding food. This comes from the labeling of foods as "good," "bad," "healthy," or "unhealthy." Dieters attempt to avoid foods that are high in calories, fat, or sugar. However, restricting certain foods in an effort to control weight often results in episodes of overeating.[2] Therefore, dieting often results in a vicious cycle that begins with restriction and is followed by a binge. Feelings of guilt often follow the binge, which ultimately leads to more restriction. Thus the cycle continues!

How does one eliminate negative eating attitudes? Give up dieting! This can be an overwhelming concept, especially for an individual who has dieted their whole lives. I've heard many clients say, "If I stop dieting, I'll blow up like a blimp." Of course, weight fluctuations are always a possibility. However, as we normalize our relationship with food and experience nutritious, consistent eating, those fluctuations seem to be less drastic than the ups and downs experienced in yo-yo dieting. Furthermore, dieting is also ineffective for most people for long-term weight loss.[4]

You may have heard of the ol' adage: All foods can fit in a healthy diet. Have you really embraced this concept? There's no mistaking it—there are foods for the body and there are foods for the soul. When we give ourselves complete permission to eat the foods we enjoy, we actually crave a wide variety of foods. Some foods are designed specifically to replenish the nutrients our body needs, and others don't do much for us nutritionally, but we eat them because they make us happy.

Consider a whole day of eating, or even a whole week. What would it look like if eighty to ninety percent of the foods you chose were mostly nutrient dense? You know— whole grains, fruits, vegetables, lean protein, dairy, nuts, beans, etc. And imagine that ten to twenty percent of the foods you ate were for your soul. What would that look like? What if you considered nutrition for your overall meal planning, but also allowed yourself to enjoy some high-fat, high-sugar foods on a regular basis?

Many are afraid that if they give themselves permission to enjoy "foods for the soul" they'll never be able to stop eating, gorging themselves on potato chips, chocolate, and fried chicken. While that may happen at first, it usually doesn't last long. When you truly pay attention to your cravings, you may find that you don't crave "soul foods" as much as you think you do. Most bodies actually crave a variety of foods. Don't believe me? Pick your favorite food. Chocolate brownies? Chips and salsa? Ok, now eat only that food for three days. Could you do it? It may seem fun at first. Chances are really good that you'd get tired of that food after just a few sittings and begin craving other foods. This is one piece of evidence that we do naturally desire variety and that the body's cravings can be trusted.

Here are some tips for guilt-free eating:

- **Body acceptance**. Developing positive eating attitudes begins with body acceptance. When specifically trying to lose weight, many find it's impossible to enjoy food without guilt. Can you really give yourself full permission to enjoy foods for your body and foods for your soul if in the back of your mind you're counting up how many calories you're consuming? It's not likely. It is time to ditch the diet, escape from the diet mentality, and embrace the dining experience. (For more information on body acceptance and improving your body image, please see chapter ??)
- **Awareness**. The first step toward guilt-free eating is awareness. Before you eat, notice your thoughts and feelings. Some find it's even helpful to do some journaling before digging in.
- **Breathe Deeply**. If you notice some anxiety or other emotion, try some deep breathing exercises before picking up your fork.
- **Focus on the food**. Savor it. Notice the flavors, textures, colors, and smells.
- **Notice your cravings**. Chances are good that if you zero in on those cravings, you'll find that they aren't as "bad" or as often as you believe them to be. It's also quite possible that you crave all sorts of foods, including the "foods for the body." Notice how many bites it takes to satisfy the craving. At times it may be two or three bites, and at other times, more may be needed.

CHALLENGE THE PICKY EATER WITHIN: FOOD ACCEPTANCE

Variety is the spice of life. In this country we are blessed with quite the selection of food. Many of us have spent a significant amount of time in the cereal aisle trying to decide on one box from a shelf of hundreds. Then of course there's the produce aisle. There are so many tastes, textures, and colors to choose from, yet so many of us choose to eat the same old foods each day.

Food rules often drive us to limit certain foods or food groups. The food hearsay can be exhausting and debilitating:

"Don't you know that carrots contain sugar?"

"Those eggs will surely raise your cholesterol."

"Traditionally grown strawberries are laden with pesticides."

"Milk has hormones."

"Don't use butter. Use margarine."

"Margarine has trans fat, use butter."

While there may be some truth to many food claims such as these, they can also be debilitating. Honestly, if you followed every food rule out there, there would be nothing left to eat. The answer? Eat a variety. Each food offers different nutrients, with different antioxidant powers, but often different pesticides or other toxins, as well. In eating a variety, you maximize the opportunity to include all the necessary nutrients while minimizing your exposure to pesticides or other toxic substances When you eat a variety, chances are greater that you'll be obtaining the nutrients you need for good health.

Many find that an enjoyable, satisfying meal includes a variety of colors, tastes, and textures. Some find eating to be an exciting adventure for their mouth, and then there are picky eaters. Perhaps you know a picky eater or you are one yourself. Picky eaters often experience great anxiety when presented with new foods.

Whether or not you're a picky eater, everyone benefits from increasing food variety. If you're looking to expand your food horizons, here is a step-by-step process to trying new foods:

- **Include the foods you love**. Start by making a list of foods you hate, foods you love, and foods somewhere in the middle (foods with which you can make do). Begin by trying the foods you put in the middle category and combine them with foods you love. As you become more comfortable trying new foods, you may become brave enough to revisit foods from the "foods you hate" category.

- **Add a delicious topping**. A topping may be needed to decrease bitterness or to add pizzazz. Sauces, butter, salad dressing, cheese, sugar, or salt may make the food more enjoyable. (Remember—now is not the time to get hung up on nutritional values. Using these types of sweet or savory toppings can help you ease into a new taste or texture.)
- **Try different ways to prepare that food**. Cooking methods often influence both the taste and texture of a food. Play around with different cooking methods until you find one that you prefer.
- **Be mindful while eating**. Focus on the taste and the texture in your mouth. See if you like it.
- **Try again later, and again later, and again later**. Multiple exposures to a food highly increase your chances of tolerating or even liking that food at some point.
- **Go on a food adventure**. Ready for a real food adventure? Visit a local farmers' market and try an unfamiliar seasonal produce. Or peruse the aisles of your grocery store looking for new and exciting produce or food products. Search the internet for new recipes or try a new restaurant. Attend an ethnic festival and experience the exciting flavors of a new ethnic cuisine.

Food can be fun. Enjoy the adventure!

GET IN TOUCH WITH YOURSELF: INTERNAL REGULATION

Your body knows exactly how much it needs … if you listen to it. There are many reasons we don't listen to our hunger and fullness cues. Hunger cues are often ignored when dieting in an effort to demonstrate self-control. At other times, hunger cues are ignored simply because of poor planning; you're out and about with no food when hunger hits.

Fullness cues are often thought of as the party spoilers. Sometimes "it just tastes so good" or the food is actually numbing out a certain emotion, making it difficult to stop. Oftentimes we're just not paying attention. Whatever the reason, it's easy to push these cues aside and use our brain to make a food decision instead of our stomachs.

So often we rely on external cues to determine when and how much to eat. We eat because it's "lunch time" even though we may not be hungry. Then there are the times when we eat because we're with people who are eating and it's the socially acceptable thing to do. Instead of listening to our fullness cue, we allow knowledge of calories or portion sizes to guide how much we eat. When you eat in response to internal cues instead of external cues, you'll eat the amount of food your body needs to feel good.

Internal regulation is about listening to your stomach instead of your brain. Your brain complicates things with thoughts, feelings, and emotions. Your stomach simply grumbles when it's empty and stretches when it's full.

We were all born with internal regulators. When you were just a baby you cried when you were hungry and you became disinterested in eating when you were full. If your parents fed you right, they continued to respect your hunger and fullness cues allowing you to eat as much or as little as you wanted at feedings. Many parents don't do it right, and pressure their child to eat at certain times or certain amounts, completely throwing off the child's internal regulation. As an adult, you can relearn how to internally regulate and return to the skills you had as a baby.

For some, the idea of no longer counting calories (externally regulating) is threatening. You may be wondering if your stomach can be trusted to guide you to eat the right amount. Dieters often try to eat the same number of calories every day. This actually doesn't make physiological sense. On the days you are more active or more stressed, your body needs more calories than on the days you are less active or more relaxed. Your body knows this. That's why you are hungrier on the days you are more active or hungrier the day after a busy day. An individual who is in touch with their hunger cues will eat more some days and less other days in response to their body's ever-changing needs.

Still not convinced that trusting your hunger and fullness cues is the way to go? Researchers have found that those who eat more intuitively are more satisfied with their bodies and perceive less pressure to be thin.[8] They are also more likely to enjoy their food and exhibit fewer food anxieties.[7]

How do you become more internally regulated? Pay attention and plan ahead. Here are some tips for paying closer attention to your internal cues:

1. **Get to know your own personal hunger and fullness signals**. What does it feel like when you're hungry? Notice symptoms such as lightheadedness, crankiness, and fatigue. What does it feel like to be satisfied? Full? Overly full? Experiment with these feelings in a non-judgmental manner and become aware of how your body responds.
2. **Provide yourself with regular opportunities for eating**. You may notice that you typically get hungry every few hours. Plan regular, satisfying meals to occur consistently throughout the day. You never HAVE to eat at those times if you aren't hungry; just be ready.
3. **Plan ahead for hunger**. When you leave the house, consider where you'll be at meal or snack time. Will there be food available that you enjoy? If not, bring a meal or a snack with you. The last thing you want is to be stuck in class or at a long meeting for work feeling overly hungry and irritable.
4. **Be mindful during the eating experience**. Notice the flavors, textures, and smells. Pay attention to your enjoyment of the meal. Find a comfortable stopping place during the meal. At some point during the meal you'll find that you're emotionally and/or physically fulfilled.
5. **You will eat again shortly**. If you plan regular, satisfying meals for yourself, then you can be comforted by the fact that another satisfying meal will be only a few hours away. If you

don't know when the next meal is coming or if it will include enjoyable foods, you may be tempted to binge. Imagine if you were on a diet and restricting your food intake and you went to a party. If you're not sure when you'll be exposed to such delicious food again, you may be tempted to scarf down every last morsel and be consumed by the abundance of options. However, if you are confident there will be another enjoyable meal in just a few hours, you can rest at a comfortable stopping place, looking forward to another fulfilling dining experience.

6. **Attend to emotions and food**. It is quite common to eat due to emotional triggers. Some eat when sad; for others it's loneliness, boredom, or procrastination. Unfortunately emotional eating has received a bad reputation. Emotional eating isn't bad. Telling yourself that you are bad for eating emotionally is only going to produce feelings of guilt and shame. When food is being used as a coping tool, remain present during the eating experience. Notice your emotions and how the food may or may not be soothing that particular emotion.

PLAN FOR EATING: CONTEXTUAL SKILLS

Are you a planner or do you prefer to be more spontaneous? If you're a fly-by-the-seat-of-your-pants kind of person, even the tiniest bit of forethought when it comes to eating can make all the difference.

Even if you enjoy a life of non-stop adventure, you can consider where you'll be adventuring and what food might be available. Having good contextual skills is about thinking ahead. Plan for eating meals and snacks at regular intervals. Find your own meal and snack rhythm. For some it's three meals and two snacks. For others it may be two meals and three snacks. What's most important is that you plan regular and satisfying meals at predictable intervals. It may be that some of your meals are at a restaurant. That's fine—a regular, satisfying meal doesn't have to be homemade each and every time.

When you leave the house, think ahead and ask yourself these questions: Where will I be at the next mealtime? What food will be available? What foods can I bring with me? By asking yourself these simple questions, you can be better prepared when hunger strikes, whether you're studying at the library or climbing the nearest mountain. Of course you don't have to eat if you're not hungry at your regular meal times.

More than just planning ahead, having good contextual skills is about developing basic cooking skills along with an arsenal of quick and easy meal and snack ideas. You don't have to be the next top chef to eat well. You simply need to learn some basic skills such as boiling water, chopping vegetables, cooking in a skillet, and heating up your food (whether it's in an oven, toaster oven, or a microwave). Fortunately, these days all of this information is at the tip of your fingertips: on the internet. There are websites and videos that will teach you whatever you need to know. "If you can read, then you can cook," says mom. She's right. Cooking is really about following directions from a recipe.

Yes, cooking takes some time, but if you stick with the quick, simple recipes, you'd be surprised what you can make in 15–30 minutes. That's typically less time than it takes to drive to a restaurant and pick up food. Plus, you'll save money. Meals don't have to be perfect. Don't get hung up on the details of fat, calories, or salt (unless you have a medical condition that requires it). Instead, focus on planning a variety of foods, and chances are good that it will be relatively balanced.

One of the biggest mistakes people make when they plan their meals is that they plan only for the main dish. If you think about side dishes when you're putting your grocery list together, then you're more likely to hit more food groups at the table.

Some prefer to go to the grocery store every day. Others like to get their shopping done at the beginning of the week and purchase groceries for the entire week. It doesn't matter which style you prefer. What matters is that you plan out meals with a few different food groups.

Here are some simple tips for getting into a rhythm of planning what you eat:

1. **Start with what you know**. Write down all the dinner meals you currently make and enjoy that are easy for you to make given the time you have available to fix the meal. What's your time limit? Is it five minutes? Or fifteen minutes? Or thirty minutes? Or an hour? Write down only the recipes that you will actually make and meet your time limit. Include quick and easy side dish ideas with each meal.
2. **Expand your list of favorites**. Grow your list by asking friends for recipe ideas, using the internet (www.allrecipes.com), or exploring cookbooks. Aim to grow your list to 20+ meal ideas. Try out EASY, balanced meals. If you like them, add the meal to your list of favorites.
3. **Choose a few meals from your list of favorites**. If you're a planner and prefer to shop less often, then make a list of 3–5 complete meals that you plan to make, including an easy side dish or two. Consider the ingredients you already have and need to use. Start small. If this is your first time to plan out meals, then aim for just making a few meals in one week. Consider time available to prepare/cook when selecting meals. Some may be for weekends when you have more time to cook and others for weekdays when you're short on time.
4. **Make a list**. Write down the ingredients that you need for that week's recipes.
5. **Leftovers make it easy for future meals**. Purchase enough ingredients so that there are leftovers. If you'd like, you can pack leftovers for lunch. Also, you can freeze the leftovers in individual containers for a quick, frozen meal in another week.

Here's an example of a week of five easy meals with side dishes and an accompanying shopping list:

Meals

1. Hamburgers (or veggie burgers) on buns with baby carrots dipped in ranch dressing and a side of baked beans
2. Tacos with ground beef or chicken, black beans, cheese, salsa, and lettuce on soft flour tortillas or hard, crunchy corn tortillas with a side of heated frozen or canned corn
3. Tuna melts on English muffins, bagels, or buns with a side salad
4. Baked potato bar with the following toppings: steamed broccoli, canned beans of your choice, cheese, salsa, sour cream, chives, bacon bits
5. Pasta with stir-fried vegetables (broccoli, mushrooms, and zucchini are good) and cut-up turkey sausage or beans with pesto sauce, marinara, or just butter and Parmesan cheese.

Shopping list

Meats
   Ground beef/turkey or veggie burgers
   Pre-cooked chicken breast or ground beef/turkey for tacos
   Sausage
Grains

   Buns
   English muffins (or you can use the buns from the hamburgers)
   Pasta
Canned goods
   Black beans
   Chickpeas, white cannelini beans, or red kidney beans
   Tuna
Dairy
   Cheddar cheese
   Parmesan cheese
   Sour cream
Frozen
   Corn
Produce
   Baked potatoes
   Broccoli
   Zucchini

   Mushrooms
   Baby carrots
   Lettuce
   Chives
Miscellaneous
   Pasta sauce of your choice (pesto or marinara)
   Salsa
   Bacon bits
   Mayonnaise

Competent eating isn't about eating perfectly. Consider nutrition when making your shopping decisions, but don't let it rule and then ruin your life. Happiness found in a certain dress size or number on the scale is fleeting. True joy is about accepting your genetic blueprint and loving your body by providing it with both nourishing foods and play foods. Pick foods you truly enjoy. Play around with food. Notice your reasons for eating in a non-judgmental, accepting manner. Focus on your food as you eat and check in with what your body is saying as you enjoy the meal or snack. No one becomes a competent eater overnight. It's a journey. Enjoy the ride.

References

1. Clifford, D., Keeler, L.A., Gray, K., Steingrube, A., and Neyman Morris, M. 2010. "Weight Attitudes Predict Eating Competence Among College Students." *Family & Consumer Sciences Research Journal*, 39, 2, 184–193.

2. Herman, C. and Polivy, J. 1980. "Restrained Eating." In A. B. Stunkard (Ed.), *Obesity* (pp. 208–225). Philadelphia: Saunders.

3. Lohse, B., Satter, E., Horacek, T., Gebreselassie, T., and Oakland, M.J. 2007. "Measuring Eating Competence: Psychometric Properties and Validity of the ecSatter Inventory." *Journal of Nutrition Education and Behaviors*, 39, S154–S166.

4. Mann, T., Tomiyama, A., Westling, E., Lew, A., Samuels, B., and Chatman, J. 2007. Medicare's Search for Effective Obesity Treatments: Diets Are Not the Answer." *American Psychologist*, 62, 220–233.

5. Psota, T.L., Lohse, B., and West, S.G. 2007. "Associations Between Eating Competence and Cardiovascular Disease Biomarkers." *Journal of Nutrition Education and Behavior*, 39, S171–S178.

6. Satter, E. 2007. "Eating Competence: Definition and Evidence for the Satter Eating Competence Model." *Journal of Nutrition Education and Behavior*, 39, S142–S153.

7. Smith, T.S. and Hawks, S.R. 2006. "Intuitive Eating, Diet Composition, and the Meaning of Food in Healthy Weight Promotion." *American Journal of Health Education*, 37, 3, 130–136.

8. Tylka, T.L. 2006. "Development and Psychometric Evaluation of a Measure of Intuitive Eating." *Journal of Counseling Psychology*, 53, 226–240.

SPOTLIGHT

The next chapter is edited from a piece that originally appeared in *Psychotherapy Networker* in 2011. It is intended to help professionals understand the HAES principles and to begin working with their clients and patients with this approach. In this article, Judith Matz discusses some of the basic ideas of HAES, the questionable science that points to an "obesity epidemic," and gives examples of how these might be used to think about your own relationship with food as well as your clients' relationships with food. Matz offers a number of client examples, and how the HAES and non-diet ideas can be used in practice.

Chapter Sixteen

Diets and Our Demons

Judith Matz

Every January, the weight-loss frenzy begins anew as the overeating of the holiday season subsides and millions of us resolve that this year will be the year that we *will* lose weight and keep it off. Dieting has become one of the great American pastimes, and no matter what our size, none of us are immune from the messages that we are too fat—or that we better start worrying about becoming too fat.

We read about the latest diet craze, enter weight-loss contests, talk about our dieting struggles, celebrate the shedding of pounds, and commiserate about their eventual return. As we stand in line at the grocery store, surreptitiously scanning *The National Enquirer*, we're filled in about the fat-thin-fat-thin-fat roller coaster ride of Oprah, Russell Crowe, Kirstie Alley, Jessica Simpson, John Travolta, and any other celebrity who puts on or takes off the pounds. As we unload our shopping cart, other magazine covers promise that we can lose weight and keep it off, that we can have firm abs and thin thighs, and that we can accomplish all of this before the spring fashion season rolls in. It's hard to miss the irony that the same magazine features recipes for delectable five-cheese lasagna and melt-in-your mouth double-chocolate fudge cake.

The 60-billion-dollar-per-year diet industry keeps offering new programs and plans. Low-fat, low-carbohydrate, and low-calorie diets get recycled with new names, claiming that they aren't a diet (since, as we all know by now, diets don't work!), but a way of life. Fitness clubs ready themselves for the onslaught of new members, counting on the fact that these exercise enthusiasts will work out religiously for a month or two and then drop out, fleeing the tedium of Stairmasters and treadmills.

The common cultural notion that anyone can successfully lose weight and keep it off with enough hard work and commitment mirrors the values embedded in the American Dream. Yet despite this collective belief—and the short-term weight loss that occurs with just about any type of weight-reduction plan—the most frequently cited statistic is that 95 percent of dieters will regain the lost pounds. Given that a few percent will maintain the weight loss, we all know someone who can claim "success," yet the vast majority will regain the weight. Although the blame—and shame—for the failure is usually placed at the dieter's doorstep, strong physiological, psychological, social, and even economic forces make dieting a losing battle.

As the New Year's resolution to diet and lose weight for good gives way to the almost inevitable cycle of overeating and weight regain, my phone begins to ring with queries from people weary of this dance. Clients struggling with compulsive or binge eating frequently seek therapy because they're aware that their overeating may have an emotional component. But, the idea that people eat to soothe or avoid painful emotions, while often true, is only part of the story. If we focus only on the emotional reasons for overeating, we neglect factors that cause the diet/binge cycle to take on a life of its own. In fact, the empirically demonstrated truth behind the pop-truthiness of "diets don't work" is that dieting—intentional self-deprivation—sets in motion automatic physiological and psychological factors that actually trigger overeating. In fact, there is growing evidence that *diets* make us fat!

WHY DIETS FAIL

The most immediate reason that diets really don't work long-term is that they promote a loss of the internal signals for hunger and fullness that are necessary for normal eating. This was the finding of a classic study conducted by Janet Polivy and Peter Herman at the University of Toronto, published in 1999. In this experiment, a group of dieters and a group of non-dieters were given the task of comparing ice cream flavors. Participants in each group were divided into three subgroups. Before getting the ice cream, the first subgroup was asked to drink two milkshakes, the second subgroup was asked to drink one milkshake, and the third subgroup was not given any milkshakes. Next, the researchers offered the groups three flavors of ice cream and asked the participants to rate the flavors, eating as much ice cream as they desired.

The results revealed that the non-dieters ate as you might expect: those who had not consumed any milkshake ate the most ice cream, those who consumed one milkshake ate less ice cream, and those who had consumed two milkshakes ate the least. The dieters, by contrast, reacted in exactly the opposite way. Those who were offered no milkshakes prior to the taste testing ate small amounts of ice cream, those who drank one shake ate *more* ice cream, and those who'd consumed two milkshakes ate the *most* ice cream!

The researchers termed what happened to the dieters "disinhibition," which occurs as a result of a "diet mentality." The milkshake preload had a different effect on the dieters than on non-dieters. Non-dieters, eating in an unrestrained and normal manner, tend to regulate their food consumption according to internal physical cues of hunger and satiety. Therefore, in the experiment, the non-dieters regulated the amount of ice cream they ate based on perceived fullness. What could be more obvious and natural?

The dieters, however, reacted in the opposite way—the more milkshakes they consumed, the more ice cream they ate. Why did they lose the capacity to regulate their intake? According to the researchers, this "counter-regulation" occurs because the milkshake preload disinhibits the dieter's usually inhibited or restrained eating, almost like a switch: "I've blown it anyway, so I might as well keep eating before I go back on my diet." This is an almost irresistible incentive to go on eating well past physical fullness.

Most of us have internalized cultural ideas about the body we'd like to have and how much we want to weigh, based on improbable models of perfection beckoning from just about every media site. But these images usually bear little resemblance to what's natural, healthy, and physically possible for our individual and bodies, because genetics plays a major role in determining our size and shape.

Weight is the result of a complex combination of factors that aren't yet fully understood. Although the question of nature versus nurture has long been debated when it comes to weight, research shows that the weight of adopted children resembles that of their biological parents, not that of their adoptive parents. When researchers looked at identical twins raised apart, they found that their body mass index was nearly identical, despite different environmental settings. This means that the influence of genetic inheritance has an enormous impact on what we weigh.

For example, metabolism plays a significant role in determining our weight. Resting metabolic rate refers to the amount of energy the body burns when not engaged in physical activity; it accounts for approximately 70 percent of the calories we burn each day. About 40 to 80 percent of the influence for resting metabolism is apparently inherited. In the journal of *Nature Medicine*, Jeffrey Friedman, director of the Starr Center for Human Genetics, writes, "The commonly held belief that obese individuals can ameliorate their condition by simply deciding to eat less and exercise more is at odds with compelling scientific evidence indicating that the propensity to obesity is, to a significant extent, genetically determined."

This inherited weight range, known as the set point, is the weight your body settles at when you are eating in response to signals of hunger or fullness and engaging in some level of physical activity. Our set point acts like a thermostat, seeking to maintain our natural body weight within a range of 10 to 20 pounds. When we take in less food as fuel, our body deals with this reduction by slowing down to conserve energy. Metabolism is lowered, reducing the rate at which calories are burned. Within 24 to 48 hours of beginning a calorie-restricted diet, metabolic rate decreases 15 to 30 percent. Our body has successfully slowed itself down to defend against this self-imposed famine. By contrast, when our body takes in more food than it needs as fuel, the metabolism speeds up and burns calories more quickly. In her book *Health At Every Size: The Surprising Truth About Your Weight*, Linda Bacon, a physiologist specializing in nutrition and weight regulation, explains that when this mechanism is working properly, it functions as a force that pulls you back to your comfortable range whenever you veer away; however, if you consistently override your body's signals of fullness, this system becomes broken. The goal is to find *your* healthy weight, keeping in mind that even if we all ate the same and exercised the same, we wouldn't weigh the same. Weight is a complicated matter, which be affected by a variety of other factors including medical issues such as thyroid problems or polycystic ovary syndrome, the side effects of medications, poverty, stress, and lack of sleep.

Beyond the psychology of dieting and our largely inherited physiology, we're still driven by the evolutionary pressures that drove our ancient hominid ancestors—hunters and gatherers who had to make the most of every bite in order to survive. Sometimes their food was plentiful, but during times of scarcity, their bodies adapted by lowering metabolism rates to conserve every calorie consumed. Following a period of scarcity, their bodies became even more efficient at storing fat in preparation for the next famine. These fat-layered bodies, better able to adapt to scarcity, were likelier to reproduce. As a species, therefore, we've inherited a predisposition to hold onto fat after each period of scarcity. Today, our bodies can't distinguish between hunger caused by famine and hunger caused by a self-imposed diet—and they react to the latter as if it were the former. The "failure" of diets is actually a "success" in terms of species survival!

When dieting for weight loss, our bodies respond to the perceived famine by feeding off fat and muscle. Muscle is the metabolically active part of our body: the more muscle we have, the more calories we can burn. Since every weight-loss attempt included the loss of both fat and muscle (but what's regained is only the fat), dieters burn even fewer calories, which makes it easier to gain weight and results in a higher fat-to-muscle ratio. Repeated dieting attempts may significantly increase the percentage of body fat over time. In fact, in 2007, Traci Mann and her colleagues at UCLA conducted a comprehensive and rigorous meta-analysis of 31 long-term studies of obesity treatment for Medicare patients. They found that despite losing 5 to 10 percent of their starting weight in the first six months, the vast majority had regained all the weight—and within four or five years, one-third to two-thirds of subjects had regained more weight than they'd lost.

In 1993, after it was discovered that less than one percent of dieters could maintain their weight loss for five years (the criterion for success), the Federal Trade Commission charged 17 companies, including Weight Watchers, Jenny Craig, and Nutrisystem, with making false and deceptive claims about the safety and efficacy of their programs. While many programs claim that they are not diets, whenever food is manipulated for the purposes of weight loss, it is, in fact, a diet, and not one of them has produced research demonstrating long-term results.

The pitfalls of diets have been known for decades. Not only does dieting make people fatter but it also affects psychological health. In a classic study during the 1940s, researcher Ancel Keys studied thirty-six men to see what would happen if they were placed on a semi-starvation diet for six months. The men were given nutritionally adequate food, with the same number of calories as most commercial weight-loss plans. The changes observed were dramatic. In addition to losing about 25 percent of their body weight, they experienced noticeable personality changes, becoming lethargic, irritable, depressed, and apathetic. They became obsessed with food, and they talked constantly about eating, hunger, and weight.

Once the men had begun the re-feeding portion of the study, restrictions were no longer placed on their eating. They binged for weeks, often consuming food to the point of feeling ill. Despite their overeating, they continued to report feeling ravenous. The weight previously lost returned rapidly as fat, and most of the men lost the muscle tone they'd had prior to the experiment. Some of them ended up weighing more than they had before the start of the study. Their emotional stability and energy returned only after they'd regained the weight.

Whether our clients meet formal diagnostic criteria for binge-eating disorder or experience similar, but less intense, patterns of compulsive eating and dieting, we must confront the role of dieting in maintaining their behavior. We need also to remember that people who diet are eight times as likely to develop an eating disorder, score higher on measurements of stress and depression compared to non-dieters, and experience greater health risks, such as cardiovascular disease and type 2 diabetes as the result of weight cycling. Perhaps most insidious of all is the shame that our clients experience, first about the perceived unacceptability of their bodies, and then about their failure to maintain weight loss after they've struggled to adhere to one or more prescribed diet methods.

THE ANTIDOTE TO DIETING

The prognosis for losing weight and keeping it off as a result of dieting is bleak indeed, yet, there's another way—a Zen-like way of eating—so natural, so intuitive, even so commonsensical that it's almost too obvious. Still, it took a consciousness-raising movement to reclaim the idea of eating in response to internal cues of hunger and fullness, rather than following external rules and prohibitions that almost inevitably lead to overeating. The notion that people who'd spent much of their adult lives following entrenched and often punitive dieting regimens should and could relearn how to eat in a more natural, normal way was introduced during the 1980s by pioneers Susie Orbach (*Fat Is a Feminist Issue*), Jane Hirschmann and Carol Munter (*Overcoming Overeating*), and Geneen Roth (*Breaking Free from Compulsive Eating*). While each has her own take on how to stop dieting and make peace with food, their revolutionary work—now increasingly supported by research—generated a movement that researchers often call intuitive eating.

Intuitive or attuned eating teaches people to reconnect with natural, inner signals telling them when, what, and how much to eat. We're born knowing how to eat. Babies cry when they're hungry, alerting a parent or caretaker, who in response offers a breast or a bottle. When satisfied, the infant turns away, indicating their fullness. They may need to eat again soon, but they're in charge of the feeding schedule.

As children grow older, numerous factors can interfere with their ability to identify hunger needs and ensure an attuned response. Parents concerned about nutrition may "force" children to eat foods they don't like, or restrict foods they enjoy. The structure of family mealtimes and school may prevent children from eating when hungry or demand that they eat when not hungry. As they become more aware of their body size and the culture of dieting, they may become caught on the dietary roller coaster, compromising their body's ability to self-regulate. Using food to manage emotions can further move them away from their own internal cues for hunger and satiation.

Attuned eating, by contrast, supports people in their journey to reestablish a natural, anxiety-free relationship with food. The first step in this process is to ask clients if they know when they're physically hungry. At workshops, I always pose that question to my audience, and find that therapists, as well as clients, are frequently disconnected from the physical sensations of hunger. Typical hunger cues participants bring up—weakness, lightheadedness, irritability, headaches, and poor concentration—actually indicate that they've waited too long to eat. Unfortunately, when we let ourselves become that ravenous, not only do we experience physical discomfort, but we also feel desperate and are much likelier to eat whatever is available. Instead, recognizing the sensations of hunger—a physically empty or gnawing feeling in the stomach—is essential for attuned eating.

After years of dieting, Lucy found herself completely disconnected from physical hunger. When she was following her diet, she ate by the clock at prescribed times, following a rigid, low-calorie food plan that had little to do with physical hunger. When she broke her diet, her eating became chaotic. She'd either skip breakfast or grab a few cookies and her morning coffee on the way out the door. For lunch, she often opted for the convenience of fast food, eating quickly in the car to save time, and then frequently continued to munch on the candy and chips available in the nearby vending machine as she tried to tame her boredom and stress of the afternoon. But on other days, she might only have a diet soda and yogurt, so that by the end of the day, she felt headachy and crabby, indicating that she'd waited too long to feed herself. In fact, she reported feeling so ravenous one day that when she met her friend at a restaurant, she consumed half the bread basket, a heaping plate of pasta Alfredo, and a hot fudge sundae.

I helped Lucy learn to check in with her stomach on a regular basis by asking herself, "Am I hungry?" every 15 to 30 minutes. If she noticed physical hunger, she needed to eat, so that she could develop the hunger–food connection that's essential for breaking out of overeating patterns. I suggested that she welcome her hunger by saying to herself, "This is terrific. I get to eat!" But after so many years of feeling guilty about food, she found it hard to believe that she was truly entitled to eat and could trust her body to tell her when to eat.

Lucy found it useful to think of a young child who was hungry, realizing that she'd never say to that little girl, "Too bad if you're hungry. I'm not going to feed you." I instructed her to carry food with her when she was away from home and take it to her office, so that even if she got caught up in a project and did not want to stop, she could take care of her need to eat. She noticed that, as learned to listen to her body's reliable internal signals, she became less focused on food and her anxiety about whether she "should" or shouldn't" eat decreased.

After so many years of deciding what to eat based on diet rules and food plans—or eating in rebellion to those rules—Lucy was surprised when I asked her in our session what she was hungry *for*. She'd had breakfast earlier in the day, but it was now 12:45 p.m., so I'd asked her to check in with herself and see whether or not she was hungry. She said she could feel some hunger, but didn't have a clue what she wanted. Usually she ate whatever was in the house, or whatever was convenient. The idea that her body could guide her in her food selection was truly novel.

Most of us have had the experience of craving something—and the wonderful feeling of actually getting it. Many of us also know the feeling of wanting something to eat, deciding we "shouldn't" have it, eating something else, and feeling deprived and unsatisfied afterward. It's this experience that often leads to standing in front of the refrigerator, grabbing and eating whatever's there.

As she sat in my office, Lucy said that she didn't have a specific craving and really didn't know what she wanted for lunch. I asked her to think about whether she wanted something hot or cold, and she quickly responded, "Hot." I then asked her if she wanted something mushy or crunchy, spicy, bland, or salty. As we narrowed down what would taste good to her and feel good in her body, she settled on kung pao chicken with noodles from a local Chinese restaurant.

Her next step was to order this dish and see if it was a good match. If she did feel physically and psychologically satisfied from the food, she'd strengthen her trust in herself and her ability to figure out what to eat in the future. If the match wasn't right, she could use it as a learning experience. What would have made her lunch more satisfying? As long as Lucy could refrain from judging herself for what she craved, she could begin to gather all kinds of eating experiences that would help her become more attuned to what she really needed and wanted to at a particular moment.

Learning not to be judgmental during this process is key. Like most clients, Lucy had a list of "forbidden" foods that she believed weren't OK to eat. Part of the journey toward attuned eating is to realize—and become comfortable with—the idea that our bodies crave a wide variety of foods. I'll frequently say to my clients that I've never met anyone who goes through this process and only wants to eat cookies, candy, and ice cream—nor have I ever met anyone who only wants fruits, vegetables, and salads.

As clients give themselves permission to eat formerly forbidden foods, they're likely, at first, to eat more than they need. After all, these foods have been off-limits for some time, and it's exciting to be able to eat them again. What helps clients get beyond overeating and eat a cookie *only* when they are hungry for a cookie, is the understanding that the food won't be off-limits again. Scarcity makes us feel anxious, needy, and greedy, while abundance allows us to feel calm, satisfied, and fulfilled. If clients believe that the next diet is just around the corner, they'll continue to overeat. If they prove to themselves that they can keep cookies available and eat them when that's what they're hungry for, they'll find they no longer need to eat them out of a feeling of deprivation.

After several sessions, Lucy told me that she'd binged on ice cream before our first meeting because she was sure I'd tell her that she shouldn't eat ice cream. Now that she understands this philosophy, she reports that she has ice cream in her freezer at all times, and eats some when that's what she's hungry for. She explains that in the evening, she often wants something sweet, and has discovered that eating ice cream when she wants a peach won't satisfy her any more than eating a peach when she craves ice cream does. Attuned eating doesn't mean eating whatever you want, whenever you want, and as much as you want. Instead, this method guides you to eat what you're hungry for, when you're hungry, choosing from a wide variety of possibilities that includes nutritious foods.

The final step in attuned eating is stopping when full. At the beginning of this process, Lucy, like most clients, frequently ate until she felt stuffed, finding it easier to recognize her signals for hunger than for fullness. Gradually, she began to notice and pay more attention to these feelings. She realized that when she made the right match in choosing a food that left her feeling satisfied, it was easier to stop. She also learned that without a physical signal to start eating—if she used food to assuage boredom, for example—there'd be no physical signal to stop: eating would be entirely disconnected from hunger and satiety. Rather than reprimanding herself for eating past fullness, she allowed herself to consciously experience how her body felt, asking herself, "Is this okay with me?" When the answer was "no," but she still made the decision to continue eating, she learned to do so without self-recrimination. As she became more attuned to her body's messages, Lucy found it much less tolerable to eat past fullness. In fact, she understood that the sooner she stopped eating, the sooner she'd get hungry and could enjoy another satisfying eating experience.

Since we live in a culture that more or less institutionalizes disordered eating, many people—who are not, or don't consider themselves, overeaters—find they can benefit from this perspective on eating. In my 18 years of using this approach, I've had many friends and colleagues tell me that just becoming more mindful about their hunger and fullness helped them build a better relationship with food. One friend commented that she used to feel bad when she had an occasional craving for a McDonald's cheeseburger and fries; now she takes pleasure in the experience, without guilt. She realized that it was worth spending money on the fresh raspberries at her grocery store to satisfy that desire.

This approach is well suited to people practicing different eating styles—vegetarian or kosher, for example—as long as their orientation to food is based on philosophical or religious principles and not on the desire to lose weight. Conscious nutritional considerations—as long as they aren't diets in disguise—are well adapted to intuitive eating. For example, one client felt that putting soy in her diet would contribute to her physical well-being and decided that a glass of soy milk in the afternoon would coincide with her body's need for protein. If your client receives advice from her doctor to make dietary changes that can positively affect a health issue, such as reducing saturated fats to lower cholesterol or understanding the effects of sugar consumption in the case of diabetes, and she's able to follow these recommendations, there's no problem. Unfortunately, many people report that a visit to their doctor in which they were instructed to restrict food triggered overeating.

Most of these clients aren't self-destructive or unmotivated to become healthy. Rather, the dynamics of the diet/binge cycle render them extremely sensitive to perceived deprivation, especially when accompanied by the familiar advice to lose weight. Additionally, if clients frequently turn to food for comfort when experiencing anxiety, the scare tactics or dire warnings used to convince clients to restrict their diets create fear that puts them at greater risk of overeating. Learning to become an intuitive eater of all foods, by contrast, makes it easier to adopt dietary changes as a means of good self-regulation, without the sense of deprivation that often triggers dysregulated eating.

EMOTIONAL OVEREATING

I believe that most clients can't begin to explore their use of food for affect regulation until they have an internal system of physiological self-regulation in place. When people are caught in the diet/binge cycle, thoughts about eating and weight create anxiety, draining mental energy and making it even harder to face the uncomfortable feelings that may drive them to binge. But once they're no longer in the throes of the diet/binge cycle and have developed a consistent and reliable structure to feed themselves, they're in a much stronger position to explore the relationship between eating and their emotions.

Sasha knew that she overate in response to a wide range of feelings—anger, sadness, loneliness, boredom, and even happiness. It wasn't the feelings themselves that activated her overeating: it was her inability to tolerate a particular feeling that prompted her to turn to food for self-soothing. Clients often use words like *numbing*, *comforting*, and *distracting* to describe how they feel when they eat. This process is often unconscious. Sasha doesn't say to herself, "I'm feeling angry with my husband but I can't tolerate this feeling, so I'll go eat something to calm myself." Instead, she finds herself at the refrigerator, reaching for food even when she isn't hungry. She may be aware that she's trying to push away her anger; or, like many clients, she may not even be aware that something is bothering her. This action sets off a chain of events that serves to take her even further away from whatever negative emotion first threatened her.

As she continues to eat, Sasha begins criticize at herself, declaring that she's out of control, fat, and disgusting. In the past, these reprimands would have led her to conclude that she must go on a diet to lose weight; however, she now understands that losing weight won't solve the real problem, though she may not yet be conscious of what that problem is. Instead of denigrating herself, she speaks to herself with compassion saying, "I'm reaching for food and I'm not hungry. Something must be bothering me, and this is the best way I have to deal with it right now. I look forward to the day when I no longer need to turn to food."

Four months into therapy, Sasha could report that most of her eating was now in response to feelings of physical hunger. She was ready to work on the emotional aspects of her overeating. Gradually, when she found herself reaching for food even when she wasn't physically hungry, she learned to ask herself, "Can I wait?" When the answer was "No," because she felt too anxious in the moment without this form of self-soothing, she gave herself permission to eat anyway, since the objective was for her to outgrow her need to use food for comfort, rather than exert control over her eating. She learned to give herself gentle nudges in the direction of waiting to eat, by reminding herself that food tasted and felt better when she was physically hungry and becoming curious about what was really bothering her at that moment. Her goal was to feel that she was in charge of her eating—to make mindful decisions that left her comfortable and satisfied—as opposed to controlling her eating, which meant using restraint fueled by guilt.

Rather than using control to stop herself from eating, Sasha learned to ask herself the following: "I'm reaching for food and I'm not hungry. I wonder what I would think about or feel if I didn't eat right now?" In the past, the moment she'd reached for food, she lost access to what was really bothering her; she'd now gained a window into her feelings. She began to identify more of the conflicts in her relationship with her husband and to talk directly with him about her concerns. As a result, the couple elected to go to marital counseling to address long-standing issues.

As the relationships among dieting, overeating, and emotions became clear, therapy helps clients develop their ability to regulate affect without automatically reaching for food. Clients who integrate attuned eating into their lives will find that their relationships to food, themselves, and the world change in profound ways.

ATTUNED EATING VS. WEIGHT MANAGEMENT

Mounting research on intuitive eating shows positive outcomes, from improved cardiovascular health, increased pleasure, and enjoyment of food to fewer dieting behaviors and food anxieties, greater body satisfaction, and better coping skills. In a well-controlled study in 2002 reported in the *International Journal of Obesity*, Linda Bacon and her colleagues compared a traditional weight-management program with a non-diet approach. Both groups showed similar improvements in metabolic fitness, psychological factors, and eating behaviors; however, the dropout rate for the diet group was 41 percent, compared to 8 percent in the non-diet group. The diet group showed short-term weight loss and improved self-esteem, but these results weren't maintained after one year; conversely, members of the non-diet group showed improved outcomes over the same time period.

In 2005, a two-year follow-up to Bacon's study appeared in *the Journal of the American Dietetic Association*. Participants in the non-diet group had maintained their weight and sustained their initial improvements while members of the weight-management group had regained the weight and showed little sustained improvement. The researchers concluded that the approach based on intuitive eating "enabled participants to maintain long-term behavior change; the diet approach did not. Encouraging size acceptance, reduction in diet behavior, and heightened awareness and response to body signals resulted in improvements in health risk indicators."

WEIGHING OUR ATTITUDES

It is ironic that with two-thirds of us moving into the "overweight" or "obese" categories, fat-bashing remains a common occurrence, and weightism (or weight stigma) arguably remains one of the last socially acceptable prejudices. Unfortunately, psychotherapists aren't immune from this bias. In his book, *Love's Executioner and Other Tales of Psychotherapy* Irvin Yalom acknowledges this prejudice. In the chapter titled "The Fat Lady," he writes, "I have always been repulsed by fat women. I find them disgusting: their absurd sideways waddle, their absence of body contour—breast, laps, buttocks, shoulders, jaw lines, cheekbones, *everything*, everything I like to see in a woman, obscured in an avalanche of flesh…How dare they impose that body on the rest of us?"

Yalom's honesty is admirable, but his observations raise a topic not often discussed in our profession. Most of us agree that the cultural ideals of thinness are unrealistic and harmful, but how do we really feel about people who are fat—or "large," or "oversized"? At workshops, I ask therapists to brainstorm the qualities they associate with "thin" and "fat." Like most others in the general population, they tend to regard thin people as healthy, successful, attractive, active, and sexy while fat people are lazy, stupid, ugly, and unhealthy.

Where does this loathing of fat come from? Charisse Goodman, author of *The Invisible Woman*, points out that "one of the most curious contradictions of weight obsession is that if a woman succumbs to it and keeps her weight unnaturally low by even the most desperate means, she is popularly considered in our culture to be an attractive person who 'cares about herself,' even if she risks her health in the process. On the other hand, a heavy woman who shuns this mania and refuses to waste her life fixated on her figure is characterized as unattractive and lacking in self-regard." In the *Obesity Myth* law professor Paul Campos considers the darker side of our disgust with fat as he explores the idea that Americans worry that we have become too big for our own good. He writes, "Nor is it a coincidence that, amid America's whirlwind of overconsumption, with its attendant anxieties about our economic, cultural, and military voraciousness, our anorexic Puritans promise that we can maintain our virtue by refusing to surrender to the most literal of our gluttonous impulses." Could it be that our own desires and fears about being in losing control are displaced onto the body of a fat person? What other unconscious dynamics might be at play?

Even as we begin to acknowledge the unfair prejudice and discrimination against overweight people, the obvious question arises: given the preponderance of evidence that people falling into the overweight and obesity categories have a significantly higher rate of health problems, how can we responsibly ignore this information? While it's impossible to explore the complexity of obesity research fully, my hope is at least to raise the possibility that there's another side to this story. Despite the bombardment of anti-obesity campaigns, a mountain of research suggests that the drastic claims that fat is killing us are more problematic than you might expect.

These findings surprised J. Eric Oliver, author of *Fat Politics: The Real Story Behind America's Obesity Epidemic.* With a background in statistics, he set out during a postdoctoral fellowship at Yale University to understand how the soaring rates of obesity and its catastrophic consequences could be handled politically. What he discovered surprised him: "Based on the statistics, most of the charges saying that obesity caused various diseases or that obesity caused thousands of deaths were simply not supported. Yet consistently, these pseudofindings were promulgated as fact." Paul Campos reports a similar experience: "When I began researching this topic five years ago, I assumed the fact that being 'overweight' was a serious health risk was so well established that this aspect of the subject was hardly worth discussing. Yet in the course of plowing through dozens of books, hundreds of articles in medical journals, and countless interviews with medical and scientific experts, I discovered that almost everything the government and media were saying about weight and weight control was either grossly distorted or completely untrue."

Consider the frequently cited statistic that 300,000 die from obesity each year—which was based on a 1993 study by Michael McGinnis and William Foege, reported in the *Journal of the American Medical Association (JAMA).* What they actually found was that "dietary factors and activity patterns that are too sedentary" contributed to 300,000 deaths per year. Inaccurate reporting by media sources and its use to validate health policies led McGinnis and Foege to publish a letter in *The New England Journal of Medicine* saying that the results of their study had been misrepresented. The researchers explained that obesity, high blood pressure, heart disease, and cancer were side effects of dietary and activity patterns, but they hadn't concluded how many deaths actually resulted from each single factor.

In 2004, the Centers for Disease Control and Prevention (CDC) presented new research, claiming that 400,000 deaths per year were attributable to obesity; however, this study was debunked for its poor research methods, and in January 2005, the CDC lowered the death estimate to 365,000. In April 2005, lead researcher Katherine Flegal of the CDC published in *JAMA* findings that put the actual annual rate of deaths due to obesity at 25,814, and determined that being overweight—or even in the lower end of the obesity range—wasn't associated with excess mortality or a shorter life expectancy. Despite this good news, the 300,000-deaths-per-year statistic continues to be used to justify treatment of obesity, and Julie Gerberding, who was director of the CDC at that time, stated that the CDC didn't plan to use the much lower obesity mortality figure in its public-awareness campaign, nor did it plan to reduce its fight against obesity.

This scenario is an example of how the concepts of causation and correlation frequently get misused in scientific research. While the popular conviction is that obesity *causes* higher mortality and health problems, it's next to impossible to establish causality in large population-based studies. When, as often occurs, weight is *associated* with health problems and mortality, it's possible that other factors, such as a sedentary lifestyle and poor nutrition, lead to *both* higher weights and higher death rates. Consider the fact that bald men have higher death rates. Does that mean that offering a toupee will decrease mortality among these men? Of course not! Instead, it's higher testosterone levels that cause both baldness and heart disease. Likewise, weight loss in and of itself isn't a panacea for the great majority of health problems. As an acknowledgment of the failure of weight-loss programs, some experts recommend that a smaller reduction in weight, of about 5 to 10 percent of body mass, can improve a variety of health conditions. Remember that the failure rate of dieting is 95 percent, and that dieting frequently launches people into a yo-yo cycle that isn't innocuous. In his book *Big Fat Lies: The Truth About Your Health and Weight*, Glenn Gaesser, exercise physiologist and professor at Arizona State University, presents the outcomes of research regarding 17,000 Harvard alumni who were asked how frequently they dieted and how many pounds they lost with each attempt. Compared to men who maintained fairly stable (even if higher) weights, those men in a yo-yo cycle, repeatedly losing and gaining weight, had an 80 percent higher rate of heart disease, and a 123 percent higher rate of type 2 diabetes, compared to their non-dieting classmates. Glaesser warns, "What we have here is a paradox, with potentially calamitous consequences. Losing weight seems to increase the chances of dying from a disease for which weight loss is frequently prescribed to help cure! This brings to mind the most fundamental canon of all helping professions: 'Above else, do no harm'" (refer to Chapter 6).

Does that mean that someone who's large must passively accept that there's nothing effective to improve health? The answer is a resounding "no!" People of all sizes can participate in behaviors that improve health and longevity. Steven Blair, former director of research at the Cooper Institute for Aerobic Research in Dallas, followed 26,000 men and 8,000 women between the ages of 20 and 90 for 10 years. He discovered that both obese fit men and lean fit men had low death rates, and that the obese fit men had death rates half that of lean unfit men. Lean unfit men who fell into the ideal weight category had twice the risk of mortality from all causes, compared to the fit men who fell into the overweight and obese categories. Blair declares that, "by tracking the health status of thousands of women and men who have had fitness tests and medical exams at the Institute over the past 30 years or so, it has become abundantly clear to me that in terms of health and longevity, your fitness level is far more important than your weight. If the height-weight charts say you are 5 pounds too heavy, it is of little consequence healthwise—as long as you are physically fit. On the other hand, if you are a couch potato, being thin provides absolutely no assurance of good health and does nothing to increase your chances of living a long life."

If there's so much evidence challenging conventional wisdom that fat is bad for us, then why don't we hear about it? Probably because we tend to view information through a thinness-bias lens, seizing upon results that favor thinness and ignoring content that doesn't support thinness as the optimal health and beauty standard. This bias was made crystal clear when a doctor was interviewed on CNN to discuss the results of two major studies in 2008, one from Canada and one from Japan, which concluded that people who fell in the "overweight" category live longer than those in the "ideal weight" category. At the end of the interview, the doctor threw in the caveat that, "It's probably still a good idea to lose some weight."

Economic issues play a role in perpetuating the hysteria around weight. Not only do people pursuing weight loss spend billions of dollars each year, but obesity researchers often have their work funded by the diet industry. A clear example of this conflict was the National Task Force on the Prevention and Treatment of Obesity, created and funded by the federal government to set national health policy. In 1996, *JAMA* disclosed that eight out of nine board members were university-affiliated professors and researchers with financial ties to at least two and as many as eight commercial weight-loss and pharmaceutical companies apiece. Laura Fraser, author of *Losing It: America's Obsession with Weight and the Industry That Feeds on It*, explains, "Diet and pharmaceutical companies influence every step along the way of the scientific process. … What it comes down to is that most obesity researchers would stand to lose a lot of money if they stopped telling Americans they had to lose a lot of weight."

What does all of this mean for clients who feel they must lose weight to become healthier and happier? As clients end their compulsive or binge eating by becoming attuned eaters, they usually hope that they'll lose weight. From the outset, I empathize with that wish, and point out that if weight loss occurs, it'll be a side effect of normalizing their eating. Since weight is the result of complex factors still not completely understood, my goal is to help clients feel more comfortable in—and take better care of—their bodies, no matter what their size.

I consider myself to be weight neutral—meaning that I don't assume anything about people's physical and mental status based on weight, and I don't use weight as a measure of a person's success or failure, a framework now commonly known as Health At Every Size. Since health relates to much more than the number on the scale, factors such as a healthy relationship with food, physical activity, good sleep habits, and regular medical care are better indicators. I encourage clients to focus on the fitness, strength, and flexibility they develop through physical activity, as well as on the joy of movement. I know that when many clients use weight loss as their motivation to exercise, they stick to a regime for a while, but as soon as they miss a day or two, they feel guilty and quit working out. This is a shame, since the reality is that exercise is a healthful behavior for all of us, and that people become healthier when participating in physical activity regardless of whether or not any weight is actually lost. As my clients focus on sustainable behaviors, normalize their eating, and work on building a more positive body image, we view any weight loss as their bodies' making an adjustment, but not as the main event.

No matter where therapists find themselves on the continuum of size acceptance, it's our duty to become more aware of this issue and familiar with the research. By increasing awareness of our own behaviors in our professional and personal lives—negative comments about weight, fat jokes, talking about being "good" or "bad" in reference to eating behaviors—we can help change societal norms. If America is truly a melting pot, it's time to throw size diversity into the mix. If we're truly interested in the well-being of our larger clients, then we need to fight the discrimination toward them, including our own. As Ghandi put it, "We must be the change we want to see in the world."

SPOTLIGHT

In the next chapter, Michelle May provides another way of thinking about letting go of the dieting mentality. May presents three possible approaches to eating; intuitive eating, overeating, and restrictive eating, and offers the "Mindful Eating Cycle" to illustrate these possible eating patterns. She discusses hunger and fullness cues, and knowing how to respond in ways that are satisfying and help avoid the often inevitable overeating that follows restrained eating or "dieting."

Chapter Seventeen

How to Break the Eat-Repent-Repeat Cycle

Michelle May

Dieting is an outdated paradigm that simply doesn't lead to sustainable changes for most people. It doesn't address the underlying reasons people eat more than they need, the counter-productive effects of restriction both physically and emotionally, and the unintended consequences of turning exercise into punishment for eating.

To understand why diets don't work, consider the differences between people who manage their eating effortlessly, people who struggle with overeating, and people on a diet. I call these eating patterns Instinctive Eating, Overeating, and Restrictive Eating.

We'll compare these eating patterns using the Mindful Eating Cycle. The Mindful Eating Cycle is a model for recognizing the conscious or subconscious decisions about eating and how each decision affects the decisions that follow. The Mindful Eating Cycle provides important information about why, when, what, how, and how much you eat, and where you invest your energy.

Why? Why do I eat? In other words, what drives my eating cycle?

When? When do I want to eat? When do I think about eating? When do I decide to eat?

What? What do I eat? What food do I choose from all of the available options?

How? How do I eat? How, specifically, do I get the food I have chosen into my body?

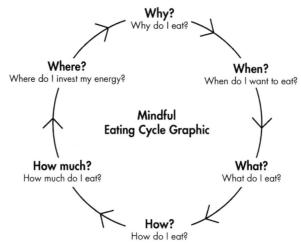

Figure 1. The Mindful Eating Cycle.

How Much? How much do I eat? How much fuel do I give my body when I eat?

Where? Where do I invest my energy? Once I've chosen and eaten food to fuel my body, where does my energy go?

THE INSTINCTIVE EATING CYCLE

Why? The cycle driver is fuel. In the Instinctive Eating Cycle, when your body needs fuel, it triggers the sensation of hunger and guides you to decide when and how much to eat.

When? You eat when you're hungry. Your body lets you know it needs fuel by sending you hunger signals. Once you recognize the need for fuel, you decide whether to eat or not depending on the circumstances, your preferences, the availability of food, convenience, and other factors.

What? You eat whatever you want. You select food from all the available options to fuel your body. Your food choices are affected by your preferences, your awareness and degree of concern about nutrition information, and which foods are available. In the Instinctive Eating Cycle, you don't use rigid rules to decide what to eat, so food doesn't hold any particular power over you.

How? You eat intentionally. When you're in an Instinctive Eating Cycle, you eat with purpose. Usually that purpose is to satisfy hunger but even when the purpose is enjoyment, eating holds your attention so you're able to experience maximal pleasure.

How Much? You eat enough to satisfy hunger. You decide how much food to eat by how hungry you are, how filling the food is, how soon you'll be eating again, and other factors. When your hunger is satisfied you stop eating—even if there's food left. You recognize that being too full is uncomfortable and unnecessary.

Where? The fuel you consume goes toward living your life. Your physical energy can be directed toward your activities during work, play, exercise, and even rest. Your mental energy can be focused on your daily tasks and goals. Your emotional energy can be focused on your feelings and relationships. Any leftover fuel is stored until it's needed. Once your readily available fuel is depleted or stored, the symptoms of hunger return, triggering a desire to eat, and the cycle repeats itself.

THE OVEREATING CYCLE

Why? The Overeating Cycle is driven by triggers. Common environmental triggers include mealtime, appetizing food, social events, and advertising. Emotional triggers include reward, love, stress, boredom, anger, loneliness, and others. Even thinking about starting another diet or stepping on a scale can be a trigger. The distraction or pleasure from eating is initially but temporarily satisfying, driving the Overeating Cycle.

When? Environmental triggers are frequently present in our food-abundant environment and you are always experiencing various emotions so you may feel like eating all the time.

What? You are more likely to choose tempting foods or comfort foods when you are eating in response to triggers other than hunger. You may be less likely to choose nutritious foods since you're not eating in response to physical needs.

How? You may eat quickly, automatically, unconsciously, and/or secretly. As a result, there is less enjoyment and satisfaction from eating.

How Much? If hunger doesn't tell you to start eating, what tells you to stop? The amount of food you eat is often determined by external factors like how much food has been served or how much is in the package. Therefore you may feel too full, miserable, or even numb after eating instead of content and satisfied.

Where? When you eat food your body didn't ask for, you have no choice but to store the extra fuel for later in the form of body fat. You might feel less energetic, causing you to be less physically active, or feel bad about your choices, leading to more emotional triggers and more overeating. When you eat in response to external and emotional triggers, the pleasure and distraction are temporary, so you have to eat again to feel better. More importantly, when you eat in response to triggers instead of meeting your true needs, those needs will go unmet and continue to drive your Overeating Cycle.

THE RESTRICTIVE EATING CYCLE

Why? The Restrictive Eating Cycle is driven by rules that determine when, what, and how much to eat. The rules may come from an "expert" or may be self-imposed.

When? The rules determine whether or not you're allowed to eat, for example, "Eat six small meals a day" or "Don't eat after 7 p.m." The rules place artificial constraints on your eating that don't necessarily honor your body's natural hunger rhythms or address the real reasons you want to eat in the first place.

What? You are only supposed to eat the "good" foods allowed on the diet. You may have to resist your favorite foods or try to avoid situations with forbidden foods you'd be tempted to eat. Since diet rules are always changing, you may sometimes feel confused about what you should eat. Choosing the right food is very important because when your choice is good, you're good. But when your choice is bad, you're bad.

How? Following the rules may require you to be very structured or even rigid in your eating. However, always having to choose good foods may cause you to feel deprived, while choosing bad foods may cause you to feel guilty.

How Much? The quantity of food is predetermined by the rules. This may require weighing, measuring, counting, or other external means to determine how much food you can have or how much food you should eat. This is to prevent you from eating too much food, or perhaps not eating enough, based on the assumption you don't have the ability to consume an appropriate amount of food without following a set of rules.

Where? The Restrictive Eating Cycle usually requires a great deal of mental and emotional energy. If you're significantly under-eating, your body may attempt to conserve as much fuel as possible by decreasing your metabolism. Furthermore, while exercise is very important for overall health and fitness, exercise is sometimes used to earn the right to eat or punish yourself for overeating or for eating a "bad" food.

EAT, REPENT, REPEAT CYCLE

It's common to vacillate back and forth between overeating and restrictive eating: when you eat what you want, you feel guilty; when you eat what you "should," you feel deprived. Either way, you're almost never at peace with your choices, so you switch cycles over the course of a week or a month, or move rapidly from one cycle to the other in the same day or even the same meal.

After overeating, you may feel compelled to compensate by restricting yourself. Even in a Restrictive Eating Cycle, you can continue to eat in response to your triggers but choose

Table 1. The Mindful Eating Cycle: Recognizing Common Eating Patterns

Decision	Instinctive Eating	Overeating	Restrictive Eating
Why? Why do I eat?	To meet your need for fuel.	In response to my environmental and emotional triggers.	According to the rules.
When? When do I eat?	When I'm hungry.	When I'm bored, stressed, lonely, celebrating, getting my money's worth, etc.	When I'm supposed to.
What? What do I eat?	Whatever I enjoy.	Foods that are convenient, comforting, free, etc.	Depends on the rules.
How? How do I eat?	With the intention of feeling better when I'm done.	Quickly, mindlessly, secretly.	Rigidly tracking food and exercise.
How much? How much do I eat?	Enough to satisfy my fuel needs.	Until the food is gone, I feel comfortable, or I'm interrupted.	I weigh, measure, and count my food.
Where? Where do I invest my energy?	Living my life—work, play, physical activity.	Any excess of fuel is stored.	Focused on following the rules.

foods that are allowed on your diet. For example, if you eat veggies instead of chips when you're stressed, you're still eating instead of coping effectively with stress. Eventually you'll begin to feel deprived or worn out by all of the time and energy it takes to follow the rules. So you cheat, feel guilty, and give up, shifting back into your Overeating Cycle, once again eating your favorite foods in response to the triggers you never dealt with in the first place.

This pattern is often referred to as yo-yo dieting, but when the Overeating and Restrictive Eating Cycles are intertwined, I call it the eat-repent-repeat cycle. You move wildly from one extreme to the other, feeling powerless to change, without understanding why. The problem is that a yo-yo is either up or down. You're either wound up tightly adhering to the rules or you're unraveling and heading toward the bottom again. Even if you decided you didn't want to spend the rest of your life in one of these two extremes, there's really no in-between.

Instead of a yo-yo, I prefer to think of a pendulum. A pendulum, while still accounting for potential extremes in your choices, will find a gentle arc somewhere in the middle as it loses momentum. When you finally stop wasting so much of your energy on overeating and dieting, you'll naturally settle into a more comfortable, centered way of managing eating. This frees up the rest of your energy for more enjoyable, productive, and fulfilling activities.

RELEARNING TO EAT INSTINCTIVELY

The way to break the eat-repent-repeat cycle is to restore your Instinctive Eating Cycle by finding the balance between the extremes. Instead of following strict rules created by experts, you become the expert in yourself. By relearning to use your hunger and satiety cues, you can determine when, what, and how much you need to eat. You'll also recognize when you want to eat for reasons other than hunger, giving you the opportunity to meet your true needs in positive and constructive ways so food can serve its proper function—to nourish you and fuel a fulfilling life.

You have the freedom and flexibility to eat the foods you love fearlessly, and the purpose and awareness to love the foods you eat mindfully. You were born with the natural ability to effortlessly manage your eating this way.

Each decision point in the Mindful Eating Cycle is an opportunity for new awareness and change.

Why do I eat?

As you become more conscious of your own eating cycles, you may notice that when you're overeating, you often feel *out of control*. When you're dieting, you finally feel *in control*—though it's usually too difficult (and boring!) to sustain permanently. When you're eating instinctively, instead of spinning out of control or trying to stay in control, you are *in charge*. Therefore, no matter what the circumstances, you are making the best choices for yourself (including occasionally eating when you're not hungry for convenience or pleasure, but *without* guilt or compensation).

When do I eat?

Am I Hungry? Hunger is a primitive yet reliable way of signaling a need for fuel and, therefore, regulating dietary intake. A very simple but useful approach is to ask, "Am I hungry?" before eating. Whenever possible, remove yourself from the presence of food and situations you associate with eating for a few moments to minimize triggers. Identify hunger by *physical* symptoms including a growling stomach, lightheadedness, irritability, and other signs that your stomach is empty and your blood sugar is dropping.

Once you're able to identify hunger, you can fine tune your awareness by determining how hungry you are. Through trial and error you'll discover that waiting to eat until you are sufficiently hungry increases satisfaction, while waiting too long can lead to overeating—no rules required!

If there are no physical signs of hunger, it is likely that the urge to eat was triggered by something in the environment or an emotion. If a craving doesn't come from hunger, eating will never satisfy it. Therefore, it is necessary to reduce and/or respond more effectively to the underlying trigger.

Decrease and Deal with Environmental Triggers: To decrease eating in response to environmental triggers, you must first become aware of their associations. When you recognize that an urge to eat was triggered by something in your environment, you can choose to redirect your attention until the urge passes, reminding yourself that you'll eat when you get hungry. You can prepare for these situations by having a variety of appealing alternative activities available such as reading, letter writing, journaling, or woodworking.

You may also decide to decrease your environmental triggers by putting food out of sight, avoiding the break room, and ordering half-portions or sharing meals. With practice, this process will helps you break the habitual association between certain activities, people, and places and overeating. Over time you are likely to find yourself eating less often in response to cues in the environment when you aren't hungry.

Respond Effectively to Emotional Triggers: All people eat for emotional reasons, including celebrating, expressing love, or finding comfort in Grandma's apple pie. In many cultures around the world, social events often revolve around eating and emotional connections to food are part of "normal" eating. Emotional eating becomes maladaptive when it is the primary way that a person copes with emotions. To be clear, this does not imply that if you overeat, you may have major psychological problems. It simply means that you have learned to use food for purposes other than energy and nutrition at times.

If you've been using food to help you cope with stress and other emotions, dieting will disrupt your primary coping strategy. If you don't learn alternative means of coping, then distress will increase and overeating will eventually return. Alternatively, when you're able to gain insight into your emotional triggers, you can improve your ability to identify feelings and expand your range of coping mechanisms. Examples include stress management, positive thinking, and setting boundaries in relationships. Often, new skills and tools are needed, so it is best to approach this as a process, seeking support or counseling when necessary.

When you learn more effective strategies for coping with your emotions and use food less often for comfort or to avoid dealing with feelings, two things happen. First, your desire to overeat diminishes. Second, and more important, you'll begin to find fulfillment in experiences other than eating and learn to meet your true needs more effectively.

What do I eat?

Eating instinctively doesn't mean eating perfectly (whatever that is). In a non-diet approach there are no rigid food or nutrition rules, because a "normal" diet consists of a variety of foods, including those eaten for pleasure. When favorite foods aren't forbidden and can be enjoyed without guilt, there's less drive to overeat them. When deprivation is no longer a factor, you won't need an endless supply of willpower and self-control.

The desire to eat healthier foods increases further through awareness and personal experience about the effects that different foods have on your body. You'll discover that it's possible to balance eating for nourishment with eating for enjoyment. You'll naturally seek balance, variety, and moderation in your diet. You will create your own "masterpiece".

How do I eat?

Mindful eating, eating with *intention* and *attention*, leads to increased satisfaction and pleasure and increased awareness of hunger and satiety.

> **Intention:** Be purposeful when you eat:
> - Eat when you're truly hungry.
> - Eat to meet your body's needs.
> - Eat with the goal of feeling *better* when you're finished.
>
> **Attention:** Give your full attention to the activity of eating:
> - Eliminate or minimize distractions.
> - Tune in to ambiance, flavors, aromas, temperature, and texture of the food.
> - Listen to your body's cues of hunger and fullness.

How much do I eat?

With increased awareness of your physical cues, you'll also begin to identify satiety and learn to stop eating before you become too full. Avoidance of the physical discomfort of fullness becomes an internalized mechanism of portion control.

When you do overeat, rather than feeling guilty (which only drives more overeating), it's important try to identify why it happened and what you will do differently next time. Then return to instinctive eating by waiting to see when you become hungry again and what you're hungry for.

Where do I invest my energy?

Diets prescribe exercise to burn calories, essentially turning it into punishment for eating. However, exercise has benefits far beyond caloric expenditure and will improve health and decrease the risk of illness even without weight loss. Exercise also helps you reconnect with your physical body and improve your sense of well-being. Therefore, exercise isn't a means to an end, but an end in and of itself.

If exercise is uncomfortable or you have other negative thoughts about exercise, it is important to start with small steps by increasing your lifestyle activity such as parking further from the building and walking to the mailbox. As your comfort increases, you can develop a physical activity plan tailored to your personality and level of fitness. Realistically, exercise must be comfortable, convenient, fun, and rewarding in order for it to become a long-term habit.

Exercise is only one place you can invest your energy. As you focus on the physical, intellectual, emotional, and spiritual areas of your life that deserve your energy and attention, you create a self-care buffer zone. When the needs of your body, mind, heart, and spirit are being met, the desire to use food to fill those holes decreases. As you satisfy these needs in more positive and constructive ways, food can serve its proper function—to fuel and nourish your fulfilling, vibrant life.

Live Vibrantly!

Relearning to eat instinctively restores your freedom and flexibility. If you're exposed to food when you're not hungry, you may take a passing interest in it, but you probably won't eat a significant amount because you'd feel uncomfortable afterward. You can eat anything you want when you're hungry, so you don't have to spend a lot of time deciding in advance what you're going to eat. You may consciously choose to follow a healthier diet, but you don't expect yourself to be perfect. You truly enjoy food because you don't feel physically or emotionally uncomfortable during or after eating. And when you're satisfied, you go on living your life without thinking about food again until your body tells you to.

When you learn to manage your eating by listening to your instincts, you'll begin to trust your ability to take charge of other areas of your life as well. When you're *in charge* instead of trying to stay *in control*, you'll feel empowered to infuse intention and attention into other areas for a more balanced, satisfying, and vibrant life.

SPOTLIGHT

Next, Michelle May presents a fanciful idea of a "meme" or "idea gene" that has spread around the western world, and is rapidly moving into many other areas as well. This idea is that dieting or restrictive eating is a *good thing*, a healthy thing to do, and the way "healthy" people should live. Dr. May argues that this idea is faulty and that we may not even be aware of how our attitudes about dieting are influenced by this "meme." She discusses ways of getting rid of the dieting meme.

Chapter Eighteen

Paint-by-Number or Masterpiece: The Difference Between Restrictive Eating and Healthy Eating

Michelle May

There is a meme* (like an idea gene) that has become so widespread, so ubiquitous, that it is accepted as normal. It has subtly integrated itself into the beliefs, thoughts, language, and behavior of American culture. It is so pervasive that it has become "conventional wisdom," so almost no one questions it.

This meme is the belief that restrictive eating is healthy. This meme is so insidious that most people who have been infected with it don't even realize it. Even the people responsible for spreading it don't recognize its potential for long-term damage. In fact, most believe that they're actually helping others when they pass along this meme. They might even feel defensive or irritated when they read this. Hopefully they'll keep reading anyway.

* What Is a Meme? A meme is a unit of cultural information, such as a cultural practice or idea, that is transmitted verbally or by repeated action from one mind to another. Memes are the cultural counterpart of genes. Like genes, some ideas will propagate less successfully and become extinct, while others will survive, spread, and, for better or for worse, mutate. Memeticists argue that the memes most beneficial to their hosts will not necessarily survive; rather, those memes that replicate the most effectively spread best, which allows for the possibility that successful memes may prove detrimental to their hosts.

DO YOU HAVE THIS MEME?

To see if you might have this "restrictive is healthy" meme, too, take a look at the following statements and ask yourself if it is true for you most, or even some, of the time. (Or, to see if you might be perpetuating this meme, ask yourself if you are intentionally or inadvertently teaching other people to adopt these statements.)

_____ I use labels to decide whether or not I can eat a particular food.
_____ I weigh, measure, or count just about everything I eat.
_____ I usually pass up foods that are high in certain ingredients, like fat or carbs.
_____ I avoid certain places or situations where there will be a lot of unhealthy food.
_____ I sometimes give in and eat bad foods but make up for it by exercising more.
_____ I answered yes to one or more of the above and I'm proud of my self-control.
_____ I answered no to all the questions but I admire people who do.
_____ I feel guilty when I eat certain foods.
_____ I feel bad about myself when I eat foods I know I shouldn't.

A "yes" answer to any of the statements above may indicate that you have this meme.

It usually starts benignly enough with information about health, nutrition, weight or trying change one's diet because of an illness like diabetes. Unlike mindful eating, which is based on choosing foods based on what we really want to eat without guilt, this meme mutates into rigid rules and restriction.

The difference between mindful eating and restrictive eating is the difference between a work of art and paint-by-number. Either way, you end up with a nice picture—until you get up close to take a look. Restrictive eating is composed of rigid lines and somebody else's choice of colors. Mindful eating is a masterpiece that reflects an individual's preferences, culture, lifestyle, health goals, and other personal factors.

Mindful Eating vs.	Restrictive Eating
In Charge	In Control
Nourishment	Diet
Fuel	Calories
Quality	Points
Healthy	Skinny
Aware	Preoccupied
Conscious	Consumed
Mindful	Vigilant
Information	Dogma
Guide	Rules
All foods fit	Good or bad
Balance	Perfection
Variety	Temptation
Moderation	Deprivation
Choosing	Earning
Deciding	Rationalizing
Flexible	Rigid
Hunger-based	By the clock
Comfort	Portion sizes
Physical Activity	Penance
Introspective	Smug
Effortless	Willpower
Trust	Fear
Learning	Failing
Self-acceptance	Condemnation
Enjoyment	Guilt
Pleasure	Shame
Freedom	Bondage

HOW IS THIS MEME SPREAD?

One of the reasons that the "restrictive is healthy" meme is so successful at replicating itself is that it initially appears to be beneficial to its host. For example, if you are concerned about your weight, everybody infected with the meme tries to pass it on to you in an effort to "help" you (or more cynically, sell you something). It is transmitted through loving advice, striking before-and-after photos, or fear-based messages.

The meme spreads vertically through advertising, television, magazines, books, the internet, and research. It is propagated by marketers, models, celebrities, reporters, experts, bloggers, legislators, and academicians. It is then spread horizontally from doctor to patient, dietitian to client, friend to friend, partner to partner, and parent to child.

This meme is also swiftly moving from the United States to the rest of the world. Countries seeing an increase in obesity rates are now being inundated with the restrictive messages that Americans have been subjected to for decades. The obvious evidence that this meme hasn't helped Americans hasn't stopped its spread attests to its craftiness.

Some people who spread the meme are carriers but don't actually manifest it themselves. For instance, some health and fitness professionals eat instinctively *without* restriction but spread the meme when they put their patients or clients on a diet or rigid exercise regimen. Others believe they are promoting "lifestyle change" and "healthy eating" when these are really just euphemisms for, "you're going to be on this diet for the rest of your life." The meme is so imbedded into the culture that health and wellness professionals can't see that restriction is at the core of their message.

This "restriction is healthy" meme is powerful because it has a built-in protective mechanism: the belief that some people are incapable of handling freedom or choice. After "catching" this meme, there are usually early signs of the promised results. However, since deprivation leads to increased cravings followed by overeating, the initial belief—some people are incapable of handling freedom or choice—appears to be true. This leads to another round of restriction, ensuring survival of the meme. This is the eat-repent-repeat cycle discussed in Chapter 17. Once caught in this vicious cycle, it is difficult to recognize the real source of the problem.

HOW TO GET RID OF THE MEME

Take a close look at the "picture of health" you're painting for yourself (or others). Is it constrained by rigid lines and someone else's choice of colors? Or does it express your individuality, your preferences, and your lifestyle? Choose now how you want to create *your* work of art. If you want to rid yourself of the "restrictive eating is healthy" meme, here are some specific steps you can take.

1. Expose the meme. Filter everything you read, hear, and say by asking, "Is this restrictive in nature?" (You might be surprised when you start to notice just how pervasive it really is!)
2. Begin to monitor your thoughts. (This meme is sneaky so it may be helpful to journal so you capture the real essence of your beliefs, thoughts, feelings, and choices.) When you notice restrictive eating thoughts from the second column above, gently replace them with true healthy-eating thoughts from the first column.

3. Remember, the meme may have you convinced that you are incapable of managing your eating without rigid rules. Find role models, health care providers, and non-diet approaches that don't propagate the meme.
4. Use nutrition information as a tool not a weapon. Remember, all foods can fit into a healthy diet.
5. Make the healthiest choice you can *without* feeling deprived. Use the simple principles of balance, variety, and moderation to guide you.
6. Let go of the belief that you need to eat perfectly. That is the meme talking. Accept that you'll sometimes regret some of the choices you make; that is part of healthy eating. When you don't get caught up in guilt and shame, you're able to learn from your experiences.
7. Repeat often: "It's just food and I *can* learn to trust and nourish myself without restriction."

With practice, support, and new mindful eating skills, you will discover joy in creating a masterpiece that reflects your lifestyle and health goals.

SPOTLIGHT

The next chapter is from Karen R. Koenig's book *The Food and Feelings Workbook*. I present this as a sample of the kind of emotional work that can be done to heal chronic dieters, people who hate their bodies, and people who struggle in general with food. Koenig offers a perspective on one's relationship to food, as well as practice exercises to help the reader learn more, and begin to change that relationship.

Chapter Nineteen

Feelings, Not Food

Karen R. Koenig

Because feelings are so complicated and we're so poorly schooled in handling them, it's easy to see why anyone might get food and feelings confused. However, if you consistently binge or reject food when you're upset rather than let your feelings flow, you are not meeting your body's needs for nourishment and pleasure or your heart's need to experience its wisdom. Very possibly you don't even realize that your eating behaviors are being driven by internal discomfort. In fact, you may be *so* out of touch with your emotions that you have no idea they even exist, simmering below the surface of consciousness. They're only a heartbeat away, but if you constantly tune them out, they might as well be on the moon!

Remember, feelings are the portal to your inner world, the key to your deepest yearnings and desires, the compass that guides you through life. Focus in on feelings as sharply you do on food and weight obsessions (maybe even *half* as sharply) and you'll get vital information that will move you toward health and authentic happiness. This may seem like a tall order to someone who's depended on dysfunctional eating to quell emotional pain. Yet, there's no other way. Food is food and feelings are feelings, and never the twain shall meet.

If you're tired of searching in supermarkets and restaurants for the cure to what ails you, if you're sick of obsessing about fats and calories or the magic number on the bathroom scale, it's time to find a better way to manage your emotions.

WHAT IS THE CONNECTION BETWEEN FEEDING AND FEELING?

One of the major reasons we focus on food when we're in distress is the powerful primitive connection that exists between feeding and feeling. It's no accident that food becomes an issue when emotional dander starts to fly. If you take a closer look at your earliest years on earth, you'll see that you come by an appetite-affect response quite naturally.

Here's what happens. Nothing is more critical for an infant than being fed. At best, a poorly nourished child will suffer malnutrition; at worst, it will starve to death. An effective parent takes the utmost care feeding an infant: The bottle must be heated to just the right temperature, the baby must be held at the correct angle, and feeding must stop if the baby falls asleep or has had enough.

Moreover, the physical and emotional bonding that occurs between parent and child during feeding is nearly as crucial as the receipt of adequate nourishment. An innate physical need gets expressed through closeness. Think how most of us like to hold hands, hug, cuddle, fondle, and have sex. Touch often reaches our hidden wounds and comforts us in a way that words simply cannot. Additionally, on a metaphysical level, touch makes us feel less alone in this vast and mysterious universe, offering reassurance that someone is close by.

As infants, we suffer from two mystifying and terrifying human conditions: We're often hungry and we hate being left alone for long. Being fed while we're held is something close to divine. For babies, it just doesn't get any better. (Sometimes for grown-ups too!) And that's where feeling and feeding first intersect or fuse. When we're lovingly held while receiving nourishment, two of our most urgent needs are gratified at once; hence, most of us begin to associate feeding with safety, security, closeness, pleasure, and comfort. From then on, the two are forever inextricably entwined—married for better or for worse.

Moreover, milk, our first meal, is a tasty source of pleasure in its own right. Containing tryptophan, milk produces a relaxing response. Even if we weren't cradled in loving arms as we drank, we couldn't help making a deliriously delightful, unconscious connection to being fed and a contented drowsiness. And, forever after, this is one of the unconscious attractions that food has for us—the blissful tranquility we felt as infants, something we still, at times, achingly long for.

Some babies, however, are not so fortunate. Their parents are out of sync with their feeding needs or fail utterly to meet them. Infants who remain hungry for too long may associate hunger with extreme emotional discomfort and distress. Or they may be handled roughly when fed, a bottle shoved into their tiny mouth, and forced to drink until it's all gone whether they're full or not. Some babies receive little, if any, positive body contact when fed. In such cases, feeding and feeling are still coupled, but in a cruel way: Nourishment is associated with punishment and/or literal intrusion, and food may eventually be perceived as discomforting.

It's essential to understand this initial, potent connection between feeling and feeding, especially if you're the kind of disordered eater who comes down really hard on yourself. You think there's something critically wrong with you, that you're defective, weird, weak, unbalanced, or depraved because of the intense, overwhelming urgency or repulsion you feel toward food. Understanding this primitive association makes it easier to suspend judgment after your next binge, or when all you've eaten all day is a lettuce leaf. The key is to recognize that you're biologically programmed to focus on food when under stress. This association is hard-wired, so, please, have some compassion for yourself.

The link goes far beyond infancy, however. Even if it wasn't the case in your particular family, in our culture (and most others), food is special and often confers specialness. Parents may serve frozen dinners every night, but when company rings the bell, they generally make an extra effort to serve a tasty and tasteful meal. Food is associated with times of high emotion—candy for Valentine's Day, homemade cookies for a sick friend, a decorative wedding or birthday cake, candy canes hung on a Christmas tree, chocolate coins for Chanukah, an array of dishes on the dining room table after a funeral, and a traditional turkey that brings family home for Thanksgiving. Everywhere we turn, food is smack in the middle of occasions that tug at our heartstrings.

In the best of worlds, our parents weren't disordered eaters or obsessed about weight and didn't use a spoon or a scale to keep their inner world from exploding. Instead, they validated our feelings, spent just the right amount of time soothing us, and handled their own feelings competently. They offered us goodies from time to time when we were unhappy, but gave us the message loud and clear that food is the appropriate response to physical hunger, and that friends and family are there for sympathy and support.

The sad truth is I've only met a handful of people who've had parents this insightful, thoughtful, sensitive, and emotionally intelligent.

If you weren't raised in the best of worlds, but like many of us, grew up in your own little world, your appetite-and-emotions connection may be faulty. You may use food to feel better, to avoid feeling worse, or to feel nothing at all. If you fixate on weight and food to avoid emotional wounds, rather than turn to people for support, you have the whole process backwards.

If you want to end disordered eating, you have to break the link between feelings and food.

This is a formidable, arduous task because this connection *is* hard-wired and because of the considerable reinforcement we receive about using food as an emotional Band-Aid.

However, take heart: *This link can be broken.* Through hard work, you can reprogram yourself to form a positive, healthy relationship with your heart and your hunger. I know you can succeed because I've done it myself and helped scores of others do it. But first you have to learn everything you can about your emotions. I mean everything!

STOP AND FEEL

How do you feel about your food problem now that you understand the powerful biological connection between food and feeling?

_____

_____

_____

PRACTICE EXERCISE:

Self-Comfort

PURPOSE: To learn to physically self-soothe

RATIONALE: Self-soothing is a necessary skill in regulating emotions, a combination of positive self-talk and receiving physical comfort (even from yourself!).

WHAT YOU NEED: something comfy to sit on

DIRECTIONS: Sit in a comfortable chair or on a stack of big, soft pillows and burrow in until your body feels just right in your cozy nest. Now wrap your arms around yourself and give yourself a gentle hug. Notice how it feels. If it's okay, rub your arms gently, give yourself a pat on the back, or stroke your hair. Say comforting things to yourself. Try to connect your gestures and words with being soothed, and relax into them. It's fine if the exercise feels silly, strange, or makes you uncomfortable. Keep at it until the discomfort dissolves and you relax.

REFLECTION (to be done after completion of exercise): What was it like trying to physically soothe yourself? Did you connect with any comforting experiences from childhood or did your attempts feel foreign or have negative associations? If your reaction was negative, try to understand why you might feel this way.

_____

_____

_____

WHY DOES FOOD TASTE SO GOOD WHEN I FEEL SO BAD?

Let's face it—focusing on food is a grand distraction from our troubles. The very activities of searching through cupboards, shopping and cooking, chewing and swallowing, and cleaning up afterwards divert your attention *away* from what's going on inside you *toward* what you're doing. The mental effort of calculating calories and fat grams wipes everything else off your slate. Not that you're necessarily aware of this diversion when you grab a snack when you're not hungry or daydream about the fantastic life you'll have when you lose ten pounds—frankly, you're probably on autopilot. You may be thinking about food not *because* you're upset, but to *prevent* yourself from becoming upset. Vaguely aware of internal alarm, you hurry to shut off distressing sensations before they erupt into consciousness.

If you're a dysfunctional eater who turns toward food when you're feeling bad, it tastes good in part because you're desperately looking for ways to ward off the blues, the blahs, or the jitters. How often do you continue to eat something that's flavorless, barely edible, or downright repulsive—dry cereal, frozen donuts, stale crackers, a tub of butter, rancid leftovers—rather than experience your feelings? Let's face it, you wouldn't order any of these foods in a restaurant, but you tolerate them because a bad taste—any taste—beats a bad feeling any day of the week. Sometimes, what you're swallowing is so horrid that it really is a toss-up; but too often, even when you're in doubt, food wins out.

Another reason that food tastes good for people who view it as a panacea is that it's meant to be eaten so that our species will survive and flourish. Food is supposed to be appetizing and appealing, delectable and divine. So when you bite into a juicy apple or a buttery croissant, it's no surprise that your taste buds cheer wildly. They're happy even if you're not. But just because something tastes good doesn't mean you should be eating it, especially if the real business at hand is attending to emotions.

Science has come a long way in understanding the complexities of appetite and affect. Research tells us that under stress our bodies crave carbohydrates, which have chemical properties to soothe and relax us, just as milk did in infancy. Not only does food taste heavenly, it's also a source of what we're physiologically lacking in moments of distress. Take carbohydrates whose chemical compounds break down in our bodies in such a way as to calm and comfort us. Food does this job extremely well—too well!

If you eat when you're in emotional distress, are you starting to see what you're up against? Is it beginning to make sense why you're drawn toward yummy when you're feeling crummy?

In spite of the fact that food is meant to nourish and be savored, if you're a restrictive or rigid non-eater, you may use food to decrease or avoid emotional turmoil because the act of saying "No" is such a huge chunk of effort and such a validation of being in charge of your life. If you're feeling proud and elated about disciplining yourself to refuse food, there's very little room for upsetting emotion to squeeze into consciousness. Moreover, by rejecting food you're putting your world back in balance as you offset internal agita with self-restraint. The very act of overpowering your innate hunger and craving for nourishment is a way of proving to yourself that you're strong and invulnerable.

As you've learned, this is an exceedingly complicated subject that involves both body chemistry and early nurturing.

STOP AND FEEL

How does understanding the link between food and feeling lessen your shame about your disordered eating?

_____

_____

_____

IS IT EVER OKAY TO OVEREAT OR SKIP MEALS IN RESPONSE TO DISTURBING FEELINGS?

There's nothing unusual or wrong with occasionally turning to or away from food or skipping meals when you're down in the dumps or overwound. It's all in your perspective—the way you think about food and its place in your life. "Normal" eaters may seek a lift in a candy bar or a cannoli, but they know that eating is no magical remedy for the downside of life. They recognize that food can be a savory treat, but will not solve ongoing problems. In fact, "normal" eaters may be terrible problem-solvers, but the one thing they don't regularly do to feel better is stuff themselves or habitually deny themselves nourishment and the pleasure of food.

Moreover, even if they eat when they're frazzled, people who have a healthy relationship with food generally remain at least minimally connected to their bodies, and therefore stop eating when they're full or satisfied. They're just as likely to consume half of what they've chosen as they are to clean their plate. Whatever happens to the food once they're satisfied is of no concern to them.

Of course, even people who are comfortable around food sometimes become so upset that they *do* disconnect from their bodies. What distinguishes them from people with eating problems is that this behavior isn't part of an everyday pattern. They don't beat themselves up, eat in secret, feel shame, or swear to eat differently tomorrow. Their self-concept, self-esteem, and general attitude have nothing to do with their behavior around food.

Most importantly, they wouldn't spend the next hour and a half (or day and a half) chastising themselves or use splurging on a treat as permission to go on a wild food binge. And they certainly wouldn't deprive themselves the next time they were hungry. If you asked what they did when they were distressed, they might not even remember that they'd enjoyed a bag of munchies or skipped an entire meal. They might have secondary emotions about what they were initially *feeling*, but not about what they'd eaten or not eaten. Plus, they'd trust that their appetite would return to normal when emotional equilibrium returned.

On the other hand, even "normal" eaters can truly lose their desire for food when hit with intense emotions. After a shock to the system, their appetite shuts down and the sight, thought, or smell of food may lose its appeal. "Normal" eaters do not intentionally deprive themselves of sustenance and nutrients as a way to cope; the response is automatic and unconscious and, except over an extended period of time, is not self-injurious. If this reaction occurs only occasionally, it's nothing to worry about.

However, avoiding food on an ongoing basis is another story. If your conscious intent is to not eat because you think you'll get fat or won't get thin, or because eating makes you physically and emotionally uncomfortable, you're imposing an unhealthy restriction on your body. Moreover, you may have discovered that one of the best detours around your messy inner world is to shift from your heart to your head by refusing food. Instead of dealing with your life, you reminisce about a thinner past or fantasize about a skinnier future.

Although it's absolutely fine to occasionally use or refuse food when you're feeling low, breaking out into a binge or going on a hunger strike on a regular basis is simply unhealthy. Your work is to trust that you'll gradually move toward eating more normally, and only rarely eat or refuse food when you're upset (with absolutely no remorse!). Which brings me to the subject of realistic expectations. The truth is you're going to need a lot of practice to sever the connection between feeling and feeding. The good news is that you can practice all day long, every day—every time you're hungry or have a craving, every time you sense inner turmoil, every time you start obsessing about food or weight. Each moment is a golden opportunity to work toward getting food and feeling right!

STOP AND FEEL

Are you worried that you'll never be able to choose feeling over dysfunctional eating?

_____

_____

_____

PRACTICE EXERCISE:

It's Only Food

PURPOSE: To recognize: 1) what it is about food that attracts/repels when you're in emotional discomfort and 2) how you confer upon food magical powers it doesn't have. (Do this exercise only when you are feeling calm and relatively comfortable with yourself.)

RATIONALE: Most of us have strong feelings about food one way or the other. Recognizing your visceral reactions is a great way to improve your relationship with eating _and_ feeling.

WHAT YOU NEED: Food that you are drawn to or repelled by when you have emotional flare-ups

DIRECTIONS: Place in front of you a food that you usually eat or overeat, or alternately, one that you intentionally avoid when you're upset. Notice how unmagical the food is, how it's merely a mix of ingredients. Pick it up, smell it, and even play with it. Focus on its composition (e.g., eggs, sugar, wheat, flour) and write what you notice about it. Take a bite and note how the food tastes and feels in your mouth. Concentrate on defusing this food's power and write your reactions to your first bite. Taking a slow second and third bite, continue to write your reactions.

_____

_____

_____

REFLECTION (to be done after completion of exercise): What did you find magical about this food? What did you find ordinary? Exactly what does this food do for you when you are in emotional distress? What tells you that it really has no magic at all?

_____

_____

_____

HOW CAN I SEPARATE FEELING FROM FEEDING?

If you're fairly accepting of and comfortable with feelings, you'll have an easier time than if you're almost entirely disconnected from them. The more disengaged you are, the earlier in the emotional process you'll have to sit up and take notice. People have varying accessibility to feelings. I've had clients whose typical response to being asked what they were feeling was an "I-don't-know" shrug, and others who could describe in minute detail exactly what was going on inside of them.

How well you separate feeling from feeding depends on where you are on the connected-to-feelings continuum. Stop and think how you'd describe yourself (and how those who know you well would describe you). Are you strongly in touch with feelings, moderately in touch, or out of touch? If you and your emotions rarely take a spin around the dance floor, you'll have to educate yourself about how your bodily sensations translate into emotions. What sensations indicate you're angry? Lonely? Sad? Disappointed? Frustrated? Helpless? Confused? Does each emotion feel the same in your body or does each arise from different physical sensations?

The first step in disengaging appetite from affect is to translate body sensations to emotions. Start by paying specific attention to your breathing, pulse, and energy level. Notice if your chest feels hollow or fluttery, your gut is a tight knot, a hundred butterflies are flitting around your belly, your shoulders are tense, your fists or jaw are clenched, you're spacey or queasy, thoughts are racing around your head, or if there's a sense of dread in the pit of your stomach.

Too often we ignore physical manifestations of emotions rather than recognize them for what they are—messengers sending out a bulletin about what's going on inside of us. Here are some examples. If every time you visit your friends Leann and Scott, they do nothing but bicker, you may feel an unpleasant clenching in your stomach as you're about to ring their bell. If at the last minute you bow out of driving your best friend to the airport because you decide to sleep in, you may suffer a gnawing, nagging feeling that you did something wrong. If you're about to read a letter from the college you're dying to get into and your sister asks you a dumb question, you may feel disconnected from reality and not even hear her. These are all examples of physical reactions that accompany internal distress.

Your response to danger is biologically programmed, and of necessity, highly attention-grabbing in order to keep you alive. When you perceive a threat, your senses automatically perk up, your breathing quickens, and blood flows to your heart, making it pound. The emotions you have when you're robbed at knifepoint are probably a good deal easier to identify than what you're feeling on Saturday night with nothing to do—antsy, mildly anxious, tired, empty, lonely, alienated, sad, or bored.

Some emotions broadcast themselves loud and clear, while others barely whisper, so you'll have to become very still and listen closely to what's going on inside of your body to discover what emotion may be struggling to surface. You can't skip this process.

If you want to disengage feeding from feeling, you have to experience the physical sensations that arise within you, no matter how uncomfortable.

PRACTICE EXERCISE:

Physical Manifestations of Emotion

PURPOSE: To connect physical sensations to emotions

RATIONALE: The best way to recognize if an emotion is stirring is to scan your body for physical sensations that you are feeling something deeply.

WHAT YOU NEED: painful memories

DIRECTIONS: Choose a disturbing incident that happened during the past week or one that's been haunting you for ages. Bring your feelings about it into sharp focus. As if you're watching TV, turn up the volume and make sure the picture is clear and bright. Label what you're feeling: dread, shock, rage, remorse, disappointment, powerlessness. Notice the sensations in your body that connect to this emotion. Also note what happens when you label what's going on, especially if the feeling worsens or eases up. Pay attention to what organs or body parts are in play and what's happening to them. Choose another feeling and go through the same process.

REFLECTION (to be done after completion of exercise): Were you able to identify the parts of your body holding your emotion? Do you usually pay attention to this kind of reaction or ignore it? What happened when you gave physical sensation the label of an emotion?

_____
_____
_____

If you're feeling the least bit unskilled at connecting to body sensations that signal emotions, take heart. You can learn more about how internal commotion is channeled into an emotion. For now, simply pay attention to physical shifts that may indicate internal distress. The next step will be to fine tune and become expert at labeling emotions. This means distinguishing guilt from shame, anger from fear, helplessness from anxiety, confusion from uncertainty.

If you are interested in learning more about what to *do* with emotions at this point, you can read more about this in *The Food and Feelings Workbook, by Karen R. Koenig.* For now, suffice it to say that you're on your way to developing a new set of skills (or behaviors) that will be sure to build and strengthen your emotional muscles!

FURTHER EXPLORATION

1. What do you think makes the connection between food and feeling so strong for you?

_____
_____
_____
_____

2. How did your childhood experiences reinforce focusing on eating or not eating when you're emotionally uncomfortable?

_____
_____
_____
_____

3. Why is food even more comforting when you're upset?

_____
_____
_____
_____

4. Why might you turn away from hunger and cravings rather than nourish yourself?

_____

_____

_____

_____

5. How would you describe the difference between how disordered and "normal" eaters use food when they're upset?

_____

_____

_____

_____

6. As you contemplate the idea of listening to both your feelings and your hunger, what inner tugs of resistance do you notice?

_____

_____

_____

_____

7. How do you feel about overcoming your emotional connection to food: hopeful, hopeless, or mixed?

_____

_____

_____

_____

8. In general, how would you rate your connection to your feelings: strong, moderate, poor, non-existent?

_____

_____

_____

_____

9. What do you need to do to increase your connection to your emotions?

_____

_____

_____

_____

10. How can you improve at tuning into physical sensations that may be precursors to emotions?

_____

_____

_____

_____

11. Where do you imagine you are in the process of breaking the connection between food and feelings? Do you feel as if you're taking your first step? Do you think you may be halfway there?

_____

_____

_____

_____

Reference

Koenig, K. The Food and Feelings Workbook, 2007, Gurze Books, Carlsbad, CA

SPOTLIGHT

Next, Alice Rosen offers a description of the use of several spiritual practices to the healing of disordered eating. She explains the compassionate means of addressing the underlying causes for such difficulties, to make way for true healing and for putting food in its rightful, very important place in our lives. Rosen describes the ways in which this work allows us to reclaim the pleasure of eating.

Chapter Twenty

Applying Spirituality to a Non-Diet Approach

Alice Rosen

The intention of this chapter is to address the application of spiritual practices to the treatment of disordered eating, as a way to foster an attuned and peaceful relationship with food and body. In so doing, the considerable energy, once directed toward maintaining an eating disorder, may be freed up to benefit oneself and the world.

Since 1980, I have been using a mindfulness-based, non-diet approach with people who have a dysfunctional relationship with food and body. I entered this field of work after my personal experience of liberation from disordered eating. Prior to that time, I had many years of meditation practice, but in 1980, I had a powerful experience when I attended a mindfulness retreat. I went there with a renewed intention to concentrate my awareness on present moment experience, not only during formal practice, but also during transitions and mealtimes. This intention came from my growing realization that time was short and that now was the only time I really had. It was during my first meal, to my utter surprise, that I discovered a point at which I had no further desire to eat, even when there was more appealing and delicious food on the plate! I discovered total contentment, where I knew that one more bite would not bring any more pleasure. Usually I felt sluggish and tired after eating, but my body felt a new lightness and freedom. I also noticed that my frequent thinking about what I was going to eat next disappeared during the whole ten-day retreat. Both my mind and body had more available energy.

I realized that I could get enough, that I needed no will power, nor did I need to listen to any external dictates. All I needed was to pay attention to my body's sensations and signals. At that time, I had no knowledge of any of the non-diet movements, so this self-discovery was very empowering, indeed. I am still impassioned with the realization, and have the mission to help others know, that *the ultimate authority about when, what, and how much to eat lies within.*

There is a way to be at peace with food. That "way" is devoid of concepts or thinking, and can be known only by experience. This is what I mean by a taking a spiritual approach.

I will continue this chapter by describing the disordered eating in the population I am addressing, and discuss the role of food in our lives. I will then talk about spirituality and examine how it is relevant to a non-diet approach. I will include clinical models, which incorporate spiritual practices into the treatment of disordered eating, and mention some essential qualities of a qualified professional in this field. Lastly I will share some useful practices, which can be integrated into clinical work.

WHAT IS DISORDERED EATING?

Eating disorders are complex, multidimensional syndromes. Simply put, they are any of a range of psychological disorders characterized by abnormal or disturbed eating behaviors, which then affect the body and health. Please note that there is no mention of weight in this definition. My focus is upon a population with binge-eating disorder and bulimia. I believe that disordered eating lies on a continuum and I therefore am including sub-clinical disorders, manifesting as yo-yo dieting, emotional eating, restriction, occasional compensatory exercise or laxative use, and mindless eating. In general, those who seek professional help, using a non-diet approach, already have a glimmer of realization that exhaustive diet or purging attempts have failed, but the diet mentality might still be very much embedded in their psyche.

It is important to understand that disordered eating and dieting exist in the service of emotional survival from very vulnerable states of mind and mistaken beliefs about oneself. Ideas of inadequacy, feelings of sadness, loneliness, rejection, anxiety, and insecurity are examples. Disordered food behaviors and dieting are well-intended protections, comforts, and distractions from these intolerable states of mind. Ironically, however, the consequences of these behaviors then increase the very feelings they are meant to eliminate.

When the medical/health/education professions and the media forces call "obesity" the problem, they are avoiding these real core issues, in our cultures as well as in our spirits, hearts, minds, and guts. This ignorance has caused even more suffering in the form of decreased self-esteem, exacerbation of disordered eating, health issues, and in misdirected time, money, and energy spent. My wish is for all concerned to wake up to the harm and misuse of power inherent in focusing upon weight loss. What we really are hungering for is *lightness of Being.*

Food as the essential aspect of the cycle of life

Let's look more closely at food and eating.

Food is an essential aspect of the cycle of life, and is part of the miracle of life itself. Its existence is directly dependent upon nature (the sun, air, wind, earth, rain) and we are dependent upon food for survival. Food is an accompaniment for human rites, passages, celebrations, and religious/spiritual practices. Infants experience safety, trust, love, and worth in being fed when they are hungry. Providing food is an expression of care and love. Food comforts and brings people together. Food feeds the heart and soul as well as the body.

All spiritual traditions hold life as sacred. That we sacrifice of ourselves and are dependent upon other life forms, people, and energy to feed ourselves is not a trivial matter. Gratitude and responsibility can come from this realization of our interconnectedness. Since the earliest cultures, hunting, growing food, harvesting, grace, eating, and giving offerings and alms have been interwoven with spiritual life.

Eating is also a very intimate act. We take food into our mouths and transmute it into the very cells and elements of our body. Our bodies also break down food to provide the energy we use to live our lives.

How can we not feel awe and have reverence when we are aware of this circle of life and our interdependence? How can we not contemplate communion and gratitude when in this awareness? How can we not see in metaphors of sweetness, bitterness, saltiness, sourness, spiciness, and juiciness, the interconnectedness of food, heart, and spirit?

But sadly, those on the spectrum of disordered eating are not in touch with this circle of life. They are disconnected from their body's basic survival instincts of hunger and satiety and the pleasure in eating. In the great design, that which is necessary for survival is pleasurable. To be deprived of this basic right is beyond sad. This disconnection causes suffering.

Chronic disordered eating and dieting, along with cultural/media messages, go against the natural order of life, (dis-order), sapping our vitality and keeping us unaware of our interconnectedness. Eating for reasons of hunger and stopping because the body indicates satiety is natural. It is an innate ability. So, to have a fear-based, conflicted, or dissociated relationship with that which we are dependent upon is a serious problem. Such a relationship affects our psyches, health, relationships, culture, and socio-economic reality. How we relate to food (the quality of our relationship with food) is indicative of how we relate to and live our lives in general. This chapter addresses the question, "How can we repair this disconnection? How can we rekindle the awareness so that we feel reverence, pleasure, peace, and gratitude in relationship to food?"

What do I mean by spiritual path?

The quest for a spiritual path arises out of the search for meaning, and the longing for happiness and connection. The universal experience of suffering and the desire to be free from suffering fuel this seeking. Spirituality is not religion or faith, and not doctrine or system of rules to follow. Even though I come from a Buddhist perspective, there are many other spiritual ways, which I do not wish to discount. Although there are teachings, directions, and supports, the spiritual path is independent of acquired beliefs and external dictates. Instead, it is a personal journey of coming back home to one's self, to self-discovery and self-determination. I say "back home," because that is our original state, which has only been obscured by our conditioning. It is still here and has always been here. It is clear and cannot be tarnished. It may be called our true nature. Here is a salient quote from T.S. Elliot:

We shall not cease from exploration

And the end of all our exploring

Will be to arrive where we started

And know that place for the first time.

– T.S. Elliot, *The Four Quartets*

This is the "who" we are without materialistic trappings, accomplishments, and ways of defining ourselves and our worth. The spiritual path fosters awakening to our innate goodness and inter-connectedness. And it points to liberation from emotional reactivity and limiting thoughts.

Spirituality practice encourages dwelling in or returning to the present moment, rather than entertaining thoughts of past or future. Living in the present is to be non-judgmentally aware of what is happening, what one is doing, and what one is feeling and thinking. It is in this present moment that one can respond appropriately, and only in the present moment that one can find true satisfaction. That is what I discovered when I ate mindfully. Those with a diet mentality are past-and future-focused, as in "I ate so much yesterday that I can't eat today," "I exercised this morning, so I can eat ice cream," "When I lose the weight, I will ....," "Tomorrow I will start my diet," "I can't wait to be alone so I can eat that cake," "I have to lose weight for the reunion," "I will always be alone." The good news is that when this kind of thinking arises, it is possible to calmly come back to the present moment. In that moment one could know what is really true. One could know if she was hungry, or what else she was feeling, and choose to respond in an appropriate manner.

All beings want to be happy and many of us look outside of ourselves for improvement, control, escape, salvation, and ways to avoid or get rid of unpleasant feelings. The Diet Mentality is certainly an example of such external dependency, and it clearly causes suffering. In the mistaken belief that losing weight is the way to achieve happiness, love, and success, many rely upon diets and experts for self-improvement. They focus upon their weight rather than address what is really going on. They try to control their body's food intake and energy expenditures, and try to eat the "right" foods in order to feel good about themselves. They entertain thoughts of attaining perfection and acceptance through weight loss. They use food rules to control themselves, but end up eating when not hungry, or restricting and purging to feel morally cleansed.

Of course, since these methods never work in the end (cue in The Rolling Stones', "I Can't Get No Satisfaction"), most people stuck in the diet mentality end up eating in an unrestrained way and using food to survive the negative self-feelings, which they could not obliterate. (Sadly, they do not understand that they do not lack in will power, but that bingeing after a diet is a natural bodily response.) I recently heard a good slogan, "Don't stuff your face. Face your stuff!" This is a suggestion to attend to what is really happening in the present. When some come to the understanding that these strategies of managing their discomfort rather than facing it not only do not work, but also invariably cause more suffering—on the physical, emotional, social and even financial levels—they may turn toward a spiritual path.

Spiritual models in clinical use today

Of all the spiritual practices, mindfulness is the one that's had the biggest impact on clinical practice. Mindfulness cultivates self-acceptance, compassion, and the ability to notice distressing events without reactivity. This practice of kind inquiry in a good way to "face one's stuff." Much credit goes to Jon Kabat-Zinn, Ph.D., for his groundbreaking work offering Mindfulness Based Stress Reduction programs (MBSR), which he started in the early 1980s. Originally targeted for those with chronic pain and disease, these groups have expanded to treat individuals with binge eating disorder, addiction, depression, anxiety, and trauma. There is research to show the positive effects of these programs[1].

The research by Jean Kristeller, Ph.D.[2], conducted with a binge eating disorder (BED) population, shows that mindfulness approaches can intervene by improving self-regulation. Obese individuals with BED who attended groups and practiced mindful eating decreased the frequency and severity of binge-eating episodes. In addition they experienced an increase in awareness of hunger and satiety cues. This shift in awareness contributed to an understanding that giving up conscious control over eating (dieting, restricting) paradoxically leads to an increased sense of self-control. In this population, there was also evidence of decreased depression and anxiety.

The prevalent mindfulness-based models in clinical use today for eating disorders are Mindfulness Based Cognitive Therapy (MBCT), Acceptance and Commitment Therapy (ACT), Dialectical Behavioral Therapy (DBT), and Mindfulness Based Eating Awareness Training (MBEAT), developed by Dr. Kristeller. Of course, since the 1970s, there are many more programs and methods that embrace the essence of mindfulness. Some of the contributors of this book, including myself, have created their own effective ways of incorporating mindfulness into their work and programs.

There is an elegant psycho-spiritual model called Internal Family Systems (IFS)[3], which has helped me to further integrate a spiritual approach into my work. Since 2004, I have been learning and practicing IFS, developed by psychologist, Richard Schwartz, Ph.D. Rather than fostering dependence upon external authorities, IFS empowers clients to trust and heal themselves. Isn't self-trust the crux of the non-diet approach? It operates from an understanding that even though we have a complex, inner system including exiled, vulnerable, protective, impulsive, and often, extreme and conflicting parts of ourselves, there is an all-abiding, essential Self, untouched by life's traumas, which is already wise, clear, compassionate, infinitely patient, and truly curious. This is our true nature, which I spoke about when discussing the spiritual path. Dr. Schwartz uses a capital 'S' to differentiate this term. The model describes a skillful access to this Self, which is available to be present to all misguided and troubled parts of the personality. The IFS process is a pathway to unburdening mistaken and limiting beliefs, and becoming harmonious, whole, and Self-led. A good analogy is to imagine an orchestra. The parts of the inner system are all the instruments, and Self is the conductor. Without a conductor it would be less than harmonious, and the drummer may get carried away.

I now use the term "Self-Led Eating" to describe my work. Please imagine a boardroom meeting. The reason for the meeting is to determine when, what, how, and how much to eat. When there is disordered eating, the seats at the table are dominated by different parts, such as diet managers, restrictors, avoidant parts, reward- and comfort-seeking parts, rebellious and impulsive parts, emotion-laden parts, critics, and so on. Not only is there no one at the head of the table, but the body is exiled from the room and demonized. In Self-led eating, Self is at the head of the table and has invited the body back to sit by its side. Self allows the body to speak to whether or not it is hungry and what would satisfy it. Due to this clarity of leadership, other parts then come forward to play their roles in the service of providing food and taking time to eat. If there are other valid concerns, Self will modulate and come up with the best harmonious decision. "Yes you are hungry and want homemade macaroni and cheese, but we don't have the ingredients, and we have hours yet before we are home. Eat this yogurt now, and when we get home, we can have a good meal. I will remember to get the ingredients next time I shop." Self listens mindfully and is the compassionate head of the table.

How apt that within the word "mindfulness," resides "fullness"; and within "mindlessness," there is "less." Learning to pay calm attention in the moment to the input of the body, to its feelings and sensations, not only makes physical fullness possible, but also adds a fullness and satisfaction to life. Supporting and teaching our clients to practice mindful eating is essential to helping them feel nourished, rather than lacking or empty. This practice includes noting the arising of hunger, focusing in to determine what food would satisfy, choosing/ preparing food, savoring the food, being aware of food entering the stomach, and noting and responding to satiety cues and other bodily responses. In this work, it is also very important to legalize all foods. Having ideas about what is "good" or "bad," deprives us of the experience of knowing for ourselves, and of course, sets up rebellion. Again, it is a natural response to want to be in charge of our food choices and it is especially offensive to be told, "you should not eat that because you are fat, and you are bad if you do." That which is forbidden becomes alluring, even if we don't really want it. If I said, "After tomorrow, you can never again have ice cream," what might you be doing tomorrow? Yes! You would be sampling ice cream.

Essential qualities for the therapist

In discussing the applications of spiritual practice, let's first consider some essential qualities for the professional:

Foremost, the professional has direct knowledge that her body is self-regulating. She can differentiate emotional from physiological hunger and has the capacity to sit with uncomfortable feelings. She may still be on her own healing path, however. "Perfection" is not essential, although she does have a practice of eating mindfully.

The professional knows and trusts that the client can have her own experience of the innate ability to feed herself and care for her vulnerabilities. Therefore she does not have to feel responsible to "manage" her client's eating. This may be experienced as a relief. It follows that she does not focus upon the client's weight or food choices, but upon HOW the client eats and relates to food. Also, and very important, she is not weight biased. This means that she refrains from judging a client for her size and remains un-triggered in the face of a client's desperate need to lose weight. I think of weight-loss desperation as a red herring. It often succeeds in distracting from the disordered behaviors we are trying to examine and the buried vulnerabilities and pain, which may feel so intolerable. I often hear about the need to lose weight, but I hardly ever hear a client say, "I really want to learn to stop eating when I am not hungry."

Finally, the professional provides spiritual tools and practices, support and encouragement on the journey to being at peace with food. This might include guided exercises, reading material, other resources, and treatment recommendations. I believe that a client is best served with a team that includes other professionals as well, such as a nutritionist, medical doctor, yoga therapist, and psycho-pharmacologist.

The application of mindfulness facilitates the direct experience of hunger and one's inherent ability to satisfy it. At the risk of being repetitive, this is the most important aspect of the journey. To that point, I offer weekend intensive No-Diet and Self-Led Eating workshops, where being present with the eating experience is the main agenda. We slow down the eating process to include noting the intention to pick up the utensil, bringing the food to one's mouth, and putting the utensil down. This is to insert awareness at every choice point.

I also offer The Conscious Café, a mindful-eating practice group where participants come hungry, bring a food they want to eat and share, and eat mindfully together. It is very powerful for folks to have a shared experience of getting "enough" and see their craving dissolve into calm, simple pleasure. We also experiment with eating foods, which are considered "bad" or which trigger uncontrolled eating. Many discover that either when they taste these foods, they actually don't like them, or that they can find the point of satisfaction, where they desire no more. In this way they come to see that these foods no longer have control over them.

In the safe space of The Conscious Café, participants can speak for, express the concerns of, and validate the parts of themselves that resist mindful eating in their daily lives, again, in the service of avoiding unpleasant feelings. They eventually get to see that being mindful does not *cause* these feelings, but instead illuminates what is already there, and is begging for attention. They then have the choice to attend in a non-judgmental way to these feelings and to their strong impulses to eat when they are not hungry. Inserting this "wedge of awareness" between an impulse and behavior is an important aspect of the practice.

Another powerful spiritual tool is the practice of gratitude as a way to remember our interconnectedness. Following is a mealtime grace I heard many years ago from poet, novelist, teacher, and healer Deena Metzger. I recite this before every group eating experience and it always touches people with its eloquence.

"We thank the sun, the wind, the earth, the rain, for this beautiful food…

All the creatures who gave their lives to feed us, and all the human effort that went into bringing it to us.

May we take it in and may it nourish us,

And may we return the energy to the world in ways which lessen suffering and bring joy."

– Deena Metzger

It is also a valuable practice to set daily intentions about a balanced relationship with food. If we are mindlessly practicing disconnection, what else can we expect to get than more of the same? We all can benefit from stopping to identify our values and intending to embody them anew each day. How would it look if I we did that each day? How would our relationship with food be if we did that?

Setting intention is best done first thing in the morning. Then, taking time at night to non-judgmentally assess the day is a way to stay connected to the intention. If a goal were followed through, one could reflect on how that felt. For example, if one prepared a snack for the late afternoon, how did that affect the tendency to eat too much while preparing dinner? Does it make sense to do that again tomorrow? One can also determine if she set an unrealistic goal, and pinpoint any resistance she may have had.

Other tools for being embodied and present in the moment are guided body scans and breath explorations, gentle or restorative yoga, and meditation. I always refer appropriate clients to yoga and MBSR courses, and offer resources about mindfulness. I explain that adding activities into their week, which support them in "coming to their senses," is integral to their work, and to an outpatient model.

I start sessions with a guided exploration and frequently check in with body sensation during the session. Many times clients are surprised and informed by experiencing shifts or arising states, which they would normally disregard. Once, in working with a 19-year-old woman with anorexia nervosa, I invited her to sit quietly with me and explore her breath for just one minute. I brought her attention to its three-dimensional quality. Afterwards she said she could see her thoughts, was aware of her breathing, experienced a new stillness, and became aware of her body on the couch feeling alive. The next week she reported that the relaxation made her feel like a child again with no worries or responsibilities ... free. She realized that she could "turn off her brain" and did not have to analyze everything. When she was feeling bored, frustrated, and lonely, and wanted to isolate in her room, she took a deep breath, "stopped thinking," and the urge went away. This was the beginning of her getting more in touch with herself and her buried feelings. She came to realize that she did not need starvation and constant calorie counting to be "in control." All this from paying attention!

It is important to offer compassionate ways to come to the table with "resistance to change." I see resistance as the parts of our clients that are very committed to their protective roles and that see their job or beliefs as the only way. For example, a client recently said, "I could not physically be in my body last night without eating a lot of food for comfort." The intention of her bingeing part is positive, (to comfort herself) although it ends up causing her more discomfort, shame, and hopelessness. I am sure that many of us have clients who have developed type 2 diabetes but no amount of convincing, scaring, or educating seems to get them to change their eating behaviors. Their binger part might say, "Eating is the only way I have to bust out and reward myself for complying with others' expectations all day. Don't take that away from me!" As professionals, our job is to model compassion, clarity, patience, and hope for such parts of our clients. We can help them see the good intentions of their "resistance" without criticism and shaming, and in that there is a softening.

Last but not least, the ancient Buddhist practice of Metta, or loving-kindness is a way to befriend rejected aspects of our being and nurture self-acceptance and self-love. This occurs through the unfolding realization that one is deserving of love and affection. What a radical concept for most of our clients! Loving-kindness is an antidote for such resistance to self-caring.

This is a practice of simply saying phrases such as: "May I be safe and protected, may I be happy, may I have ease of mind"; as a way of directing loving-kindness toward oneself. I often hear, "I don't believe that about myself, and I certainly don't deserve that." But just saying this can be enough. Traditionally, one starts with oneself and then moves out to include all beings, but it is appropriate for this population to maintain a practice of befriending oneself. The Buddha said, *"You can search throughout the entire universe for someone who is more deserving of your love and affection than yourself, and that person is not to be found anywhere. You yourself, as much as anyone in the entire universe deserve your love and affection."*[4]

When clients come to an awareness of parts of themselves, which they fear will take them over, or toward which they feel criticism or shame, extending loving-kindness to that part is a way to make more space for non-judgmental awareness. Sometimes I combine using loving-kindness with the IFS process. I often recite these powerful phrases during a session with my clients.

The Buddha taught that suffering was based in craving, aversion, and delusion. Not to be simplistic, but the manifestation of disordered eating can be condensed into these three words. Being anchored in the present moment is a powerful antidote to the "practices" of craving, aversion, and delusion. If we want to be free from such suffering, it makes sense that examining one's relationship with food is an excellent inroad.

In conclusion, applying spiritual practices to the treatment of disordered eating is a compassionate and skillful means to address underlying causes, makes way for true healing, and for reclaiming the pleasure of eating.

May we all have a peaceful relationship with food and with the body.

References

1. Kabat-Zinn, J., Massion, A.O., Kristeller, J., Peterson, L.G., Fletcher, K.W., Phert, L., and Santorelli, S.F. 1992. "Effectiveness of a Mindfulness-Based Stress Reduction Program in the Treatment of Anxiety Disorders." *American Journal of Psychiatry* 149, 936–943.

2. Kristeller, J., Baer, R., and Quillian-Wolever, R. 2006. "Mindfulness-Based Approaches to Eating Disorders," in Baer, R. (ed.) (2006) *Mindfulness and Acceptance-Based Interventions: Conceptualization, Application, and Empirical Support.* San Diego: Elsevier.

3. www.selfleadership.org for resources and training and learning.

4. Salzberg, S. 1995 *Loving-Kindness: The Revolutionary Art of Happiness.* Boston: Shambhala Publications. P. 31.

SPOTLIGHT

While this book discusses the ways in which diets don't work, there are many practical things that people can do to improve their health. In this next chapter, Jon Robison provides ten practical things that people can do *now* to improve their health. These include *celebrating* freedom from dieting and from body hatred. Robison's approach is to appreciate the body and use its wisdom to eat intuitively and move it in ways that feel comfortable and healthy. These ideas are central to the Health At Every Size model.

Chapter Twenty-One

10 Things You Can Do Right Now to Ease Concerns About Your Weight and Improve Your Health

Jon Robison

G iven the focus on weight by the health establishment, the government, and the media, it is not surprising that so many people in this country are anxious about their weight and their health. And there certainly is no shortage of recommendations out there directing people to lose weight with this or that diet, lifestyle program, or eating regimen.

Unfortunately, the research over the last 25 years is quite clear. There is no evidence that any of these approaches result in long-term weight loss for the vast majority of people who engage in them. **There are no exceptions** and none of the approaches (low fat, low calorie, low carb, etc.) work any better than any of the others.

Even more unfortunately, however, this complete lack of evidence does not stop people from being seduced into trying to lose weight with the latest incarnation of these approaches. Yet, despite the huge time, money, and emotional investment, successful long-term weight loss is achieved by only a handful of people. The result is widespread confusion and anxiety about food and widespread weight cycling—people losing and regaining weight over and over again. Furthermore, the relentless pressure, particularly on women and children, to lose weight increases the likelihood of eating disorders, disordered eating, and body hatred.

Is there no solution to the weight-related struggles so many people are having? Is there nothing people can do to ease their concerns about weight and health? The good news is that there is indeed. By substituting a **Health-Centered Approach** for the traditional

Weight-Centered Approach, people can reduce their anxiety about food and weight while at the same time promoting good health.

The **Health-Centered Approach** targets lifestyle factors such as physical activity, quality of diet, and stress. It is **weight-neutral** because it treats weight as an outcome of these factors combined with genetics and environment rather than as a direct target for treatment. While this differs substantially from the traditional wisdom about weight and health, please keep in mind that the traditional wisdom in this case is clearly not working or helping and is likely causing considerable harm.

The following 10 suggestions, based on this **Health-Centered Approach**, can go a long way toward helping people to ease the concerns about their weight, while at the same time improving their health and the quality of their lives. References for further reading on each suggestion can be found at the end of the chapter.

1. SAVE YOUR TIME AND MONEY

Don't spend another minute or another dime on anything (book, clinic, TV show, etc.) or anybody (doctor, dietitian, relative, talk show host, etc.) who even remotely suggests they will help you lose weight permanently.

Nothing in the health and medical fields has been proven more soundly, over and over again, for as long a period of time as the fact that focusing on weight loss is unlikely to lead to permanent weight loss and more likely to lead to weight cycling and weight gain. People who diet repeatedly over the years end up weighing more than they would have if they had never dieted. Weight cycling can make all the health problems weight loss supposedly helps (diabetes, hypertension, lipid abnormalities, etc.) worse.

NOTE: If you are a health professional, read claims made by weight-loss researchers with great care. The National Institutes of Health says 5 years should be considered long-term success for weight-loss programs. Anything less should be viewed with suspicion. Just as importantly, be sure to check and see how many people started in the study and how many people's data were actually used in the final analysis. It is not unusual for weight-loss studies to claim as a success a relatively small amount of weight loss in a small subset of the people who began the study. This is bad science at best.

2. JUST SAY NO!

Do not use (or let anyone else use) your weight or BMI or any other measurement of body size or composition as an indicator of health.

None of these has been shown to be strongly related to or predictive of health. People can be healthy at a wide range of weights, BMI's, body fat percentages, etc. Similarly, people with "normal" or "optimal" body composition measurements can have the same health problems that are often referred to as weight-related.

3. ASK FOR ANSWERS

If you have a health condition commonly considered to be "weight-related," (most likely candidates are hypertension, abnormal cholesterol, abnormal blood glucose) and a health professional recommends weight loss as a solution, ask her/him the following questions:

1. What is the success rate of the approach you are suggesting? (What is the likelihood I will regain the weight I lose?)
2. What is likely to happen to my health condition if I lose the weight and then regain it?
3. Is there any way to treat this condition that does not involve a focus on weight loss? (How would you treat a thin person who had this condition?)

The answers given by your health professional to these questions should look something like:

1. The success rate is no better than 5%, so it is quite likely that you will gain back all of the weight that you lost and perhaps a bit more.
2. It is quite possible that your health issues (high blood pressure, diabetes, abnormal cholesterol, etc.) will get worse after you regain the weight.
3. All of these conditions can be helped through lifestyle changes with little or no weight loss. (**A Health-Centered Approach**) The best treatment for a fat person for any of these conditions is the same treatment that would be recommended for a thin person.*

Note: If you don't get something like these answers, consider seeking help elsewhere.
For the special case of diabetes, see section at the end of the article.

4. USE YOUR IMAGINATION

If you do not have a health condition but you are worried that you will develop one if you don't make some lifestyle changes to lose weight, try the following:

Imagine that you are, right now, at the weight that you believe will be healthier.

Work out a plan (with a health professional if desired) of the kinds of lifestyle changes you think you might be able to sustain to remain healthy at that weight.

Implement that plan, right now, at your current weight.

Be sure your plan **does not** include any type of externally determined caloric intake or food restriction, since these have been proven not to work for most people. Steps 5–8 below refer to the kinds of changes that are most likely to help prevent and ameliorate these so-called weight-related health conditions. They will also help your body to settle around its natural (genetically programmed) healthy weight.

5. CONSIDER MOVING YOUR BODY

If you are relatively sedentary and you think engaging in more physical activity would help you to be healthier, find ways to move your body that feel good to you.

The most up-to-date information on exercise is encouraging, especially for people who have been sedentary and have had difficulty trying to live up to the ever-changing, complicated, and demanding exercise recommendations from the government and health establishment.

> For the vast majority of people, **fitness is a much more important indicator of health than fatness.**

> The greatest gains in health-related fitness are achieved when people go from being sedentary to getting even small amounts of physical activity.

> Physical activity does not have to be done all at once to achieve significant health benefits—3 ten-minute periods of exercise are as good as one 30-minute period.

> All kinds of movement count, including walking, gardening, dancing, sports, and running after your kids.

6. DECLARE YOUR INDEPENDENCE

Don't let anyone (that's right—anyone!) tell you what or how much to eat to lose weight.

Our bodies have wonderful, intricate mechanisms to help us to know how much to eat to maintain a healthy weight. No set of rules, guidelines, or regulations provided by experts can come close to the precision of the complex interactions among hunger, appetite, and satiety that naturally help us regulate our food intake and our weight if we pay attention to them. Ignoring these internal cues by following endless sets of external ones (Weight Watchers, Jenny Craig, The Food Pyramid, etc.) is likely to result in more rather than less disordered eating. A growing body of research suggests that adults and children who diet are more likely to gain extra weight as they get older than those who don't.

7. LISTEN TO YOUR INTERNAL WISDOM

Learn to eat according to your internal signals: appetite, hunger, and satiety. By paying attention to these signals, you can avoid having to pay someone else to tell you what and how much to eat.

NOTE: For some people, eating can become a stand-in for other hungers that are not being satisfied. These may be related to a search for life balance, connection or meaning, and purpose. Sometimes, there may also be deep-seated struggles with depression, anxiety, and trauma that get played out with food. It is critical that these underlying issues be addressed. It is even more critical that no matter how much of a problem food and weight have become for an individual, with few exceptions, external food restriction will almost certainly cause more harm than good.

8. CONSIDER DR. ROBISON'S SIMPLIFIED DIETARY GUIDELINES

The original Four Food Groups were designed to help us to get the nutrition we need to grow and thrive. Over the years The Dietary Guidelines for Americans have become too complex, too prescriptive, and too focused on disease prevention and weight control.

Some people may have a medical condition that requires them to eat or not eat particular foods. But, for most people, the following guidelines can help establish the foundation for a nutritious diet while at the same time minimizing the constant worry about everything we put into our mouths—a seemingly ever-present stressor that is decidedly unhealthy! Here they are:

Enjoy Your Food

Eat a Wide Variety of Food

Pay Attention to Internal Signals Whenever You Can

Share Your Food with Someone Who Is Needy—Gratitude Is Deeply Nourishing!

Bon Appetit!!

9. TAKE NOTICE OF WHAT REALLY MATTERS

Notice any changes that occur over time with this approach. Ask yourself:

What health-related changes have I experienced?

Do I feel differently about food?

Do I feel differently about myself?

Am I spending less time and energy worrying about my weight and what I am eating?

10. CELEBRATE

That's right! Congratulate yourself! It is very likely that you have:

Ended your time on the frustrating roller coaster that is dieting.

Increased your self-esteem and body image.

Taken charge of your eating by paying attention to your body instead of paying someone else to tell you what to do.

Helped your body settle near the weight it is genetically programmed to achieve.

Opened up potentially significant amounts of time and energy that you used to spend worrying and fretting about your weight and food.

Ameliorated or normalized any of the so-called weight-related health conditions you may have had whether or not you experienced any change in weight.

THE "SPECIAL CASE" OF TYPE 2 DIABETES

But Dr. Robison, don't we need to recommend weight loss for people with type 2 diabetes? The answer to this question is a resounding **No!** Here is why:

There is no evidence that weight-loss interventions work for people with type 2 diabetes (most likely they work even less well than for the general weight-loss-seeking population).

Losing weight and then gaining it back can cause blood glucose problems to get worse. Since the vast majority of people will gain their weight back, this is a major issue.

The good news is that research clearly demonstrates that problems with blood glucose can be helped greatly by using **A Health-Centered Approach** without significant weight loss and even in people who gain body fat during the course of the study.

NOTE: Diabetes is a serious disease that causes great hardship and suffering for those who have it. However, the idea that we are currently experiencing an "epidemic" of diabetes has been oversold. According to the **U.S. Centers for Disease Control**, during the 1990s, when the "explosion" of overweight and obesity was said to occur, the most accurate data suggest only a small increase in the incidence of diabetes. Similarly, despite a good deal of fear-mongering to the contrary, type 2 diabetes remains a rare occurrence in children. Statements to the contrary are often based on physician's anecdotal reports or large phone interviews, neither of which can substitute for representative population data.

FINAL THOUGHTS

Because the concepts that *thin equals healthy* and *weight loss equals better health* are so deeply ingrained into the fabric of our culture, after examining this different approach people will often still ask this final question: **If I do all of this, will I lose weight?** The answer to this question goes straight to the heart of the difference between the **Health-Centered** and **Weight-Centered Approaches**. The answer is that, if people follow the suggestions outlined here, there are three and only three possibilities:

1. They will lose weight
2. They will gain weight
3. Their weight will not change

What is wonderful about this answer, unlike almost any other answer related to this topic, is that it is undeniably scientific and unarguably true. If people are above their natural weight, they may lose some weight. If people are below their natural weight, they may gain. If people are close to their natural weight, they may stay the same. Which one of these outcomes will occur is often not predictable. What is predictable is that people will end up healthier and much less concerned about their weight and their health.

References

1. **Success and Safety of Dieting For Weight Loss**

   Mann T, Tomiyama J, Westling E, Lew A, Samuels B, and Chatman J. 2007. "Medicare's Search for Effective Obesity Treatments." *American Psychologist*, 62(3):220–233.

   Aphramor. 2010. "Validity of Claims Made in Weight Management Research: A Narrative Review of Dietetic Articles." *Nutrition Journal*, (http://www.nutritionj.com/content/9/1/30).

   Matz, Judith and Frankel Ellen. 2006. *The Diet Survivor's Handbook: 60 Lessons in Eating, Self-Acceptance and Self-Care*. Naperville, IL: Sourcebooks Inc.

2. **BMI and Health**

   Franzosi MG. 2006. <www.thelancet.com>368:624–625.

   Wildman RP, Munter P, Reynolds K, McGinn AP, Rajpathak S, Wylie-Rosett J, and Sowers MR. 2008. "The Obese Without Cardiometabolic Risk Factor Clustering and the Normal Weight with Cardiometabolic Risk Factor Clustering." *Arch Intern Med*, 168(15):1617–1624.

   Dr. Keith Devlin. "Do You Believe in Fairies, Unicorns, or the BMI?" http://www.maa.org/devlin/devlin_05_09.html.

3. **Improving Health Without Weight Loss**

   Gaesser, GA. (2002). *Big Fat Lies: The Truth About Your Weight and Your Health*. Carlsbad, CA: Gurze Books.

   Campos P., Saguy A, Ernsberger P., Oliver E., and Gaesser G. 2006. "The Epidemiology of Overweight and Obesity: Public Health Crisis or Moral Panic?" *International Journal of Epidemiology*, 35(1):55–60.

4. ***The "Special" Case of Diabetes**

   Bjorntorp P et al. 1970. "The Effect of Physical Training on Insulin Productivity in Men." *Metab Clin Exp*, 19:631–638.

   Lamarche B et al. 1992. "Is Body Fat Loss a Determinant Factor in the Improvement of Carbohydrate and Lipid Metabolism Following Aerobic Exercise Training in Obese Women?" *Metab Clin Exp*, 41:1249–1256.

   Centers for Disease Control, *Morbidity and Mortality Weekly Report*. 9/5/2003; 52(35):833–837.

   Armstrong D and King A. 1993. "Demand Feeding as Diabetes Treatment." *Obesity and Health* 1, 109–110, 115.

5. **Physical Activity, Weight, and Health**

   Gaesser G. 2006. "Fatness, Fitness, and Health: A Closer Look at the Evidence." *WELCOA, Absolute Advantage*, 5(3):18–21.

   McAuley, Blair. 2011. "Obesity Paradoxes." *Journal of Sports Sciences*, 29(8):773–782.

6,7. **Easting According to Internal Cues**

   Satter, Ellyn. 2008. *Secrets of Feeding a Healthy Family*., Madison, WI: Kelcy Press.

Tribole E and Resch E. 2010. "Intuitive Eating: A Revolutionary Program That Works." 2nd edn. New York: St. Martin's Griffin.

8. **Dietary Guidelines**

Satter, Ellyn. "Dietary Guidelines and Food Guide Pyramid Incapacitate Consumers and Contribute to Distorted Eating Attitudes and Behaviors." www.ellynsatter.com/resources.jsp.

Marantz PR, Bird ED, and Alderman MH. 2008. "A Call for Higher Standards of Evidence for Dietary Guidelines." *American Journal of Preventive Medicine*, 34(3):234–240.

9,10. **Evaluating Outcomes**

Bacon L, Stern JS, Van Loan MD, and Keim NL. 2005. "Size Acceptance and Intuitive Eating Improve Health for Obese, Female Chronic Dieters." *J Am Diet Assoc*, 105(6), 929–936.

Bacon L and Aphramor L. 2011. "Weight Science: Evaluating the Evidence for a Paradigm Shift." *Nutrition Journal*, **10**:9 doi:10.1186/1475-2891-10-9.

CPSIA information can be obtained at www.ICGtesting.com
Printed in the USA
BVOW11s1408210116

433327BV00003B/53/P